Therapeutic Exercise

Exercise Techniques for Patients with Common Orthopedic Conditions

Doug Creighton MS DPT OCS FAAOMPT

Oakland University

Program in Physical Therapy

School of Health Sciences

Rochester, Michigan

To: Kris, Karleigh, Katie, Cam, Lilo, Koa, Akamu, and Stitch

Copyright© Doug Creighton 2012
Second Edition - 2016

Published by The Educational Publisher
Columbus, Ohio
www.EduPublisher.com

ISBN13:978-1-62249-359-3

Preface

Therapeutic exercise has been and I suspect always will be the foundation of physical therapy intervention. It is our profession's primary form of intervention and is what distinguishes physical therapy from other health-related disciplines. I have been a certified orthopedic manual physical therapist for over 34 years. I feel that providing skilled joint and soft tissue manipulation is one of the most important interventions that can be provided to a patient seeking our help. Nevertheless, I also feel the prescription of therapeutic exercise is the most important intervention we provide.

There are many different modalities and intervention techniques associated with physical therapy. The popularity of numerous modalities and interventions has risen and fallen over the years. Therapeutic exercise has stood the test of time. In fact, I like to tell my students, when all else fails to help your patient, therapeutic exercise will not. At some level most patients, many of whom come to us in pain, lacking mobility, lacking strength, lacking balance, have minor instabilities, or are just deconditioned, benefit in some way from exercise.

The primary purpose of this textbook is to assist entry-level students. Students seeking advanced clinical competencies in orthopedic manual physical therapy will also find that this text offers a nice review of basic exercise concepts and many creative exercises that even seasoned therapists may not have considered. While the title of this book relates to patients with impairments and functional limitations associated to common orthopedic conditions, many of the exercises shown in this text can assist patients in other practice settings as well.

The exercise techniques found within this text seek to reduce pain, and facilitate, not retard tissue healing by modifying speed of therapeutic motion, arc of therapeutic motion and providing assistance or partial assistance to joint movements when necessary. Further, the exercises shown within this text seek to enhance muscular strength and stability, soft tissue mobility and human locomotion without significant provocation of symptoms or damage to joint cartilage and other sensitive joint tissues.

This is the preface, so I will not speak to this a great deal now but I would like to briefly expand on the idea of damaging to joint cartilage or other joint-related tissues during the performance of therapeutic exercise. I think if we are not careful it is possible to overstretch, irritate, and possibly damage muscular and more importantly capsuloligamentous stabilizing structures, including the intervertebral disc, with the prescription of certain self-stretching and self-mobilization exercises. This damage may have occurred when patients complain of increased soreness or achiness after repetitively performing these types of exercise motions. Further, I think it is possible to over load joint cartilage with closed kinetic chain single leg stance strength building exercises if prescribed to the wrong patient, or if performed for too long a period of time. I am not saying to not prescribe these things just consider who is doing them, how large and how loaded the motion is, and how long are you going to have the patient perform them. Many of the exercises in this text are prescribed with an eye on the patient's future years. The movement patterns and exercise positions shown in Chapters 10 -18 challenge musculoskeletal structures but they also support and control load the soft tissues, joint cartilage, and spinal segments. In other words, the musculoskeletal structures that commonly degenerate and become painful during life. I believe, that a good therapeutic motion or a good therapeutic exercise can be performed for the better part of one's life span. Meaning, the therapeutic motion, and the resultant load that motion causes, is not so great, that it would damage supportive musculosketeletal structures that might be is various stages of decline or degeneration.

We should encourage our patients to get and stay as strong and as flexible as possible, but not at all costs. For example, many of our patients can build a reasonable degree of spinal, upper extremity, and lower extremity strength by performing reduced load and reduced arc of motion exercises. For example, if a lower extremity lunge (spilt stance squat) strength building exercise causes pain secondary to injury or degenerative change, be clever and make a simple load modification. Have the patient stand between and press down on the backs of two chairs. This will often allow a patient with symptomatic hip, knee, or ankle-foot injury or arthritis to perform this strength building motion. In Chapter 14 we term this assisted lunge training.

This book is simply organized into nine foundational chapters, which review basic exercise definitions, types of therapeutic motion, various exercise positions, posture, tissue healing, arthritis, and basic aspects of patient examination and intervention planning. For example, in Chapter 6, Musculoskeletal Injury and Repair, and the Application of Therapeutic Motions; students will note numerous guidelines regarding exercise application in relation to general tissue healing time frames. The guidelines presented in this foundational chapter are very conservative and will serve clinicians particularly clinicians new to the profession in terms of minimizing adverse reactions to prescribed therapeutic exercise therapeutic motion. A chapter dedicated to each upper extremity joint, each lower extremity joint, and all three spinal regions follows the foundational chapters.

Starting with Chapter 10, the text will have a large number of digital photographs of self-stretching, self-mobilization, assisted movements and stabilization exercise. Each photograph will note a key position for therapeutic exercise performance and detailed legends will describe the therapeutic motion and clinical applications particularly in relation to common orthopedic conditions and commonly associated pain and movement impairments. In certain sections of some chapters, readers will note a sequenced progression of strength building such as the Swiss Ball Supported lumbar stabilization exercises (Chapter 18) and sequenced progression of therapeutic movements and resisted motion (Chapters 3 and 10). Clinicians will find useful updates in terms of creative patient positioning and creative arcs of movement that will add to their current repertoire of therapeutic exercise intervention.

Acknowledgments

I would like to thank my friends, family and colleagues, particularly my colleagues at Oakland University in Rochester Michigan where I have had the pleasure of working with and learning from many talented individuals. I hesitate to name any names at all for fear of leaving out a good friend or colleague but that being said; an acknowledgement page would not be complete without listing as many talented people as I can think of. I have learned a great deal from all who are listed below and without these people, projects such as this text would not be possible.

Olaf Evjenth

Jeff Annis

Stanley Paris

Robert Rinke

John Krauss

Michael Moore

Bjorn Svensen

Lasse Thue

Contents

Chapter 1 — 1
A Brief Overview on the History of Therapeutic Exercise

Chapter 2 — 5
A Review of Basic Forms of Resistance and Endurance Exercise Training

Chapter 3 — 13
Therapeutic Motion and Movements

Chapter 4 — 21
Advantages and Disadvantages of Various Exercise Positions

Chapter 5 — 27
Thoughts on Pain and Posture

Chapter 6 — 31
Musculoskeletal Injury and Repair, and the Application of Therapeutic Motions

Chapter 7 — 45
A Few Comments on Osteoarthritis and Exercise

Chapter 8   51
Thoughts on Examination and Evaluation of the Orthopedic Patient

Chapter 9   57
Matching Impairments to Exercise Intervention

Chapter 10   63
Therapeutic Exercise for the Shoulder

Chapter 11   123
Therapeutic Exercise for the Elbow

Chapter 12   139
Therapeutic Exercise for the Wrist-Hand

Chapter 13   161
Therapeutic Exercise for the Hip

Chapter 14   199
Therapeutic Exercise for the Knee

Chapter 15   237
Therapeutic Exercise for the Ankle-Foot

Chapter 16 — 265
Therapeutic Exercise for the Cervical Spine

Chapter 17 — 309
Therapeutic Exercise for the Thoracic Spine

Chapter 18 — 333
Therapeutic Exercise for the Lumbar Spine

Epilogue — 405

References — 407

Chapter 1

A Brief Overview on the History of Therapeutic Exercise

Historically or at least as far back as I can remember which by the way is 32 years at the time of this writing and now revision; orthopedic physical therapy seemed to focus a bit more on measuring and attempting to improve, alleviate, or lessen dysfunctions. Dysfunction was an interesting term. Back in the 1980's it seemed to count for everything but really meant nothing or it meant something a little different to most everyone. I am glad not many of us use such a general and generally meaningless term any longer.

The term impairment is so much better and happily, our profession has smartly moved toward finding impairments during our examination, treating those impairments, and hopefully improving (reducing) functional limitations and associated disabilities along the way. Just to review, impairments can be thought of as a loss or abnormality in psychological, anatomical, or physiological structure or function. A functional limitation as the term would seem to indicate can be thought of as a limitation in one's ability or abilities. Said another way, it is a limitation in the ability of a person to perform an activity or activities. Lastly, the term disability brings society and social roles into play. In effect, disability principally refers to how impairments and functional limitations adversely affect a person's ability to perform socially defined roles.

So, that is a quick review of and one way to define the terms impairment, functional limitation, and associated disabilities. Speaking of definitions, a word or a topic could have more than one good or even correct definition. I like it when a word or a topic has a simple and easy to remember definition. For example, the words mobilization and manipulation has historically been defined as a "skilled passive movement." I think of these two terms as skilled passive therapeutic motions Either way, this is a short, simple and easy to remember definition. Well how about therapeutic exercise, the best definition I have ever read is credited to Licht who defined therapeutic exercise as motions of the body or its parts to relieve symptoms or improve function.[1] I think that definition sums things up pretty nicely. It is short and simple and it notes how therapeutic exercise, which is really therapeutic motion, can relieve pain and improve function. There, I sort of re-worked Licht's definition. Licht came up with this definition way back in the 1960's. Seeing as how I was brought up the 60's, which is ancient history, let's look at some other historical aspects of therapeutic exercise.

MY HISTORY

My personal history with therapeutic exercise started at Oakland University (OU) in the 1980's. What a great decade! Bought my first Camaro in the 1980's. But that does not have anything to do with therapeutic exercise. In undergrad at OU I learned many of the important basics regarding the prescription of therapeutic motion. Simple basic movements like passive oscillations which can be used to reduce pain impairments and simple strength building motions that can be used to correct weakness impairments. These basic aspects of therapeutic exercise/movement still apply today. In fact, to this day, I often say to my students the following thing; "show me a PT clinician who is well grounded in the *basics* and I will show you a good clinician." I believe that statement applies to consistently prescribing the correct therapeutic exercises/therapeutic motions. In the 1990's I was fortunate enough to meet and learn from numerous talented clinicians who through the efforts of Kornelia Kulig and John Krauss came to OU to teach different pieces of course work in our Orthopedic Manual Physical Therapy Program. People like Olaf Evjenth, Freddy Kaltenborn, Michael Moore, Robert Rinke, and Bjorn Svensen and Lasse Thue. These people were excellent clinicians and they really had a great handle on how to therapeutically self-stretch, self-mobilize, strength train (stabilize), and unload musculoskeletal tissues. My work in this text is in part a reflection of these talented individuals.

ANCIENT HISTORY

Seeing as how I have been name dropping, how about a few more names just so we can legitimize the title of this chapter. If we step into the "Way Back Machine," (1960's cartoon reference), and I do mean way back, all the way to around 400 or 500 BC a physician named Herodicus claimed to have used therapeutic exercise to cure himself of a terrible disease. That probably did not happen, not real critical thinking if you ask me, but this person was also credited for developing exercises for the athletes of that time. Who knows, maybe that is when pylometrics first started? How about Hippocrates? His name seems to come up fairly often and he was a student of Herodicus. Hippocrates wrote about the beneficial effects of therapeutic exercise in terms of strengthening muscles, improving mental outlook and reducing obesity. So, you see, most of your PT instructors and exercise gurus are not talking about anything new!

MORE RECENT HISTORY

There are so many important names associated with therapeutic exercise, names like Codman who in the 1930's developed therapeutic motions to relieve pain in the shoulder.[2] There was Delorme who is credited with advancing and refining ideas regarding resistance training or progressive resistance exercise.[3] We shouldn't forget Kabat who took the *"straight"* out of therapeutic exercise and introduced the idea of moving in diagonal movement patterns. What a great common-sense idea seeing as how humans typically don't move like robots![4] And one of manual therapies, greatest clinician's, Olaf Evjenth, his career has spanned more the five decades. I maintain there is still no better stretching text then his, Autostretching, a book which he published in the 1980s.[5] Well, I doubt that it is possible to credit everyone or maybe it is but I don't want to take the time, I would rather write this book. Just remember, we should not forget history and the people who worked hard trying to originate and refine something in order to help others out.

Chapter 2

A Review of Basic Forms of Resistance and Endurance Exercise Training

As PT clinicians, we frequently need to address strength or a lack thereof with some form of resistance training. In Chapter 1 I mentioned that there is usually more than one way to define something. That applies to the term strength too. Strength could be defined as the maximum force that a muscle can develop during a single contraction. I like that definition; it fits my short and simple rule for defining things. However, seeing as how strength is important, how about another definition? How about: the maximum voluntary force that can be produced by the neuromusculoskeletal system? Well, I think that definition does not really get to the point. Therefore, I prefer to define it as: the maximum weight a person can lift one time, otherwise known as the famous One Repetition Maximum. (1RM). In all seriousness now, impaired muscle performance is commonly seen and is a real problem for many of our injured, sedentary, aged, and metabolically impaired patients. The great news is that most all of the research now demonstrates many patients with various musculoskeletal impairments and other medical conditions will benefit from correctly prescribed muscular resistance training.[6]

ISOMETRIC

Seeing as how the first paragraph discussed strength and resistance training, let's look and review some of the other terms associated with resistance training. How about the term isometric exercise? No, how about just the term *isometric*? That word alone means same or constant. In particular, *iso* means the same or constant and *metric* is a word that describes length among other things. Now let's get back to isometric exercise. This form of exercise is commonly used to address muscle strength impairments. As a muscle contracts isometrically, tension develops within that muscle but no change in joint angle occurs and the change in the length of the target muscle in minimal.

You might ask, does this really help our patients who typically need and want to move better and with less pain? Moving, from what I can recall, requires changes in joint angles. Well, I like to think that isometric muscle strength building provides a platform upon which we can further build our patients muscular strength with additional isotonic exercises. Further, isometric muscle contraction can be a valuable clinical intervention for our patients who cannot move their joints though certain portions of a range of movement due to injury, degeneration, pain, or the constraints of post-injury and post-surgical immobilization.

Still don't believe me that isometric muscle contraction is important? Well, we should also consider all those postural muscles that work isometrically the better part of their day. These postural muscles have feelings too and they happen to like training with this form of muscle contraction. The deep spinal extensor muscles are an example of this. Remember, if attempting to build a platform of strength with isometrics, before you prescribe other forms of dynamic muscle contraction, isometric strength building is pretty much range specific give or take 15-20 some odd degrees. Lastly, because I really want to move onto isotonic muscle training, isometric exercise should be used with care in our hypertensive patients, cardiovascular patients, and any spinal patient with radiculitis. Tell all your patients, "no fair holding your breathing" while performing isometric muscle contractions. "If you do your BP will go up!"

ISOTONIC

The definition of *iso* has not changed, but what about the word *tonic*? Tonic has a number of definitions, but the one that fits here is tension. So strictly speaking, an isotonic exercise or muscular contraction is one that produces the same (iso) amount of tension in order to move some form of resistance. The truth is muscle tension will vary over an arc of joint movement when lifting a constant resistance. This all has to do with the angle of muscular pull on a bony lever that is changing position in space, but let's not get to technical. Instead, how about we expand the definition of isotonic and stay in keeping with the title of this chapter, which I think is "Basic Forms of Resistance and Endurance Exercise Training." Do you remember the term concentric? This is a type of isotonic contraction where the internal forces generated within the target muscle or muscles exceed the resistance being lifted and the muscle(s) is able to shorten. Yes, the other term to review is eccentric and this refers to a type of contraction in a muscle that is not fully lengthened, somewhat slackened, and now the external force affecting that target muscle is greater than the internal force it is able to generate. This will produce a lengthening of the muscle as it continues to maintain tension. Manual resistive exercise (MRE), something we will practice a lot of in class is great for eccentric muscle training for our patients. It is easy too. Just start moving the patient limb and tell him or her to "slow you down." Before you know it, you are strength training the patient with eccentric muscle contractions.

ISOKINETIC

Are you ready to review the last *iso* term? As you most likely know, the term is isokinetic or in our case, isokinetic exercise. Let's look at isokinetic exercise from the perspective of what isokinetic devices or machines are able to offer our patients. An isokinetic device is able to provide passive range of motion, concentric resistance at a fixed speed, eccentric resistance at a fixed speed and multi-angle isometric resistance. There are several nice clinical (patient oriented) features of isokinetic training. First, the fixed or set speed resistance can accommodate to a patient's changing muscular abilities throughout a given range of movement. This accommodating resistance may convey a greater degree of safety to a patient's tissues if pain is encountered during a particular arc of motion. In other words, if the patient reduces their muscular contraction, the isokinetic device will reduce the resistance it is providing. While some might argue that this is not what happens in the real world of lifting objects and overcoming gravity, it can still be important during certain phases of tissue healing after an injury or after a flare up of a chronic condition. Further, in terms of protecting a patient's tissues, some feel, and I agree, that higher speed isokinetic resistance training promotes reduced muscular torque or force production and therefore reduced joint compression loads.

Above are some of the positive attributes of isokinetic training; there may be some disadvantages as well. Many if not most isokinetic devices offer single plane muscular training only, are most typically open kinetic chain, and clinically it is difficult for a clinician training a patient in this type of device to really know exactly where in a range of movement their muscular strength impairment is. So, regarding these disadvantages let me make the following two points very clear. Patients with strength impairments should receive more than just one form of resistance intervention as they progress through a program of rehabilitation. Moreover, in my opinion, there is no better way to deliver multi-angle, variable, and accommodating or progressive resistance than with your own hands. MRE intervention allows a clinician to determine where in the range of movement the muscular impairment lies so that the intervention becomes much more specific. MRE intervention is an important aspect of orthopedic and orthopedic manual physical therapy training and one that should continue to be emphasized in all PT curriculums.

OTHER FORMS OF RESISTANCE

So that is a brief review of isometric, isotonic, isokinetic and a quick comment or two on MRE. Regarding patients with muscle strength impairments, there are two other important forms of resistance intervention to review. The first is Free-weight exercise. Free-weight exercise training is typically performed with various sized bars and plate weights. This is the exercise of choice for healthy weight lifters and athletes, but is this form of resistance training OK for patients with orthopedic conditions? The answer is both yes and no. If there is not a significant degree of cartilaginous degeneration or soft tissue injury free weight can be easily adapted for the injured and the non-injured side of the body. For example, hamstring curls could be performed with 40 pounds on the non-injured side and 15 pounds on the side of a healing muscle tear. In addition, free-weights offer the advantage of exact incremental progression of resistance as a tissue heals or as a patient becomes stronger. A possible negative aspect to using free weights includes the potential for greater loading of joint cartilage and the potential for movement errors once a particular therapeutic range is demonstrated to the patient. Lastly, let's not forget elastic bands and elastic tubing. These therapeutic tools are also a form of free-weight and similar to a plate-weight pulley system, elastic resistance has many positive attributes such as multi-plane movement patterns, and both balance and spinal stabilization requirements when performed by our patients in certain positions.

I mentioned that there were two last forms of resistance to review, and the second one is plyometrics. Clearly, most daily movement patterns do not call for a pure isometric or isolated concentric isotonic muscular contraction. It is understandable to all therapists that many daily movement patterns require that muscles work both concentrically and eccentrically. Plyometric exercise training allows for quick shifting between concentric and eccentric muscle work. In addition, plyometrics have been described as quick, powerful movements. I like to think of them as quick transitioning muscle contractions. This form of training is typically thought of as closed chain movements such as mini-hops, jumps and other explosive bounding types of lower extremity movement. It is also important to consider that quick shifting of concentric and eccentric muscle contractions, an attribute of plyometrics, can also be applied in an open kinetic chain environment. This can be accomplished with creative patient positioning and the application of MRE training. That being said, plyometric exercises are more "advanced" exercises and often are a necessary part of athletic rehabilitation and return to sport. Lastly, with regard to plyometrics, when transitioning a patient who has been successful in the performance of other basic therapeutic motions, please keep the following general guidelines in mind. Make sure that your patient's tissues have had the right amount of time to heal (see Chapter 6) and confirm that the patient can walk, squat, jump, and stand on one lower limb without discomfort before starting too many full load plyometric exercise motions.

EXERCISE DOSAGE

Before we conclude this section on various forms of resistance, we should review an important related concept termed exercise dosage. The concept of exercise dosage is pretty simple to understand, but there are some unanswered questions as to which method of strength building is most effective. A dose of exercise can be easily increased by increasing the amount of weight lifted (intensity), increasing the number of sets, increasing the number of repetitions, increasing the lever arm length, or changing a patient's position relative to gravity. Clearly, reducing any of the above, assisting a movement, or changing a patient's position so that gravity is eliminated would reduce the exercise dose.

Now regarding the exercise dose, there are three important terms to remember. First, as just mentioned, is the term intensity or amount of weight lifted. Research regarding this parameter of dosage has been extensive and dates back to some classic work in the 1940's by DeLorme[7] and in the 1950's by Zinovieff.[8] Both researchers established strength-building parameters with multi-set repetition maximum (RM) programs in non-injured individuals.

The second parameter of exercise dosage is duration. Duration can be considered the number of sets or repetitions in an exercise program. This parameter also concerns itself with the all-important rest phase that is necessary during resistance training. It probably is obvious but, we should remember that as the intensity (weight) of a training program increases the duration (sets and reps) will often decrease.

The third and final parameter regarding exercise dosage is frequency. As you probably guessed, the frequency is the number of times an exercise is performed during the day or week. The frequency of resistance training can depend on a number of things including your patient's medical (health) status, their strength, the rehabilitation goals, and the type of exercise or muscle contraction being performed. Isometric and light, unloaded, and non-weight-bearing isotonic exercise training can be performed daily, while heavier isotonic training should often be performed every other day. In addition, the intensity of endurance training is typically low, and in some cases, endurance exercises can be performed every day. Walking programs and postural exercise are example of low intensity activities, which can be performed each day.

Our patients performing resisted training should exercise three or four times a week. If we are responsible for building strength in athletes, "split lifting routines" can be effective and help minimize overtraining. A split routine involving training three to four major muscle groups one day and then training a different set of three to four major muscle groups on the next day. Obviously, this allows for consecutive day training with a one-day rest break for the groups of muscle trained on the previous day. I would like to make one last comment with regard to exercise dosage. This textbook contains exercises for people who have pain due to an injury or who are predisposed to developing pain during movement due to degenerative changes. There are some exercises demonstrated in this text where the figure legend below makes reference to performing the exercise with equal work-rest ratios.

I have found this an effective way to minimize the development of painful symptoms both during and after the therapeutic motion/exercise if the patient is in the acute phase after an injury or if exercise motion(s) are being performed through a significantly degenerated joint surface or spinal motion segment. During the rest break, the patient is to report whether or not they have developed any discomfort. If so, the therapist can then change the intensity (weight) of the exercise, which typically means reduce, the arc of the exercise motion, change the speed of

Therapeutic Exercise

the exercise motion, or change (increase) the amount of assistance given to complete the exercise motion. In addition, if pain is encountered the clinician can reduce compressive loading on the joint cartilage or intervertebral disc during exercise performance. If we control these parameters mentioned above, (arc, speed, load, assistance, resistance, ect.) requires patient cooperation, professional ingenuity and diligence during the monitoring of the exercise we stand a good chance of prescribing an exercise that will increase tissue strength or flexibility without provoking our patient's symptoms.

ENDURANCE

Thus far in this chapter we have focused a bit more on strength and the different types of resisted motion exercise. Another important therapeutic exercise concept is endurance and we should probably review it. How about a general definition first? Endurance could probably be defined as sufficient aerobic capacity to perform and control various movements for a sustained period of time.[9] Endurance is a important aspect of our patient's lives. I believe endurance becomes even more important as people age. If you think about it, there are some daily and some recreational activities that require brute strength, but there are many more daily activities, which require endurance.

We started out with a general definition of endurance, how about we define the term further and relate it to some of the body systems. When looking at endurance, it makes sense to start with the cardiovascular system. This system really runs the show when it comes to delivering oxygen to the muscle groups, which are required to perform activities for an extended period of time. In simple terms our lungs need to extract oxygen from the blood and the heart must be sufficiently strong to deliver an adequate supply of that oxygenated blood to the working muscles. On the musculoskeletal system side of things, the working muscles need to have a sufficient capillary network in order to make use of the blood delivered by the cardiovascular system.

Various traumas causing injury to muscles, surgery, and a whole host of various cardiovascular and neuromuscular diseases can cause muscular strength and endurance impairments. Luckily, muscles typically respond well to therapeutic endurance training exercises. Endurance training can improve a muscle's metabolic capacity, including its mitochondrial size, number and enzymatic activity. This will better allow a muscle to use the delivered O_2.[10]

It is not my intent to write an exercise physiology text but we do need to complete a couple of important points. Regarding endurance training, things have not changed very much. To build muscular endurance, high-repetition, low-intensity (resistance) training at about 25% of a muscle's voluntary contraction ability will produce improvements in muscular endurance.[10] Aerobic exercise endurance training needs to occur for 20-30 minutes at least four times a week. In order to protect injured joints, arthritic lower extremity joints, or degenerated spinal segments with narrowed disc, patient positioning for aerobic training and other exercises often needs to be modified. This idea will be demonstrated throughout the text. Note, for our much-deconditioned patients, breaking up endurance training into two 10-minute segments or four 5-minute segments throughout the day can still be helpful. Do we need to take care when prescribing endurance exercise training to our patients? Yes, that goes without saying. This is particularly true in patients with cardiovascular conditions. Know what type of cardiac medication your patient is taking, where his or her nitroglycerin is and what the pill looks like. Above all, monitor vital signs as your patients' exercise. One last thing, don't think of endurance exercise training as just improving a patient's aerobic capacity. It is our job to build or improve endurance or tolerance if you prefer, for things like standing, sitting and walking.

Chapter 3
Therapeutic Motions and Movements

Strength and endurance were the focus of the last chapter. Strength and endurance impairments are two of the most common activity limiting impairments encountered by our patients. In this chapter we will detail other forms of therapeutic motion, but before we do, let's go back to a definition from Chapter 1. Licht defined therapeutic exercise as *motions of the body or its parts to relieve symptoms or improve function.* In keeping with that definition, we reviewed common types of resisted motion in Chapter 2. Resisted forms of therapeutic motion has been shown to improve function and relieve symptoms for some patients with certain orthopedic conditions. In addition to resisted motion, there are other forms of therapeutic motion that can do the very same thing, and with regard to symptom relief, part of Licht's definition, often need to be prescribed before or in place of resisted motion.

In this chapter we will review these commonly applied therapeutic motions and their effects on pain, circulation, contractile and non-contractile tissues. Usually a discussion along this line begins with passive motion and ends with resisted motion with active assisted motion and active motion thrown in between. That is a good way to sequence this discussion because it mirrors the typical progression of movement intervention that is applied to a patient whose musculoskeletal tissues have been injured, are degenerated, surgically repaired, or are otherwise irritated and painful due to a flare up in a chronic condition. Chapter 6 will cover the application of motion intervention in relation to phases of tissue healing in greater detail. This chapter will highlight the various attributes of therapeutic motion. So, let's get rolling with passive range of motion (PROM).

PROM

PROM is a form of joint movement that is performed and controlled by an external force without the incorporation of any muscular contraction. The external force can take the form of a clinician, a family member, a machine, a pulley system, elastic bands or the patient himself. PROM has many important attributes. This form of motion can assist circulation, assist synovial fluid movement, decrease pain, and minimize and prevent the numerous negative effects of immobilization including minimizing scar tissue formation, adaptive tissue shortening and joint contracture. PROM cannot prevent muscle atrophy, increase muscle strength, or increase cardiovascular (CV) endurance. Does it take skill, training, and experience to perform PROM effectively? The answer is a resounding yes! A clinician's manual contacts must be relaxed and tailored to the patient and the patient's anatomy. Patient positioning, the speed of the passive movement, and the arc of the passive movement must be performed in a way that allows the patient to relax so that pain and reflex muscular contraction does not prevent effective movement intervention. Repeated arcs of passive motion including passive oscillatory motion is an important form of manual intervention when we are dealing with both extremity and spinal pain impairment. After an injury or after a flare up of a chronic condition, I like to deliver PROM with small arcs of oscillatory angular and translatory (joint traction) motion, fashioned after both the Maitland and Kaltenborn-Evjenth systems of manual therapy. These small oscillatory therapeutic motions are performed with the injured joint close to its resting position. This is a simple form of therapeutic motion that can really reduce your patient's discomfort. You see, that is a good reason to memorize the resting position for each upper and lower extremity joint.

AAROM

Active assisted range of motion (AAROM) is the next movement intervention to discuss. AAROM is joint motion performed and controlled in part by voluntary muscle contraction and in part by an external force. A clinician, a family member, a machine, a pulley system, elastic bands or the patient himself, may give the assistance. This form of intervention is indicated when a patient is able and allowed to lightly contract his or her their muscles. The amount of assistance can vary greatly dependent upon the patient's strength, pain intensity level, or stage of tissue healing post injury or surgery.

This intervention is often used when a patient lacks the strength to perform a movement without substitution, a full arc of movement, or when active movement is painful potentially damaging to a healing muscle or tendon. AAROM can maintain the physiologic properties of a muscle, but it is unlikely to significantly strengthen a muscle. Muscular contraction, even sub maximal contraction will enhance circulation more than PROM and similar to PROM will facilitate synovial fluid distribution. AAROM will enhance coordination by providing sensory feedback to the nervous system and will maintain bone and joint tissue integrity. Further, this type of movement, again similar to PROM can be used to demonstrate a desired motion. In fact, given the level of muscle contraction with active assisted motion, this form of movement is typically favored over passive motion when attempting to improve an individual's proprioception and kinesthesia. Regarding cardiovascular capacity, small gains may occur if many repetitions are performed. Clinic based exercises that incorporate weighted pulley systems and elastic bands to assist active muscle contraction a is great way to protect, that is reduce load, on degenerated cartilage while still achieving a mild muscle strength building effect. Lastly, clinicians must carefully consider their manual contacts when performing AAROM. When possible and when needed, given a patient's strength level or pain intensity, contacts should be on one side of a body part. Grips on both the flexor and extensor surface are desirable for PROM but will not give a tactile cue that is understandable to the patient when muscle contraction is called for by the clinician. Consider this comment regarding manual contacts when performing manually resisted range of motion as well.

AROM

Active range of motion (AROM) is an intervention performed by voluntary muscle contraction. I am sure you already knew that. AROM is often prescribed for many of the same reasons as AAROM is prescribed. Clinically, the patient who may have been receiving AAROM is now stronger or contraction of the target muscle-tendon unit is no longer painful so progression to AROM can now occur. In addition, this intervention can be applied if a previously injured or surgically repaired muscle or tendon has now healed sufficiently.

In Chapter 2 we discussed strength and endurance. A lack of either will affect a patient's ability to perform a full arc of movement against gravity. Prescribing AROM as an intervention requires that the movement pattern in question can be performed fully against the resistance of gravity, and is both symptom and substitution free. AROM can maintain a particular range of movement, improve neuromuscular coordination if performed well, improve endurance, and possibly make small gains in strength if many repetitions are performed. Remember, and this is important, active motion causes muscular contraction. Muscular contraction causes joint compression and that muscular induced compression can further damage cartilage and cause subchondral pain. So, if a particular arc of AROM seems to be causing joint pain, that arc of movement should be avoided! Remember this too, muscle contraction produces a tensile load on tendons. In some cases, this can be beneficial in terms of improving tendon strength. In other cases, if there is a significant tear in said tendon, higher load muscle contraction (resisted range of motion or RROM) could make the tendon tear worse. Keep this mind, when implementing a plan of care for your patient, and when transitioning him/her from one form of therapeutic motion to another such as PROM to AAROM, AAROM to AROM, or AROM to RROM it may be necessary to reduce the arc or speed of the newly prescribed therapeutic motion in order to protect the joint cartilage, painful tendons, and other periarticular tissues.

STRETCHING

The last therapeutic motion to discuss in Chapter 3 is stretching. Muscle stretching seems like an easy concept. It is such an important intervention whether we as clinicians are applying this type of therapeutic motion passively to one of our patients or whether we are prescribing a self-stretching exercise. Funny, it seems like there should be very little disagreement or variation with an intervention we have been applying for so many years. Guess what, there seems to be! Not a day goes by where I don't observe an exercise guru on TV, a trainer in the gym, and even physical therapists and other health care practitioners in various types of clinics placing extremity joints or spinal regions in poor or even dangerous positions all for the sake of stretching. It does not have to be that way! Similarly, I have observed for years' clinicians unnecessarily tensioning peripheral nerves, overly compressing articular cartilage, and overloading the intervertebral disc joints with excessive amounts of spinal flexion, unnecessary hyperextension or worse yet large amplitude spinal rotation while performing manual muscle stretching and when prescribing various self-stretching procedures. We need to think about loading! Is the load on joint cartilage and supportive ligamentous structures, including the disc, which is a ligament by the way, worth that additional little bit of extra flexibility? I know how I feel about it, and clearly, or at least it is clear in my mind, there are many in our profession and other similar lines of work who have not made the simple connection that joints and spinal motion segments need to be protected when manual stretching is performed or when self-stretching is prescribed. As we progress through the text, I will discuss certain key self-stretches at various joints and spinal regions and I will offer up some thoughts regarding the right and safest way to perform these selected stretches. I will also show you the "bad" stretching motions, the ones that should be avoided.

VERY BASIC ANATOMY AND NEUROPHYSIOLOGY

Well, that was slightly controversial. Why don't we get back to the facts, and if not the facts maybe some important definitions and a review of some basic anatomy and neurophysiology relevant to muscle stretching. First, how about muscle flexibility? What is that really? *How about the ability of a muscle and its tendon to lengthen over all the joints they cross allowing full reversal of that muscle's actions.* That works for me and I hope it also works for you. Next, let's review some of the basics regarding the neurophysiology of muscle stretching. Neurophysiology, that's a big word and a little scary too, but here goes nothing. Do you remember an anatomical structure called the muscle spindle? This structure is in essence a unique set of muscle fibers (intrafusal fibers) along with sensory and motor nerve endings. This structure connects directly to the regular (extrafusal) muscles fibers. Here comes the simplification. When a muscle is lengthened or stretched the muscle spindle sends an impulse to the central nervous system, which signals that same muscle to contract. Sounds counterproductive with regards to stretching, but it is an important protective mechanism and there is a balancing mechanism that we will review in the next paragraph.

How about that, the next paragraph is here already and the anatomical structure that sort of balances the effect of the muscle spindle are the Golgi tendon organs (GTOs). That by the way was also a great car made way back in the 1960s. The Pontiac GTO, which was one fast car! But I am showing my age and we need to get back to the role of Golgi tendon organs and therapeutic stretching. These little guys attach into the myotendinous junction and are sensitive to length changes in the muscle tendon unit. The GTOs are most sensitive to tendon elongation whether it is passive elongation or tendon elongation secondary to muscle contraction. Either way, if a muscle is passively stretched or an isometric contraction produces tendon lengthening, the GTO will send an impulse to the CNS which allows the muscle to relax. Studies in muscle neurophysiology seem to show that the impulse sent to the CNS by way of the GTO can "override" the impulses coming from the muscle spindle. For example, if the quadriceps muscle is placed in a lengthened position for a sustained period of time, maybe somewhere in the neighborhood of 30 seconds or more, the GTO's signal to the CNS will allow the muscle to relax and elongate.

That is probably enough on our quick review of muscle neurophysiology. How about just a bit more review, this time on the anatomical structure of skeletal muscle. If you recall, there is well over 400 voluntary muscles in the body, all of which consist of different layers of connective tissue. Muscle fibers lay next to each other and are wrapped in a tissue called endomysium. On average, 150 muscle fibers are bundled together by perimysium. The entire muscle is then encased by, you know it, epimysium. So, that is the macroscopic arrangement of a muscle. Regarding the microstructure of a skeletal muscle, we should briefly look at the sarcomere. The microstructure of a skeletal muscle really consists of two progressively smaller anatomical structures. Each muscle fiber consists of smaller fibers called myofibrils, and the myofibrils are made of small little threads called myofilaments. These myofilaments are in essence made of two proteins called actin and myosin.

Now without going into a lot more detail, let's talk just a bit more about the microstructure of the muscle fiber in a way that as clinicians we will always be able to recall. The myofilaments that we just mentioned are arranged in a repeating and consistent structural pattern. That pattern runs from Z line to Z line and that is your sarcomere. So, what should we try to remember about the myofilaments? Just this, they play a key role in the mechanical process of muscle contraction and as a result muscular force development.

So now that we have briefly reviewed the structure of muscle, let's get back to muscle stretching and look at some of the effects of this therapeutic movement. There are numerous studies that have documented the importance of muscle stretching and injury prevention[11, 12]. I am in agreement with these studies and feel that good muscle flexibility can not only reduce injury risk but also enhance athletic performance. Reduced muscular flexibility may be the result of adhesions in the epimysium, perimysium, endomysium or in the contractile elements of the muscle fibers and tendon.[13] Clinical application of muscle stretching can promote both immediate and short term lengthen effects on the connective tissue components of the target muscle. Long term application of stretching such as immobilization in a lengthened position will result in sarcomere addition.

OLAF Evjenth

Lastly, let's discuss correct clinical application and duration of muscle stretching. Olaf Evjenth, the master of manual muscle stretching and self-stretching has spoken for years on how the effectiveness of muscle stretching relates to force and time. A long time before research papers were written Olaf stated that effective muscle stretching needed to be applied slowly and held for 30 seconds at least and in many cases up to two minutes.[14,15] Further, he stated that a mild to moderate stretching sensation should be felt in the target muscle only. In other words, extremity joint and spinal segmental pain should not be felt during muscle stretching. Similar to me, Olaf also felt that we should not overload support structures such as the IVD or principal extremity joint ligaments in an attempt to elongate what we believe may be a shortened muscle.

A couple more points related points, Olaf noted that when possible stretching should occur over the largest and most stable extremity joint when stretching multi-joint muscles. In other words, pre-position the smaller joints first, make sure they are comfortable and then elongate the muscle over the larger joint that it crosses. Readers of this text will see how this applies to many of the self-stretching procedures in the various extremity chapters. In addition, and I made a similar point in the previous paragraph, the spinal segments should be kept close to mid-position when prescribing self-stretching. See the Swiss Ball supported self-stretches in Chapter 18. We seem to understand that the spine should be held in an in a neutral and stable position while lifting but many seem to forget that the spine should be held in that same position while stretching. If we don't do this, we run the risk of damaging stabilizing structures during a self-stretch procedure.

Chapter 4
Advantages and Disadvantages of Various Exercise Positions

This chapter looks at certain biomechanical considerations for choosing different exercise positions. Some of the attributes of certain exercise positions may seem obvious, but having your patient in the correct position for the performance of their therapeutic exercise is very important. Correct exercise positioning can protect adjacent extremity joints and soft tissues and keep spinal motion segments from being injured. The right patient position facilitates full elongation of soft tissues and gives us the best chance at making muscles stronger. So, let's look at the different exercise positions we commonly use when prescribing therapeutic exercise.

SUPINE

Our first stop is supine. Clearly, a patient's base of support (BOS) is going to be large and their center of gravity (COG) low. This makes the supine position ideal in terms of patient stability.[16] Another important attribute of the supine position is patient relaxation and therapeutic unloading. All upper extremity (UE) and lower extremity (LE) joints as well as spinal segments are unloaded and in this open kinetic chain (OKC) position. Therapeutic unloading or something I like to call "restless bed rest" is an important aspect of therapeutic intervention for patients with load sensitive arthritic LE joints and spinal segments. Restless bed rest unloads LE cartilage and subchondral bone and reduces load on narrowing intervertebral discs. Patients with degenerated discs, and poor hyaline cartilage may experience upright load intolerance and resultant pain while standing and walking. Restless bed rest can be prescribed for 10-15 minutes several times daily to unload discs and articular cartilage. Make sure that your patients rest with their lordosis reduced and extremity joints positioned close to the resting position. Next, in terms of strength building, the supine position offers gravity resisted movement in the sagittal plane for both the upper and lower extremities. So, small strength gains can be achieved in this position. Further, numerous manual resistive exercises (MRE) for both the UE and LE musculature can be provided in supine. Regarding the spinal segments, important postural reinforcement exercises (Chapter 17) and trunk flexor muscle training (Chapter 18) can be performed in this position. It is important to keep in mind however, that some patients with cardiopulmonary difficulties may find it difficult to breathe well in this position and that strength gains, particularly LE strength gains made in supine, may not result in a great deal of functional improvement when in the upright position.

SIDE LIE

Stop number two is the side lying position. Compared to supine, in side lying the BOS is smaller and the COG is slightly higher. That being said the BOS would vary depending on the placement of a patient's LE joints. Movement of the shoulder in the frontal plane is easily achieved in this position making side lying ideal for strength training of the cranial portion of the rotator cuff and the proximal hip abductor muscles. Side lying is a great position to apply MRE concentric and eccentric training to the hamstrings, quadriceps and ankle dorsiflexor muscles. Low back pain can usually be controlled in side lying with anterior and posterior lumbopelvic positioning and MRE for cervical flexor and extensor muscles can also be provided in this position (Chapter 16). While circulation may be diminished to one lung, as compared to supine, most patients find it easier to breathe in side lying. Lastly, while side lying may compress the glenohumeral and hip joints on the undermost side, many of our patients with load sensitive spinal segments and osteoarthritic LE joints will find this position acceptable for performance of many therapeutic exercises (Chapter 13).

PRONE

The third therapeutic position to discuss is prone lying. When patients are positioned well and correct support is provided to the spinal segments this position, or a version of this position over a Swiss Ball, prone lying is typically the best position for improving spinal and proximal hip extensor muscle strength. The superficial spinal muscle layers and the dorsal portion of the rotator cuff can also be therapeutically strengthened in this position. The problem with prone lying is the prone progression. While prone progression is a necessary part of childhood developmental progression and an important aspect of adult neurological rehabilitation, carry over into orthopedic management of lumbar spinal pain patients' needs to stop. What I am referring to is the overuse of the prone on elbows and the prone on hands (press up) position. These two positions are only tolerated well when there is little to nothing wrong with a patient's lumbar segments, in other words, when there is little in the way of degenerative change. As our patient's disc degenerate and narrow, their ability to tolerate this position without the development of lumbar pain will diminish. These two positions, prone on elbows and the prone press up, passively move the lumbar segments into a great deal of hyperextension without allowing the necessary and associated anterior pelvic tilting to occur. Later in the text (Chapter 18), I will demonstrate how lumbar self-mobilization (self-stretching) in the direction of extension is best performed in the hook lying position. This hook lying lumbar extension self-mobilization gently eases the lumbar segments into extension. Further, the cervical hyperextension which often seems to occur in the press up position has no therapeutic value for the neck (Chapter 16) and if performed often enough, will over time contribute the very common occurrence of discogenic based segmental hypermobility.

QUADRUPED

Well guess what, I will have more to say on the topic of lumbar hyperextension later and how eventually if performed as an exercise motion repetitively enough, it will cause our patients' spinal segments more harm than good. Let's discuss something less controversial. Quadruped is our next therapeutic position to consider. The BOS is still large with four points of reference in contact with the ground and COG is higher than prone but certainly less high as compared to standing. This makes quadruped a good position for certain balance activities as the number of points in contact with the ground is easily changeable. In addition, this position is ideal for numerous spinal and hip extensor muscle-training exercises. Similar to prone, spinal extensor and proximal extensor (Gluteus Maximus) muscles can also be trained in this position and if a neutral position of the spine is maintained, the compressive loading on the IVD is minimal.

So, the four point or quadruped position is a great initial strength building position of deep lumbar and deep cervical extensor muscles. Unfortunately, the quadruped position can cause uncomfortable loading of the anterior knee and wrist joints. Also, if we don't position our patient's carefully, gravity and the weight of the trunk will tend to force the cervical and lumbar region into extension which can be problematic if there is advanced grade disc degeneration. Luckily with the hip joints positioned around 90 degree of flexion, lumbar hyperextension with occurs in the prone position during the press up exercise is not possible.

HOOK LIE

Next, let's review the hook lying position. The COG is raised slightly for the LE joints, but the BOS is large making this is a very stable position. Hook lying is a very good exercise position for initial strength building of the hip adductors, abductor, extensor, flexor and deep rotator muscles. (Chapter 13). In fact, with the LE joints in a non-weight bearing (NWB) position and with the lumbar lordosis flattened this is often the most well tolerated position for our patients with advanced osteoarthritic changes in the hip and lumbar segments. Further, hook lie is an excellent position for training of the abdominal and pelvic floor muscles. Similar to supine, this is a great position for patients to rest and reduce load on their weight bearing joints. Also similar to supine, patients with cardiopulmonary impairments may find it difficult to breathe in this position.

HALF-KNEELING

Now let's get the trunk into an upright position and discuss half-kneeling. This position is not used quite as frequently for exercise training in outpatient clinical practice. From a more functional perspective, half-kneeling is a transitional position often attained in route to standing up from the floor. The BOS is reduced and the COG is higher therefore your patients will need good balance responses. From an orthopedic point of view, this may be the best position to perform a common hip flexor self-stretching exercise. In terms of strength building for more advanced patients, half kneeling is essentially the end range position for a deep lunge (split-stance squat) position/movement. Patients with degenerative conditions affecting their lower extremities will find this position difficult to tolerate.

SITTING

Sitting keeps the trunk in an upright position, so let's deal with that position next. The BOS can vary greatly depending upon the size of the sitting surface and the amount of the LE in contact with that surface. In orthopedic practice, sitting is usually a position that most patients can assume and it is incorporated into many daily activities. UE and LE strength training can occur against gravity or with the incorporation of weights, pulleys, and elastic bands or tubing. Proper (improved) sitting posture is a goal for some orthopedic patients. Let's discuss sitting posture and therapeutic exercise. To my way of thinking, an exercise performed in a seated position has little therapeutic value if spinal posture is poor. Therefore, when strength-training exercises are prescribed and weight machines or pulley systems are incorporated, clinicians should make a big effort to support the spine with pillowing and when possible assure that the pelvis is in a vertical position. This is particularly important in patients with a history of low back pain. Promoting a vertical position of the pelvis will improve spinal posture, and this is reasonably easy to do if a patient is seated in an elevated position. Elevating the hips higher than the knees will usually improve a patient's lumbopelvic position. That being said, the seated position will still load the lumbar discs, in fact it loads them a lot. If your patient has a history of backache, particularly backache that worsens when sitting for some period of time, do not have them exercise in this position. Be creative, take the vertical compressive loads off the lumbar spine and accomplish your training goals in different or modified positions.

STANDING

Well our last stop in this chapter is standing. Obviously, the COG is high, the BOS is small, and the LE joints and spinal column are in a weight bearing (WB) position. Clearly, your patient's balance responses must be good if exercise training is to occur in this position. Standing is a great position for many functional activities, tasks and of course ambulation. For patients with neuromuscular or orthopedic conditions causing balance impairments and in some cases for our elderly patients, skilled professional supervision is necessary for many important balance exercises many of which require the standing position. There are many closed kinetic chain (CKC) rehabilitative and sports performance exercises that can be performed in a standing position. In addition, we can utilize this position for our patients in need of balance training. Here is what our profession needs to get better at, unloaded standing! With simple modifications, we can reduce compressive load on the IVD, articular cartilage, and subchondral bone. All we need to do is have our patient's stand between two chairs, lean over a table, or use things such as parallel bars, unloading frames, and harness systems and all of a sudden CKC exercise motions can be performed with less loading and less pain!

Lastly, here is a simple thought to keep in mind. Exercise training in the standing position works best for individuals with healthy LE joint cartilage and well hydrated intervertebral discs. That may seem simple, but that thought is often forgotten or ignored. When a patient's lumbar spine, hips, knees, or feet become more painful, and I don't mean a little soreness in their muscles, but rather a reproduction of deeper joint pain or perhaps a sharp pain as a result of performing an exercise in standing, guess what, they should not have been performing that exercise! Support (unload) these patients in an unloading frame, a harness system, or let them use their upper extremities to support themselves between two chairs and reduce weight bearing through their legs. Regarding load sensitive lumbar pain and in particular lumbar stenosis, support your patient's lumbar segments and strengthen their core muscles in positions other than standing.

Chapter 5
Thoughts of Posture and Pain

I often ask students if they think of posture as a static or a dynamic concept. By show of hands, typically their responses tend to favor the notion that posture is static. Historically, posture tended to be viewed as more of a static concept or position. Usually a patient's posture was examined and evaluated in a standing or a seated position, and that was about it. More recently and particularly in relationship to the therapeutic concept of muscular based spinal stabilization, posture has become more of a dynamic concept. Posture should be examined and evaluated in a number of different positions, during all transitional movements, ADLs, and during all stages of lifting.

The American Academy of Orthopedic Surgeons has defined posture something like this: *Posture is the relative arrangement of the parts of the body. Good posture is the state of muscular and skeletal balance that protects the supporting structures of the body against injury or progressive deformity.* That is a pretty good definition, especially the second sentence. Good posture does protect the body's support structures such as the intervertebral discs and other important ligamentous structures. Poor posture can lead to unbalanced loading of these structures, possibly accelerate degenerative changes and in some cases may be associated with enhanced pain perception.

The American Physical Therapy Association defines posture as a *state of musculoskeletal balance that protects the supporting structures of the body against injury or progressive deformity.*[17] That's a good definition too and it looks a lot like the previous one. Note that both emphasize protection for the supportive anatomical structures of the body and both contain the word balance. Well, what does the word balance mean and how is it achieved? To me, balance or the musculoskeletal balance associated with good posture means fairly uniform loading of passive restraint structures like the discs and other ligaments as well as fairly equal length tension and tone of antagonistic musculature. Also, musculoskeletal balance requires an intact nervous system providing accurate sensorimotor feedback to all of the anatomical structures including the muscles which constantly battle gravitational flexion and extension moments. Musculoskeletal balance has also been likened to postural control. Good postural control requires coordination between a number of different systems. In addition to correct sensory input and exacting motor response, the central nervous system must also analyze input from the eyes, ears, soft tissues and joint proprioceptors.[18]

ABNORMAL POSTURE

Now let's move forward to a brief discussion on postural abnormalities. Abnormal or poor posture may be the result of congenital conditions, degenerative changes, lack of postural awareness and in my opinion lack of correct postural exercises to perform. Here are a couple of common examples that illustrate how postures can become less than ideal. Abnormal spinal posture may result from abnormal vertebral segmentation. Block vertebra and hemivertebra are examples of congenital abnormalities that are associated with changes in the frontal plane spinal curvature. Said another way, failure of full segmental formation or failure of full segmental segmentation are development disturbances that are responsible for postural impairment that we will not be able to correct with therapeutic exercise. Variance in the size of the femoral head or the angle of the femoral neck will cause pelvic obliquity and resultant changes in spinal posture as well. Too often, and this is just a side note, physical therapists and osteopaths see a sacrum that looks tilted downward and immediately call it a "sacral torsion." That, in my mind is non-sense! Usually the cause of this fictional sacral mal-position is an orthopedic growth abnormality at the hip joints or the sacrum itself and any pain in the lumbosacral area is coming from the L4 or L5 disc. OK, sorry about that, let's get back to spinal posture. Thoracic disc degeneration is the most common cause of excessive thoracic kyphosis and is an example of an acquired degenerative change. Lastly, some folks, patients that is, just seem to have a better sense or awareness for their posture. This may, in part, relate to body type and whether or not good posture was a point of emphasis or at least occasionally mentioned during their formative years. Earlier in this paragraph I mentioned that the lack of correct postural exercise(s) also plays a role in poor posture. In this text we will discuss spinal strengthening, self-mobilization and postural reinforcement positions (Chapters 16, 17, 18). All of these therapeutic exercises relate back, at least in part, to improving and maintaining better posture.

PAIN AND ABNORMAL POSTURE

Pain and abnormal posture; are the two linked together? I think the answer is, sometimes they are and sometime they are not. Over many years of clinical practice and patient observation, I have noted individuals with very poor posture but no associated symptoms. This should make a clinician question whether given someone's genetic background and in particular his or her body type, is the reason for the development of less than an ideal posture for that person. Asymptomatic age-related degenerative changes causing postural abnormalities are an example of this last point as well. Sometimes these changes appear to be associated with pain and sometimes they are not. There are situations though when abnormal posture does appear to be associated with pain. Take for example a sciatic scoliosis. In this case, a person develops an abnormal spinal position or posture in an attempt to lessen the pain of an acute nerve irritation. Similarly, a painful flare up in a cervical segment is typically associated with the adoption of an abnormal cervical posture.

Part of the idea behind pain leading to an impaired posture, impaired movement, and impaired strength relates to an abnormal mechanical load or perhaps an abnormal chemical process sensitizing nociceptors in the involved tissues. Now, I am not a neuroanatomist so don't be too critical of the generalizations that are about to follow in the next section. This is a text that deals with therapeutic movement intervention, and one of the big reasons for movement intervention is pain relief. Therefore, we need to review some of the causes and types of pain as well as pain pathways. By the way, some generalizations are not bad if they facilitate lasting knowledge that we can impart to our patients. Simplifying important concepts such as mechanisms of pain perception can help us teach our patients in a way that will reduce concern and anxiety regarding their pain impairments.

PAIN FIBERS

Pain receptors (nociceptors) convey impulses to the spinal cord and higher levels of the central nervous system. This type of receptor is activated by abnormal mechanical load and chemical irritation. Nociceptors in many different tissues convey pain information by way of small, fast, myelinated A-delta fibers and slow unmyelinated C fibers. The fast A-delta fibers are likely involved with pain perception and acute injuries, whereas the slow C fibers are likely to be involved with deeper, dull, and more lasting pain perception. Now, I am really going to generalize. **A**-delta fibers are associated with **a**cute pain; **C** fibers are associated with **c**hronic pain. That is general, and certainly not complete, but very easy to remember and carry forward forever. Now, let's bring this back to therapeutic movement intervention. Therapeutic exercise motions can effectively reduce certain types of pain experienced by our patients. Joint motion stimulates joint afferent receptors whose signal travels along a third and different nerve fiber called A-beta fibers. The A-beta fibers are fast conducting fibers and much faster than the nasty old unmyelinated and slow C fibers. It is important for us to understand that the impulses from the A-beta fibers can block (close the gate) to the transmission of pain impulses from the slower conducting fibers. This blocking of pain transmission occurs in the central nervous system. Note, what you just read was an extremely simplified version of the Gate Control Theory. This is a very important pain theory and it has important clinical application for us. It was originally proposed by Melzack and Wall way back in 1965 and updated significantly in 1982.[19] We can incorporate the Gate Control Theory into our prescription of various therapeutic motions including short amplitude assisted motions (AAROM) and passive oscillatory exercise motions. These types of motion can serve to reduce our patient's perception of pain.

In the next chapter titled; *Musculoskeletal Injury and Repair, and the Application of Therapeutic Motion* we will discuss acute trauma and flare ups of older chronic (degenerative) conditions. But, before we look at injury, repair and movement intervention, we should briefly review two of the most basic types of pain: acute and chronic. Acute pain typically results from some type of tissue trauma or irritation. The trauma may result in some type of chemical irritation or mechanical deformation of nerve receptors with the result being nociception that reaches a cortical level of perception. Chronic pain, on the other hand, is nociception that continues after the painful stimulus has been removed. It includes pain that continues after tissue healing has taken place. Theories for continuation of discomfort include increased sensitization of nociceptors and perpetuating positive feedback loops at the spinal cord level. Again, one of our roles as it relates to the management of both types pain, acute and chronic, is to select and prescribe therapeutic motion, and to control compression and tension loads on joints and soft tissues in a way that does not perpetuate pain input into the nervous system.

Chapter 6

Musculoskeletal Injury and Repair, and the Application of Therapeutic Motion

In this chapter we will look at musculoskeletal tissue injury and some of the characteristic time frames for tissue repair. Within this context, different types of therapeutic motion will be presented with an emphasis on the promotion of tissue healing. Additionally, we will look at a simple examination procedures, such as over pressure testing and end feel testing, which will assist clinicians in choosing the correct form of therapeutic movement. To expand on that just a bit, if an overpressure test is positive, it tells a clinician that a particular joint or region of the spine is currently painful. If that is the case, therapeutic exercise/motion prescription should be gentler, perhaps non-weighting, unloading, short in amplitude and performed close to the joints resting position or the spinal segments mid-position. If an end feel test is not painful and it demonstrates short tissue shortening (stiffness impairment) then our exercise/motion prescription can likely be a bit more aggressive in so as to elongate tissues with tension loads and greater arcs of movement. Finally, this chapter will also take a brief look at the microanatomy of connective tissue and connective tissue loading.

I have always felt that applying therapeutic intervention to injured musculoskeletal tissues was fairly straight-forward given the predictable way these tissues tend to heal. If a clinician respects tissue healing time frames and patient response to basic examination movements, we should be able to assist and not retard or delay tissue healing. Now, I mentioned that musculoskeletal tissues, also referred to as connective tissue, heal in a predictable way, but we should keep the following thoughts in mind. The rate of healing will be affected by age, personal habits and overall medical health. For example, don't expect the connective tissues to heal as well if your patient smokes or abuses alcohol. Further, conditions such as diabetes mellitus, systemic or local soft tissue infection, stress, and nutritional status can affect the rate of connective tissue healing.[20] Next, let's take a quick look at the microanatomy of connective tissue.

Bone, cartilage, ligaments, muscle and tendon are the principal connective tissues in the body. In short, connective tissue is made up of fibers, ground substance, and cells. Collagen and elastin are the two types of connective tissue fiber, glycosaminoglycans (ground substance) is in effect the tissue fluid, and the fibrocyte is the principal cell type of connective tissue

Cartilage gets about 80% of its weight from water and is primarily type II collagen. The proteoglycans in cartilage attract and bind the water. Regarding ligaments, water makes up about two thirds of their weight with collagen being approximately 75% of the dry weight. Ligaments are made up of 90% type I collagen. Tendons are two thirds water, one third collagen and 2% elastin. So, you can see that there are quite a few similarities in that our connective tissues are predominately water and collagen with some minerals thrown in. Now we should move on to the each of the main types of connective tissues and the other principal portion of this chapter which is musculoskeletal tissue injury, repair, and the application of therapeutic motion. [21].

BONE

Bone is composed of both solid and liquid components. Type I collagen and proteoglycans (a form of glycosaminoglycan) make up about one third of bone's volume and minerals constitute about half of bone's dry weight Now, how about we break some bones? It is not real fun when it happens, but on balance, bones tend to heal well so that's good. The first day or two after a fracture, hematoma formation and necrosis of loose bony fragments will occur. The initial inflammatory process will continue for approximately 2-5 days until the necrotic bone is removed. Early repair of the fracture site consists of a soft callus consisting of fibrous tissue. This begins anywhere from 4 to 12 days' post injury and correlates to the reduction of initial pain as swelling. A more mature and dense callus forms as the soft callus is replaced by bone anywhere from the 3-4 weeks post fracture up to approximately 12 weeks post fracture. At around the 6-week mark, a return to normal structure can be seen as cortical bone forms between the ends of the fracture site.[22]

Provision of therapeutic exercise movement after a fracture relates to a number of factors such as patient age, type of fracture, severity of fracture, stability of the fracture, site of fracture and of course the number of days' post fracture. For example, stable impaction fractures at the upper end of the humerus can be therapeutically moved right away with limited movement arcs by carefully applying slow passive and active assisted motion through the shoulder joint. Similarly, a surgically fixated tibial fracture can be moved and can weight bear right away. On the other hand, only passive motion is allowed for a newly fixated patellar fracture to prevent traction loads from the quad tendon across the fracture site. We don't want the patient pulling the fracture line apart. Otherwise, the principals of therapeutic motion intervention for fractures are the same as treating other soft tissue injuries. Just follow these bony tissue healing time frames discussed in the previous paragraph and begin with short arcs of slowly applied PROM and progressing to AAROM, followed by AROM, and finally RROM to strengthen weakened muscular tissues around and adjacent to the newly formed hard callous.

ARTICULAR CARTILAGE

The next and perhaps most vital structure associated with the joints that we treat is articular cartilage. There are two broad classifications of cartilage injury and unfortunately neither one heals very well. So unlike bone and other connective tissues, the healing of injured cartilage follows a much less consistent time frame and if fact may not heal at all. The first type of injury is disruption of the proteoglycan matrix. In this first classification there is little or no damage found in the cartilage cells or collagen fibril network.[23] That being said proteoglycan degradation can cause irreversible cartilage damage. Aging, trauma, surgical disruption, infection, inflammatory disease and prolonged immobilization all may stimulate degradation of the proteoglycan matrix. Regardless of the initial cause, quick resolution of joint swelling and inflammation is extremely important. This is best accomplished with load reduction and motion modification for all of the initial therapeutic exercises. Later in the course of care and with an eye on long-term support for the cartilage, increased local muscle support for the joint in question can be important. Therapeutic muscle strength building for the muscles that move a joint with degenerated cartilage should be pain-free during the exercise, and by pain-free I mean no joint (subchondral) pain. In addition, there should not be any post exercise swelling or painful reaction to therapeutic strengthening. If a patient with some level of cartilage degeneration needs to ice after performing "therapeutic" exercises you as the clinician made them do too much. You have not correctly controlled joint motion and joint compression during the therapeutic exercise/motion.

The second classification of cartilage injury is mechanical damage. This may take the form of blunt trauma, penetration injury, frictional abrasion, cortisone injection, or sharp concentration of weight bearing forces as commonly seen when there is unequal load distribution within a joint. Examples of this include joints with varus and valgus alignment abnormalities, and joint instability. Over time, this can injure chondrocytes and disrupt the matrix.[23]

In a clinical situation where cartilage cell (chondrocyte) damage has occurred, significant adaptation of all therapeutic exercise movements will be required. The therapist must be creative in terms of selecting a patient position that facilitates load reduction (minimize compression), and both the speed and arc of therapeutic movement must be pain and noise (crepitation) free. Here is a big question to think about and hopefully research. Can physical therapists prescribe exercises for patients in a way that will correctly load their joints, and joint cartilage and promote healing without damaging this vital structure particularly if the prescribed exercise is carried out for a long period of time?

LIGAMENTS

Now we have to consider ligamentous connective tissue. Ligaments tend to follow a more predictable pattern of healing, so the three phases of healing can be discussed within the context of ligamentous injury. Clinicians need to understand all aspects of the Inflammatory Phase (Phase I), the Repair and Regeneration Phase (Phase II), and the Remodeling and Maturation Phase (Phase III) in order to correctly load connective tissues with therapeutic motion.

When ligamentous connective tissue is injured, cells release chemicals that initiate an inflammatory process. Local bleeding in torn tissue is filled with blood cells and platelets. This attracts other cells to the injured site where bacteria and cellular debris is processed through phagocytosis. In this phase as tissue is removed, fibroblasts are recruited to the area and weak hydrogen bonding begins to occur between collagen fibers. Phase I is approximately the first 72 hours after injury and is characterized by hematoma formation and acute inflammation showing itself as redness, swelling, increased temperature and pain. Movement examination will often show voluntary muscle guarding and a complaint of pain prior to the end of normal range of movement or normal end feel. In some circles this might be called a high level of tissue or joint reactivity when pain is encountered before a normal end feel. If this is your patient's response to passive movement testning consider immobilization of the joint and surrounding ligamentous tissue. For LE ligamentous injury, crutches are a must! Instruct the patient in supporting an UE joint in the resting position with a sling. Therapists need to respect this first 72 hours and unload and immobilize the injured ligamentous tissue. If it is a spinal soft tissue injury, use collar, corsets, and don't be afraid to prescribe bed rest for 48 hours. As a profession we do not prescribe this nearly enough. Remember, rest and unloading is sometimes a much better prescription than exercise!

The second phase of healing lasts from 48 hours after injury to the 8-week post injury mark. This is the repair and regeneration phase, and while many things are happening, the main thing to remember is that new collagen is being synthesized. It is even more important to remember that the new collagen is not strong. The fibers are small, disorganized, and lack solid cross-linking. Consequently, this makes the injured, but healing tissue, very susceptible to re-injury. From a clinical perspective, observation and palpation will show reduced swelling and reduced tissue warmth. From an examination movement perspective, less muscle guarding will be noted and improved range of motion will be seen. The clinician will be able to move the joint and surrounding periarticular soft tissue closer to its end range (end feel). Again, in some circles this is considered a moderate level of joint/tissue reactivity. A moderate level of reactivity clinically correlates with a full range of motion and the patient's perception of pain staring right at the first stop (end feel). Lower levels of tissue/joint irritation or reactivity typically means that we can now prescribe larger amplitude and increased speed of therapeutic motion. Note, we may still need to stay away from a full range of movement and we likely still need to control (decease or minimize) loading. The next paragraph will discuss some of these motion and loading ideas.

During the first half of Phase II a clinician should consider OKC LE motions, and progress toward unloaded or partial weight bearing LE exercises performed in closed kinetic chain (See examples of this concept in Chapter 14). CKC LE exercise must be pain free during the second phase of healing. Generally speaking, the first part of this phase should incorporate pain free and reduced arcs of passive and active assisted motion. Remember, early and careful passive and active assisted motion is necessary to prevent soft tissue adhesions and to increase collagen synthesis. To repeat, early in phase II passive and assisted motion should not be painful and should not place excessive tensile load on the healing tissue.

During the second half of this phase, so somewhere around 4 to 8 weeks after injury, weight bearing can be increased as LE load tolerance improves. Note, LE CKC exercise must be non-painful both during and after exercising. If a patient's skin temperature increases, if joint swelling increases, and as mentioned previously, if a patient needs ice to reduce discomfort after CKC LE exercise training, you as the clinician have made a mistake. The exercise is no longer therapeutic and you have in fact set the patient back. Causing pain in this phase will only neurologically inhibit already weakened muscle. Here are some other generalities regarding therapeutic motion during the second portion of phase II. AAROM can transition to AROM and then to light RROM, the speed of therapeutic motion can increase and directional changes may be acceptable. For example, UE PNF patterns can now be incorporated and low speed LE ladder training, cone (obstacle course), and other upright agility and balance exercises may be integrated. Again, full tensile loading should still not be placed on torn ligamentous tissue at this point.

Phase III is termed the Remodeling and Maturation phase and it is generally taken to begin around the 8week mark after an injury and lasts for one year. In terms of the microanatomy of the repair process, less synthesis and cellular activity is occurring and the collagen fibers continue to organize and are becoming more tightly held together with covalent bonding.[24] Examination movements will demonstrate a low level of joint/soft tissue reactivity. In other words, a clinician will typically be able to move the injured joint and associated soft tissues to the end of their normal range of motion and evaluate the tissue end feel without patient reaction and voluntary muscle guarding.

Therapeutic loading of connective tissue becomes important in this third phase. Generally speaking, weight bearing, speed of movement, directions of movement and amount of resistance and tensile loading can all increase. Partially torn ligamentous tissue, particularly after 12 or more weeks, has now likely healed up to 80% by primary intent. Given this, the ligamentous tissue will need increased and challenging forms of therapeutic motion and loading stimulation. To end this section on the three phases of healing and to complete our discussion on ligamentous injury, let's review ligamentous sprain classification. Ligamentous sprains occur on a continuum of over stretching and tearing of ligamentous and capsular fibers. The severity of a sprain can be diagnosed through both clinical examination and magnetic resonance imaging. Grade I sprains are in effect an over stretching of the ligamentous tissue without tearing and without resultant joint hypermobility. A grade II ligamentous sprain includes over stretching and partial tearing of fibers. Resultant joint hypermobility in one or more directions of movement will occur. A grade III sprain is a complete or near complete ligamentous tear and there will be a greater chance of joint instability in one or more directions of movement.

CAPSULAR TISSUE

It is difficult to discuss ligamentous injury in isolation without also discussing injury to the joint capsular tissue. Ligaments, as you most likely are aware, often blend with and thicken joint capsules. Injury to a joint capsule is often in the form of excessive tensile loading causing tearing and resultant capsular effusion. The severity of capsule injury and subsequent effusion may take the form of synovitis, a less severe injury, or hemarthrosis, a more severe injury.

Synovitis secondary to injury may be associated with tearing of capsular fibers. This level of injury is relatively harmless to the joint itself but a day or two of immobilization is usually always a good thing before moving the injured tissues.[25] Synovial irritation due to capsular fiber tearing will cause the surrounding muscle tone to be inhibited. Note, complete therapeutic strength restoration will not be possible until the synovitis has resolved. Remember, when providing movement intervention in this situation, light PROM and limited arc AAROM should be pain-free. Therapeutic movements should not make the patient more sore or more swollen. So, address the swelling associated with synovitis with pain-free motion first. I often use limited arcs or movement and a pulley system or elastic band to assist movement (AAROM) when a joint is swollen and the joint musculature is inhibited.

Hemarthrosis is associated with a more significant tearing of capsuloligamentous fibers due to a more significant injury.[25] Other soft tissues may be injured as well and this condition is associated with bleeding within the joint. This bleeding can be very destructive to intra-articular structures. Fibrinogen may cause breakdown in the collagen networks, and destroy articular cartilage; therefore, blood needs to be taken out of an injured joint right away. Injuries which cause hemarthrosis are typically high energy injuries and initial therapeutic intervention should most likely incorporate immobilization for a period of time. After a period of immobilization, the muscles controlling movement for the injured joint will have weakened and therapeutic strength training should begin. Also, after a period of immobilization, the injured joint should be examined for flexibility impairment and if found, therapeutic tissue lengthening (self-stretching) should prescribed. Both of these interventions should begin in a controlled fashion by initially minimizing arcs of movement and minimizing loads placed across the injured tissue.[25]

TENDON

Our next tissue to discuss is tendon, and we will focus on when tendons become painful. I see tendons becoming painful in three different ways. The first way tendons become painful often relates to overwork, or an extra or unaccustomed activity. Repetitive loading of a tendon without sufficient rest time can incite an inflammatory reaction. Inflammation often involves the paratenon which is the outer most layer of the tendon itself. In terms of clinical examination, an inflamed tendon will demonstrate palpatory tenderness, pain with resisted isometric contraction and possibly pain with passive elongation. This form of tendinopathy is typically referred to as tendonitis and in our younger patients without tendon degeneration, this pain impairment is usually temporary. Discontinuing the offending activity and a short course of immobilization is all that is required to successfully manage this condition.

Intratendinous degeneration is a second type of tendinopathy. This condition is often termed tendinosis and it too may be associated with repetitive over loading framed around aging, tendon atrophy, tendon micro tearing and vascular ischemia to the tendon itself. Typical inflammatory response is not found and pain may be associated with vascular and nervous tissue in growth which may represent the body's attempt to heal the symptomatically degenerated tendon. Active cessation or modification, intermittent use of bracing for immobilization or motion control and a trial of eccentric muscle-tendon strengthening may help in this situation.

The third type of tendinopathy is an acute tendon tear. Most daily activities, sports, and therapeutic exercises do not come close to ever reaching the ultimate failure point of a tendon. Heavy overuse, high energy (high load or velocity) injury, or a sudden quick movement in a loaded position perhaps superimposed upon pre-existing tendinosis will tear a tendon. An acute tendon tear is typically quite painful and may require surgical re-attachment depending on the tendon and the extent of the tear.

Therapeutic intervention for tendinopathies should be based on the type of tendon injury, the results of ultrasound testing, the phase of healing, the age of the tendon (patient) in question, the daily demand that the patient will be placing on the tendon, and of course the resultant functional limitations. In my opinion most acute tendon injuries should be immobilized with a brace, splint or cast. Remember; respect the first phase of healing, immobile and don't exercise! Also, and while there is debate about this in the literature in an acute tendon paratenon inflammation in a young patient with young tendons, a short course of anti-inflammatory medication may help.

If the tendinopathy is very painful when examined, prescribe and have the patient perform PROM and non-symptomatic AAROM which does not overly lengthen the tendon. As the painful tendon symptoms improve, and particularly if the tendon in question is required to lift heavy loads or perform quick and strenuous movements, then resisted muscle training including eccentric strengthening is typically needed. Next, we should consider stretching. If a muscle-tendon unit needs to lengthen as part of its typical daily or sports related function than manual and self-stretching should be applied. Painful and degenerated tendons (tendinosis) likely do not need manual or self-stretching exercise. Degenerative tendinopathy essentially represents a weakened structure which more likely need strength building. You will find numerous resisted (strength building) exercises in this text including a number of eccentric loading (ball dropping) exercises for the rotator cuff. Next, let's briefly review the cellular response associated with a tendon tear.

A tendon tear is often associated with acute injury; the anatomy of the healing process parallels the discussion on ligamentous injury. During week 1 and 2 the injured site fills with blood and cellular debris. By day 3, fibroblasts invade the injured site and begin to synthesize type I collagen. The orientation of the collagen will be affected by the therapeutic motions applied. Carefully applied PROM is necessary to prevent adhesions to surrounding structures, and to increase collagen synthesis. PROM should move but not fully lengthen the injured tendon during the first two weeks after a tendon repair.

During weeks 3-4, fibroblast invasion and collagen deposition continues in the injured area but the tensile strength of tendon is still poor at this point. Consider this when therapeutically applying PROM, AAROM, and AROM 3-4 weeks post injury. Remember, newly forming collagen tissue aligns itself in response to the loading it is subjected too. Therapeutic loading of the healing tendon tissue is necessary, but do not over load or over stretch the tendon at this point. AAROM and AROM should be applied in limited movement arcs that do not cause the muscle to pull too strongly on the healing tendon.

During weeks 4-6 the tensile strength of the injured tendon is improving. Collagen fibers will continue to align and organize in relation to both daily and therapeutic motion intervention. Full range active movement is allowable at 4 weeks. Light RROM is allowable at week 5 and 6. During weeks 6-8, the tensile strength of tendinous tissue has improved, and at week 8 post injury most arcs of RROM are now acceptable. In other words, it is safe in most circumstances for the muscle to "pull on" its own tendon. Also, light passive manual stretching is typically allowed at 8 weeks after a tendon tear/surgical repair. Now that we have discussed some of the guidelines for therapeutic intervention after surgical repair of a tendon, let's look at muscle tears similar to the ones our athletic patients might suffer.

MUSCLE

The muscle injury we are speaking of here is the result of strain or excessive muscular loading, rather than direct blunt trauma or contusion to the muscular tissue. A muscle tear at week 1 will show fiber disruption and hemorrhage. During the first four days there is a typical cellular inflammatory response with swelling, and fibroblasts invading the area. Ischemia due to vascular disruption can lead to scar tissue formation. Clinically, the patient will demonstrate pain with active contraction and a reduced ability to generate force. The patient should use crutches for the first 48 hours to reduce demand on a torn LE muscle. Compression wrapping is also a good idea for at least the first several days. During week 1 PROM in the pain free range is the intervention of choice.

By the end of the first week, macrophages clear away necrotic tissue and blood vessels invade the injured area. Healing is now underway. By week 3 the patient will have much less discomfort, but the muscle tissues still lack strength, and are very vulnerable to recurrent strain.

Keep this in mind when giving an athlete or a worker the "O.K." to return to their activities if they are non-symptomatic at 3 weeks after a tear. Therapeutically, we should apply AAROM and AROM possibly moving toward the application of light RROM toward the end of week 3. From a passive movement perspective, clinicians should transition from PROM that repetitively slackens the torn muscles tissue to PROM that begins to lengthen and stretch the muscle as healing occurs.

During weeks 3-5, satellite cells continue to differentiate into myoblasts, these structures fuse to form myotubes. The injured area in the muscle is continuing to get stronger and better able to withstand tensile loading. RROM can continue to incrementally increase from week 3 to week 5 and muscle stretching can also be incrementally increased. From about the fifth week after a muscle tear until around 6 months post tear, myotubes continue to fuse and form into muscle fibers that continue to grow and mature. If a muscle tear is massive some permanent loss of function will occur. Surgical repair is required if a large palpable gap exists between ends of the muscle tear. Motion intervention for return to sports competition should include manual concentric and eccentric muscle training and high-

NERVE

The last tissue we will look at is nerve tissue and the following comments pertain primarily to nerve laceration. During the first week after a nerve laceration, the nerve cell bodies respond to injury by increasing their metabolic activity. The axon distal to severance undergoes Wallarian Degeneration. Unmyelinated axons degenerate within this first week. With a sharp traumatic laceration injury, axonal sprouting may begin after about four days. With extreme trauma this may by delayed be as much as 3 weeks. Schwann cells will form tubules for regenerating axons. New nerve fibers pass down through these new endoneurial tubules. This process is not tremendously specific resulting in variable sensory and motor return. During weeks 2-8 the axon and myelin sheath degenerate, the Schwann cells and macrophages remove the necrotic debris. Fascicular cross-sectional area will continue to decrease over a long period of time. Laceration injury will result in skeletal muscle atrophy and progressive destruction of motor end plates.[25] Therapeutic movement intervention for the purpose of strength restoration is questionable and likely of little value. PROM to maintain the integrity of periarticular tissues is indicated.

The final section of this chapter will look at a clinical concept quite similar to the three phases of connective tissue healing. This concept relates to musculoskeletal injury and repair, but also encompasses painful flare ups of older more chronic conditions. These flare ups do not necessarily have to be associated with an injury.

STAGE OF A CONDITION

In essence, what we will be looking at here is the level of irritability of a clinical condition. The traditional thoughts associated with this concept dealt with the acuity or stage of a clinical condition and the terminology used was acute, subacute, and chronic. From a pain intensity, tissue injury, and clinical management perspective, this terminology is probably not quite adequate. Stan Paris PhD PT, an orthopedic manual physical therapist of long standing was the first person I know of to expand upon the traditional three prong approach to classifying the level of acuity.

Stan felt that right after an injury or right after a flare up of an old chronic condition, the patient could be classified as being in the immediate stage. This stage correlated to the first few minutes after an injury, misuse, overuse or poor position or posture causing pain to reach a threshold level. Many orthopedic movement impairments that we see in a clinical setting are reoccurrences of past conditions or flare ups of older more chronic conditions. If this is the case, we can educate a patient in what to do or not to do should the immediate stage (flare up) reoccur again. The correct intervention in this stage can significantly improve the final outcome of a given condition. Intervention in this stage may include first aid, protection, support; unloading, immobilizing or even teaching a constrained movement pattern (neuromuscular re-education) to the patient and his/her injured tissue in an effort to minimize further damage. A clinician working with a sports team may see this stage most frequently.

The second stage is now classified as the acute stage and it is typified by a condition that is still worsening. The injury or flare up is still pretty recent. Both patient symptoms and clinical findings indicate a condition that is increasing in intensity. Intervention in this stage should assist and not retard healing of the injured tissue. Immobilization, reduced weight bearing and perhaps small oscillatory passive movements (therapeutic motions) with the body part supported close to its resting position are examples of correct intervention in this stage. Remember, often the best intervention is no intervention. In this situation, we should respect the inflammatory cycle and prescribe rest, support and immobilization for the tissue or joint in question. Examples of this include a soft collar for the cervical spine, taping or bracing for an extremity joint, taping or corsetry for the lumbar spine, a sling for an upper extremity injury, crutches or a cane for lower extremity injuries and LE arthritic flare ups.

In the third or sub-acute stage, symptoms have reached a plateau. The condition is no longer worsening, but this is where the clinician must continue to be careful. Many forms of manual or exercise intervention while temporarily relieving symptoms may actually retard the healing process if these interventions are too aggressive and overload the fragile healing tissues. For the spinal segments, exercise positions that unload the discs and minimize motion through injured segments can help healing to continue to occur. For the upper extremities, therapeutic motion should include exercises assisted by a therapist, a gravity reduced plane of motion, a pulley system, or elastic bands which assist motion. The arcs of exercise movement should be short and weight bearing status controlled and minimized with canes, walkers, unloading frames, parallel bars or positioning a patient between two chairs to provide unloading of LE joints during CKC exercise movements.

In the fourth or settled stage, the injury or flare up has reached a point where the patient can now be evaluated more fully, and intervention can be a bit more aggressive owing to the fact the patient is less painful. Overpressure and end feel testing will be less painful (reactive) because the patient's tissues have more fully healed. Manual intervention such as functional massage, manual muscle stretching and manual joint mobilization may begin lengthening tissues. Therapeutic exercise intervention can now be more aggressive in terms of weight bearing status, longer arcs of movement further away from the joints resting position; gravity resisted planes of movement, increased weight bearing, reduced elastic and cable assistance and increased exercise dosage.

The last stage is the chronic stage and is characterized by a lack of progress. The pain associated with the initial flare up has now been present for more than three months. Part of the reason for describing this stage as chronic is based on clinical observation with some scientific correlation regarding the rate of primary healing. Studies show that 50% of primary healing occurs in 2 weeks, 80% of primary healing occurs in 8 weeks, and 100% of primary healing occurs in 12 weeks. Note, improvement in a patient's condition can occur after this time frame as a result of tissue remodeling. Treating pain impairments in the chronic stage should still consider how fragile the tissue may be or how degenerated the joint cartilage or intervertebral disc maybe. If a weakness or stiffness impairment exists in this stage, the exercise intervention can be more aggressive, but still should still not cause a painful flare up or joint swelling. Remember, it is not our job to damage tissues by prescribing exercise motions that overload tissues if those tissues are degenerated and structurally less sound.

Chapter 7
A Few Comments on Osteoarthritis and Exercise

Many of the exercises within this textbook consider individuals who have developed or are developing osteoarthritis. It is estimated that between 40 and 60 million Americans have some form of arthritis. This is a large range, and as of today these numbers above may actually be low. Without question these figures will continue to increase over the next ten years as the baby boomer segment of society continues to age. Each day in most every clinical practice setting, physical therapists assist patients with impairments and functional limitation due to osteoarthritis (OA). Arthritic impairments in strength, flexibility, mobility, pain and endurance are well documented in research.[26] Aging and osteoarthritis, injury and secondary arthritis, or infection with some form of acute arthritis is not fun for anyone to deal with. For certain types of OA, therapeutic exercise is right in the forefront of management for patients experiencing various impairments associated with this condition.

EXAMINATION

Before we discuss some of the aspects of therapeutic exercise management for arthritis, let's briefly review some of the key things to look for during the examination of a patient with symptomatic arthritic changes. First, look at the patient's joint and soft tissue structure and note for any deformity, swelling, atrophy or alignment changes. Second, examine the patient's active and passive motion. If your patient demonstrates active and passive movement loss in a similar direction with an overly firm or hard end feel that arrives earlier than normal, arthritic joint restriction (calcium build up, cartilage loss) and capsular shortening are likely present. On the other hand, increased active and passive motion (excessive joint mobility) with end feels that arrive late and feel soft indicate arthritic change that has caused capsular laxity and resultant joint hypermobility and instability. Third, look at the muscular strength around the joint in question. Strength loss is typically associated with chronic OA and muscular inhibition is usually seen with acute flares of arthritic pain. Forth, determine how irritated your patient's joint and related tissues are by noting whether or not active and passive examination motions reproduce pain. Reflecting on pain response to active and passive examination movements will assist you in terms of exercise selection and dosage. Keep this point in mind! Fifth and last, you should note for palpatory findings around the symptomatic joint including tissue temperature, tension and tenderness. If a patient's soft tissues overlying an arthritic joint are tender, your exercise selection (motion) will need to be gentle This paragraph was brief and certainly did not detail examination technique, but you just read over five important aspects of musculoskeletal physical examination and some things to keep in mind regarding impairments that OA can cause how your exam findings might relate to exercise prescription.

TYPES OF ARTHRITIS

There are many different types of arthritis, and the patient history can assist as an initial step toward determining which type a patient may have. With acute forms of arthritis, joint pain begins very rapidly over several hours or within just a few days. Note whether or not the history includes fever, chills, or sweating. Consider infection in this case and make sure the patient is referred to a medial colleague for laboratory investigation. Some forms of arthritis begin gradually and increase in severity over a period of several weeks to a few months. Regarding this time frame and if inflammation is present in just one joint (monoarticular) consider infection again and see that an appropriate referral is made.

Polyarthritis demonstrates a gradual onset is characteristic of several different forms such as rheumatoid arthritis, psoriatic arthritis, Reiters syndrome, and systemic lupus erythematosus. The primary symptoms of chronic polyarthritis include more diffuse joint pain, stiffness, and fatigue. Migratory joint pain and skin changes are also seen. Arthritis with an insidious onset begins so gradually and may progress so slowly that some patients have a hard time knowing exactly when their joint(s) became problematic. Early on in the course of chronic degenerative arthritis the affected joint is typically painful with use and improves with cessation of the pain producing activity. Later in the course of this condition pain may continue after the provoking activity is stopped and associated stiffness and weakness impairments become more problematic.

This form of chronic arthritis is typically degenerative in nature and is characterized by the breakdown in articular cartilage. Degenerative arthritis is associated with aging and affects well over 50% of people over age 65. Predisposing factors for chronic degenerative arthritis include obesity, trauma, generalized hypermobility, and certain genetic factors.[27] So how should we manage our patients with acute flares of arthritis, flare ups of chronic forms of arthritis, and what about longitudinal prescription of exercise for patients with arthritis or for those with the potential for developing this condition.

RESEARCH AND ARTHRITIS

How much does the research help clinicians when considering individualized exercise prescription for this condition? Unfortunately, larger research studies and systematic reviews of the literature rarely give us a glimpse into treatment success or failure for the individual. Large reviews don't let us know who became painful with exercise and what type of exercise was applied. In clinical practice, prescribing therapeutic exercises that make even one patient painful is not acceptable. The statistical work up in a large study has a way of washing individual treatment failures away. Further, it is my contention that most patients participating in larger studies are in the settled stage (Chapter 6) of an arthritic flare up or perhaps only have a low level of chronic discomfort.

That said most all research demonstrates that the majority of patients benefit from both endurance and resistance exercise training. For example, in a systemic review of the literature, Roddy, Zhang and Doherty concluded that patients with knee OA showed reduced pain and reduced disability after participating in an aerobic walking program and home-based quadriceps strengthening program.[28] In a community-based study of 439 adults over age 60 Ettinger et al found that older persons with OA demonstrated modest improvements in disability, physical performance, and pain with either a resistance training exercise program or an aerobic exercise program.[29] Similarly, in a systematic review of the literature, land-based exercise was found to reduce pain and improve physical function in people with OA of the knee.[30]

Other studies have actually examined the effect of exercise on the joint's most important structure, the cartilage itself. Bautch et al found that 30 elderly patients with knee OA did not demonstrate negative changes in synovial fluid glycosaminoglycan (GAG) concentrations after 12 weeks of weigh bearing exercise.[31] Similarly, Roos and Dahlberg demonstrated positive effects on GAG content in the cartilage in 45 somewhat younger subjects (mean age 46 years) after moderate exercise training.[32] Unfortunately, these two studies cannot be considered as longitudinal analysis of the structural response of cartilage to exercise, and that is the real question. If our patients continue to follow our exercise prescription over many years, it is possible that modifications in weight bearing, resistance, speed of movement and arc of movement will have to occur. Regarding that last comment, longitudinal analysis of individual exercise programs is one of the reasons why physical therapists should establish long term therapeutic relationships with their patients.

EXERCISE AND ARTHRITIS

Keep in mind that joint cartilage is not the only tissue affected by degenerative osteoarthritis. Other tissues are affected by osteoarthritis and the loading that occurs during exercise. Joint capsular tissue, adjacent bursal tissue, and the muscles which generate joint motion are all subject to the effects of exercise and arthritis. Too much loading, too many repetition and overly large amplitudes of exercise motion can irritate any of the tissues just mentioned. Further, and regarding muscles, painful arthritic inflammatory episodes can cause muscular weakness and inhibition. Muscular inhibition and resultant changes in movement patterns (reduced movement) due to arthritic discomfort can all lead to further muscle atrophy.

Should we prescribe therapeutic exercise in our patients with osteoarthritis? The answer is yes, but as I mentioned before, pain intensity, signs and symptoms tissue irritation and lack of load tolerance must be respected. When a patient is suffering with a painful flare of arthritis in his/her joint(s), therapists must be creative in their exercise design and dosage in order to assist the patient through the painful flare up without overloading the irritated tissues. As noted in Chapter 6, clinicians need to respect the inflammatory cycle, the various phases of tissue healing. We need to recognize which stage of flare up our patient is in. If we are respectful of these foundational concepts and utilize sound movement-based examination which correctly determines the type of impairment(s) our patient presents with, then prescription of movement intervention to reduce pain and swelling, protect tissues, lengthen tissue, and strengthening tissue and unload tissue should be very straight-forward. If we incorporate therapeutic exercise features such as short arc pain- free motion, gravity or equipment assisted motion, open kinetic chain motion and assisted or reduced weight bearing closed kinetic chain motions and exercise motions and positions with reduce intra-discal pressure, our therapeutic exercises should be able to assist in reducing inflammation, promote a degree of tissue healing, minimize the chance of recurrent flare ups and assist in improved tolerance for other activities.

In terms of exercise management of our patients in the settled and chronic stage of arthritis, in other words, the patient is currently not painful, prescribe strengthening exercises for weakened muscles, prescribe self-stretching for shorten extremity capsular tissue, and prescribe controlled spinal self-stretching mobilizations for segmental stiffness. But remember, just because the patient is not currently experiencing pain, does not mean that his or her extremity cartilage or intervertebral disc has magically healed. Continue to control arcs of resisted movement and creatively unload cartilage and intervertebral discs during the exercises you prescribe. For some patients with LE arthritic, partially unloaded closed kinetic chain exercises may improve function to a greater degree and still minimize the compressive loading on the cartilage and subchondral bone well enough that the exercise can be performed for many years. In our patients with reduced joint and spinal segmental motion secondary to arthritic degeneration, our extremity self-stretching and spinal self-mobilization exercises must improve and maintain joint and segmental motion without damaging extremity capsuloligamentous tissue, the intervertebral disc and other important ligamentous stabilizing structures. Remember, we need to protect our patient's tissues and IVD from sustained tissue overload due to poor postures while stretching (many Yoga positions) and excessive motions and loads on key stabilizing structures. Any of which can happen with loaded large amplitude and repetitive stretching motions.

Chapter 8
Thoughts on Examination and Evaluation of the Orthopedic Patient

This is a textbook on therapeutic exercise for patients with common orthopedic conditions and associated impairments and functional limitations. So why should we discuss orthopedic examination? Well, here are a couple of thoughts. First, I have always felt very strongly that expert clinical practice should be firmly based in a comprehensive understanding of anatomy, biomechanics and orthopedic pathology or conditions. Second, a comprehensive understanding of pathology as well as research evidence is necessary in order to make correct clinical decisions regarding the application of examination procedures and the prescription of exercise. Orthopedic physical therapists who cannot correctly diagnose orthopedic pathology by way of clinical examination cannot, in my opinion practice and prescribe exercise at an expert level.

The correct clinical diagnosis is very much dependent upon the foundational knowledge I just mentioned and the ability to correctly interview, examine and evaluate an orthopedic patient. Keeping in mind that this is not a physical examination text book, let's briefly look at some of the key aspects of the orthopedic physical therapy examination and try to relate a portion of the examination and evaluation process to therapeutic exercise.

KEY ASPECTS OF AN EXAMINATION

First off, it is not a bad idea to develop a friendly professional rapport with the patient during the examination. Be empathetic and try to understand their orthopedic condition from their own perspective. Figure out how their impairment(s) are limiting what they need to do or would like to do now and in the future. Remember, projecting empathy is important but it is also important to be in charge of the entire examination process. So, in addition to being empathetic, it is a good idea to project confidence. Gain the patient's confidence by demonstrating a confident demeanor in the way you take and direct a patient interview. If you do this, patient adherence to your prescribed exercise program will likely improve.

NATURE AND SEVERITY OF THE CONDITION

During the course of the examination, determine the nature and severity of the patient's problem. Here are some examples to illustrate these two concepts. As a clinician you will need to determine if the nature of the patient's primary concern focuses on pain or lack of function. If the patient is very concerned about their level of pain, therapeutic exercise intervention may initially need to be directed toward pain control measures. On the other hand, if the patient's primary concern relates to a lack of physical function, exercise intervention should be immediately geared toward reduction of functional limitations. Regarding severity, note whether a patient's condition is so severe that they need to lie in bed several times a day or is the level of severity just reducing their activity level by a small amount. Exercise dosage and type of therapeutic motion will likely be very different given these two differences in severity.

IMPAIRMENT IDENTIFICATION

During your examination of the patient, identify if there are movement (hypomobility and hypermobility), strength, neurological, or pain impairments and determine if the impairments are truly musculoskeletal in nature. Looking at each of these impairments in slightly more specific terms, determine whether or not your patient's extremity joint or spinal movement impairment is hypermobile or hypomobile. Correct diagnosis of hypermobility verses hypomobility will clearly impact your selection of therapeutic exercise intervention. Next, through observation, palpation, and clinical testing determine whether muscular strength impairment is present. If present, some form of resisted motion should be prescribed. Regarding the nervous system, clinicians must determine if nerve irritation or nerve compression is involved. If either of these two nerve impairments is present, therapeutic positioning, unloading and decompression exercises should be prescribed. Lastly, in the area of pain impairments, the chosen therapeutic exercise motion will need to reduce and certainly not worsen the pain complaint.

Therapeutic Exercise

VISCERAL PATHOLOGY AND THE PLAN OF CARE

Our physical examination should rule out the potential for more serious visceral pathology. Clinicians must at the very least, know the signs and symptoms of visceral pathology. If a patient presents with any of these signs and symptoms and if we are unable to find impairments or provoke mechanical based pain, then exercise intervention should not be rendered. In cases such as this, the patient should be referred back to his or her referring physician.

So, by way of a quick review, listed below are the common signs of symptoms of visceral pathology. First, a clinician should note the appearance of the patient and determine if they:

- Look unwell
- Look Pale
- Appear Anxious
- Have notable skin lesions that have recently changed
- Demonstrate diaphoresis
- Demonstrate Dyspnea

During the patient's history did you hear any of the following?
- A description of a recent, sudden and unexplained onset of symptoms.
- A complaint of a recent weight loss

Did the patient report?
- That their pain is awakening them from a sleep
- That their pain seems to come in waves
- That their pain is not load/position dependent
- That their reported symptoms are becoming more progressive.
- That their symptoms are changing from dull to more severe or sharp

Was the character of the patient's pain?

- Knife-like from inside to out
- Boring, which is a deep (internal) aching type of pain

- Unrelieved by rest or change in position

Other Symptoms Indicative of Visceral Pathology:

- Syncope
- Excessive Fatigue
- Night Sweating
- Fever, chills
- Chest pain
- Changes in bowel/bladder
- Pain not aggravated by movement

Examination Findings (Signs) Related to Visceral Pathology:

- Elevated temperature.
- Elevated Blood pressure
- Elevated heart rate.

Intervention Response and the Possible Presence of Visceral Pathology:

- Pain that is unaffected by intervention
- Pain that is made worse by intervention
- Symptoms that are better one day and worse the next despite movement re-education, load modification and other forms of PT intervention.

Guess what, clinicians must commit the information just listed to memory. Lastly, develop a plan of exercise intervention based on the evaluation of your examination findings. The operative word in the last sentence is *"your"*. The Plan of Care and the selection of movement (exercise) intervention(s) are not written on or based upon the prescription form you may receive when a patient first visits your clinic. The plan of care is developed based on the evaluation of the tests and measures applied by the physical therapist during their examination of the patient.

Therapeutic Exercise

PROFESSIONAL LATITUDE

This paragraph speaks to a somewhat related point. Depending on your state's practice act, you may receive a patient by way of a prescribed referral from a medical physician. The medical prescription that accompanies your patient may state shoulder pain, but if based on your interview with the patient you feel the cervical spine needs to be examined, hopefully all physical therapists have all reached the level of clinical practice where we would examine that patient's neck without hesitation. This same idea applies if you receive a patient with a diagnosis of hip pain. Certainly, examine the patient's hip, but if you feel their lumbar spine is involved, you should give this area of their body your complete and full attention during the initial examination. One more example before we wrap this up. If a prescription states that there is a muscle problem such as tendonitis or tendinosis, don't just examine the contractile structures; examine all associated joints and nerves as well to determine if pain is being referred into the muscular tissues. This line of conversation was somewhat controversial 25 years ago, still necessary 10 years ago and hopefully not necessary at this point in time. Most young physical therapists with their doctoral entry-level education and older more experienced therapists as well, function as independent and autonomous thinkers and practitioners. Clearly, if we don't fully examine a patient including all necessary body regions and systems, there is little chance of prescribing the most correct and helpful exercise program.

FINAL THOUGHTS

Some physical examinations take about 30 minutes. Some examinations take a little longer, some take less time. The point is, never feel rushed. Things get missed when you do. If needed, spread the examination out over more than one visit. Don't treat the patient the first day if it means rushing through an examination. That's right; don't treat the first day unless the patient is in a great deal of discomfort. In this case, the examination will likely be fairly short and there will be time to offer up pain-relieving interventions. If the patient is not too painful, structure your exam so you can offer up a piece of supportive advice such as postural instruction or movement reeducation at the conclusion of the examination. Otherwise, take time to reflect on your examination findings and put some meaning to those findings before starting into treatment. I learned this from Stanley Paris back in the 1980s, and it is one of the most important pieces of advice I have ever received. One additional thought, in the time you have with the patient during the initial examination it is often a good idea to explain the orthopedic condition (pathology) and prognosis to your patient. This goes a long way toward effectively handling the psychological component of a patient's pain experience. Believe it or not, helping your patient to better understand their condition often improves the result of your exercise or manual intervention.

Once the examination is underway, give the patient your complete attention and be observant of all patient movement patterns and postures including gait, changing positions on the exam table, dressing and undressing, and transitional movements such as sit to stand and rolling. This goes a long way toward developing your initial thoughts as to what type and what intensity your exercise program may need to be. Next, and this is a good point to always keep in mind, ask yourself does my patient generally look healthy or do they look ill? In other words, should I really be treating this person? Finally, does my patient appear to be in any real discomfort and how does this correlate to their perceived level of pain? Your exercise dosage may need to reflect this.

Chapter 9

Matching Impairments to Exercise Intervention

Chapter 8 looked at some important aspects of patient examination. Once the patient has been examined and the clinician has had time to reflect upon the examination findings, goals are set, and then a plan of care is developed. Clearly performance of a thorough and skillful examination and accurate interpretation of the clinical findings is the most important step toward making the correct decisions in terms of exercise selection. Selection of the best exercise for your patient can also be enhanced with a sound philosophical foundation regarding the biomechanical and neurophysiological attributes of the therapeutic exercise that will be prescribed.

In this regard, the philosophical foundation I am speaking about is matching the primary attribute of an exercise to the primary attribute of an identified impairment. In other words, and this is very simple, hypermobility impairments are treated with stabilization exercise, hypomobility impairments are treated with self-stretching and self-mobilization exercise, nerve impairments are treated with nerve decompression and positional exercise and pain impairments are treated with unloaded, passive, assisted, and reduced motion arc exercises. Now, let's look at the principal musculoskeletal impairments, and matching therapeutic exercise to the impairment in a little more detail.

Extremity joint or spinal segmental injuries commonly arise due to trauma, surgical repair, overuse and misuse of the body. All injuries, depending upon their severity, require a certain amount of healing time. This was discussed in chapter 6. Also discussed in chapter 6 was a concept that looked at the stage of a painful flare up. Arthritic degeneration secondary to aging is an example of an orthopedic condition that is prone to intermittent flare ups. Orthopedic injuries and orthopedic conditions often have commonly associated biomechanical, neurological, strength and pain impairments. Some neuromusculoskeletal impairments will be symptomatic, and some will not.

BIOMECHANICAL IMPAIRMENTS

Let's discuss biomechanical impairments first. Biomechanical impairments in this context relate to the development of hypermobility and hypomobility. Certain injuries and various forms of arthritic and disc degeneration can produce connective tissue laxity and resultant hypermobility. For example, early grade intervertebral disc degeneration is most always associated with resultant segmental hypermobility and instability. Upon examination, if the clinician finds this particular type of impairment the prescription of stabilization exercises along with other interventions such as taping, bracing, collars, corsetry, postural and movement re-education which utilizes deep stabilizer muscles, and minimizes joint and segments motion is the likely recommendation and prescription we need to make.

If on the other hand, an advanced level of degenerative change or perhaps a course of immobilization after a fracture produces hypomobility impairment, then the prescription of self-mobilization exercise, self-stretching exercise, assisted, active assisted, active and other neuromuscular reeducation movement interventions that encourages improved and increased movement patterns is likely to be indicated. If the examination of a patient demonstrated nerve impairments in the form of irritation or compression, then the prescribed exercise should seek to unload the nerve in question and otherwise seek to unload the spinal segment(s), or open an intervertebral foramen with therapeutic positioning. Note, nerve root irritation and or compression should be given your first priority in terms of exercise prescription when developing your plan of care. Therapeutic exercise intervention for nerve impairments may include postural training (spinal elongation), soft and inflatable collars, spinal corsetry, self-traction, and positional based foraminal opening exercises (Chapter 18).

Therapeutic Exercise

STRENGTH IMPAIRMENTS

If strength impairment is found then various forms of resisted exercise training (chapter 2) are indicated. Remember, in the presence of cartilaginous degeneration, early phases of connective tissue healing, or an acute flare up of chronic condition, resisted motion strength training should not increase pain or swelling. This statement relates to a point made earlier in the text and that is, if you have to provide an ice or heat treatment to your patient after a therapeutic exercise, that exercise or exercises was not therapeutic. In fact, you have overloaded that patient's tissues and actually caused harm. Pain generation, increased swelling, and increased tissue temperature are all signs of tissue, joint, or spinal segment overload and will only serve to further inhibit the muscle(s) with impaired strength.

PAIN IMPAIRMENTS

Orthopedic conditions and associated movement impairments may predispose an individual to the development of pain, perpetuate painful symptoms, cause pain at the beginning or during an impaired motion, or cause pain toward the end of an impaired motion. When pain impairment appears to be dominating the clinical picture, therapeutic exercises should be prescribed in a way that reduces constant pain and the exercise should be performed within a pain free movement arc and with a degree of resistance that does not provoke any symptoms.

Matching principal impairments to exercise type is really pretty logical. Choosing the correct exercise dosage is also based on a number of other considerations, and as we begin to wrap up this foundational chapter, here is a list of points and questions to consider when prescribing the intensity, frequency and duration of a therapeutic exercise.

1. Patient age; don't make too many age-related judgments regarding a person's ability to perform an exercise but do have a sense for exercise dosage and advancing age.
2. Arthritic and degenerative change; try to advance and progress exercises, seek to improve patient function but think of long-term protection of your patient's joint cartilage and intervertebral discs and don't overload and over compress these structures.
3. The phase of tissue healing; when was the tissue injured and how well or how much time has the tissue had to heal?

4. Painful flare ups; is the flare up of an orthopedic condition in an immediate, acute, sub-acute, settled or chronic stage?
5. The patient's prior and current level of physical activity; In other words, is the patient's tissues used to exercise (physical) activity?
6. Potential for recovery given other medical co-morbidities; Always consider this and adjust your exercise dosage appropriately given the overall health of your patient.
7. Personality factors affecting desire or motivation to exercise; don't make too many personality judgments but don't forget to evaluate this because desire and motivation does affect rehabilitation potential.
8. The long term functional goals for that patient; Make sure you know what your patient's goals are. Have that discussion during the history and interview.

Neuromusculoskeletal injury, the body's ability to heal, and interventions that deal with injury and facilitate healing are still a focus of research in the PT profession. The physical therapy clinical and research community still have a way to go in order to prove that we can structurally and functionally change the status of a patient's neuromusculoskeletal tissues for the better and not hurt, injure, or otherwise retard the ongoing healing process when prescribing exercises for the symptomatic or impaired joints or injured soft tissue. That said, our profession has really made some impressive strides in the area of neuromusculoskeletal management and the research on the benefits of therapeutic exercise continues to grow. Sill, questions remain as to whether physical therapists through exercise prescription, can facilitate healing of injured tissue and delay or stop the process of joint and segmental degeneration through load reduction, improved movement performance, controlled strengthening and controlled self-mobilizing (stretching).

So, one of the recurrent themes of this text, is that as clinicians we need to correctly exercise/stimulate the patient's tissues and enhance tissue healing without causing further tissue damage. In order for this to happen and before we move onto chapter 10, let's review some important points again. Be flexible with your therapeutic exercise prescription and be willing to do any of the following when prescribing movement intervention.

- Modify loads as necessary during exercises to protect injured and degenerated tissues
- Modify the patient's position during exercises

Therapeutic Exercise

- Modify the type of motion during an exercise
- Modify the arc of motion during an exercise
- Don't always exercise, instead immobilize
- Decompress pain sensitive tissue intermittently during a patient's waking hours.
- Decompress pain sensitive tissue during and between sets of certain exercises.
- Stay close to a joint's resting position when exercising in early stages of a flare up or early stages of tissue healing
- Reduce segmental loading and segmental motion
- Use taping, bracing, corsetry (partial immobilization) to protect tissue and facilitate healing.
- Respect the inflammatory cycle early on after an injury.
- Strengthen tissue, and at times do so with reduced joint and tissue loading
- At times, do less with a patient in a given treatment session in order to prevent painful flare ups.

Now let's move on to the shoulder and Chapter 10. Chapters 10 – 18 will look at some of the best exercises that I am aware of. There are many other exercises in addition to the ones I have chosen to place in this text. Also, there are many different variations of similar exercises most of which have merit and would also successfully address the impairments or limitations concerning your patient. Over many years of clinical practice, I have evaluated a lot of different therapeutic exercises. The following nine chapters discuss the orthopedic therapeutic exercises that I feel have the greatest clinical usefulness and have the least risk of causing painful reaction or tissue damage both during the performance of the exercise and if the exercise is performed on an ongoing basis for many years.

Chapter 10

Therapeutic Exercise for the Shoulder

Time to get to the actual exercises. Chapter 10 will look at a number of different exercises for patients with various shoulder impairments. Here is a bulleted list of some of the more important topic covered in this chapter.

- Pain management for the shoulder
- Keeping the humerus vertical and down to our patient's side for early movement therapy and initial strength building
- Moving the UE out and into elevation
    - Assisted and resisted exercises for the cranial portion of the rotator cuff
- Improving shoulder external rotation
    - Assisted and resisted exercises for the dorsal portion of the rotator cuff
- The rotator cuff and glenohumeral stabilization exercises
- Scapular stabilization
- Select shoulder self-stretching exercises

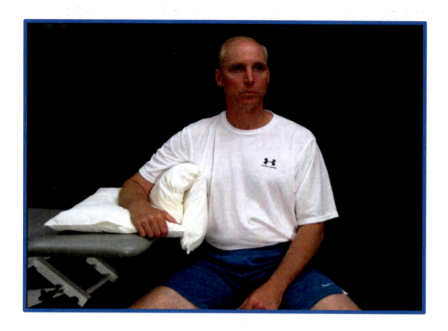

Figure 10-1: Glenohumeral Resting Position:

Supporting the shoulder joint in this position will slacken the cranial portion of the rotator cuff, enhance blood flow to the cuff tendons, and often reduce joint related pain. The Numeric Pain Rating Scale (NPRS) can be applied to determine if placing the shoulder in this position reduces the patient's reported pain intensity level. On a related note, and regarding rest for the glenohumeral joint and associated soft tissue structures, if the shoulder has been recently injured or if there has been a flare up of a chronic condition, respect the inflammatory cycle, immobilize the shoulder in a sling for several days and use this resting position intermittently during the course of the day to reduce pain and facilitate soft tissue healing. Lastly, the position shown above is an excellent position to apply heat and cold treatments both in the clinic and at home.

Therapeutic Exercise

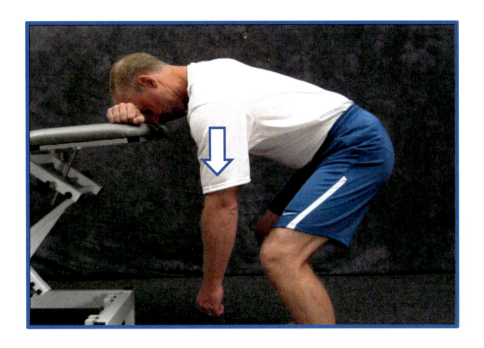

Figure 10-2: Codman's (Pendulum) Exercise:

This is an old-time classic exercise that in my opinion is often underutilized. The two primary purposes of this exercise is pain relief and light capsular stretching. Regarding pain management, this therapeutic motion could be applied between sets of muscle strength training, between sessions of manual stretching for symptomatically shortened connective tissue, and during or after sports competition involving overhead motion. Also, this exercise should be liberally applied for the management of flare ups associated with degenerative conditions and painful morning stiffness affecting the shoulder. Make sure that the patient keeps their neck and the remainder of their spine as straight as possible. Have the patient place their forehead on their forearms. Also, make sure that the patient's knees are bent to reduce tension on the sciatic nerve. The angle of trunk and hip flexion will determine where the U/E swings in relation to the trunk. This movement should be initiated by the patient's trunk making the UE primarily passive in nature. Transition to AAROM can occur when the patient is able and allowed to move the UE in that way given tissue healing time frames and pain status. Use the uninvolved UE to assist a painful involved UE (shoulder) when transitioning into other positions or back into a sling at the conclusion of this exercise.

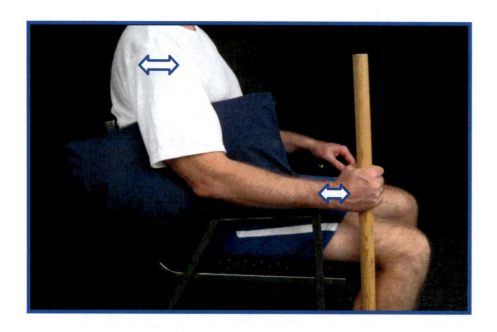

Figure 10-3: Gear Shift-Oscillatory Flexion and Extension-Pillow Support:

This exercise has many useful purposes and may apply in a number of different clinical situations. If a patient's shoulder is painful keep their glenohumeral joint close to the resting position., support the joint with a pillow, and instruct the patient to perform an active small amplitude oscillatory flexion and extension motion. The UE should remain close to the patient's side, the shoulder girdle elevator muscles should remain relaxed and the arc of motion should be quite small (oscillatory). Grip the stick or cane at a height that provides some support to the entire shoulder girdle. This exercise may be applied in a post-op situation such as a rotator cuff or labral repair, after an injury that has had several days to rest, for a flare up on a chronic arthritic condition and for chronic shoulder pain management.

Therapeutic Exercise

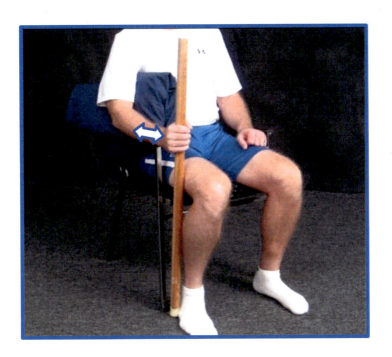

Figure 10-4: Gear Shift-Short Arc Flexion and Extension Motion:

If a patient's shoulder is painful keep his/her humerus close to vertical and his/her glenohumeral joint as close to the resting position as possible. Support the joint and associated soft tissues with a pillow during the oscillatory (10-3) or short arc (10-4) motion. Note how the patient's arm is kept close to his/her side. During this short arc motion, it is important that the humerus stays is a vertical position and slightly in front of the patient's torso. Ensure that the patient is performing a short pain-free motion. Again, this exercise may be applied in a post-op situation such as a cuff or labral repair, after an injury that has had day to or two of rest/immobilization, after a stable humeral head fracture, or for a flare up of a chronic arthritic condition, and for chronic shoulder pain management. I often prescribe several reps and sets of this exercise performed for 10-30 seconds.

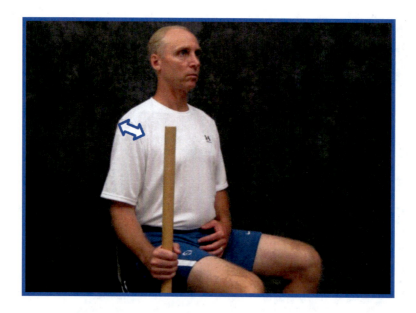

Figure 10-5: Gear Shift Short Arc Flexion and Extension:

If the shoulder is now less sensitive and able to move in a larger arc of motion without discomfort, remove the pillow and allow the patient to move into a greater degree of flexion and extension. Note, the patient should be instructed to relax their shoulder girdle muscles, keep their shoulder girdle depressed, and also have a relaxed grip on the stick. Have the patient move their arm in pain free arcs for 30 seconds and then rest for 30 seconds. If there is no increase in shoulder pain, continue this exercise for several minutes. Note, and this is important, we can control the degree of shoulder elevation by where we have the patient grip his/her stick. In the picture above, I have taken a very low grip position on the stick. Note that the end point of this therapeutic motion is only about 40 degrees of elevation. If you have a patient grip the upper portion of a stick, the end point of elevation can be 90 degrees or more depending on the length of the stick.

Therapeutic Exercise

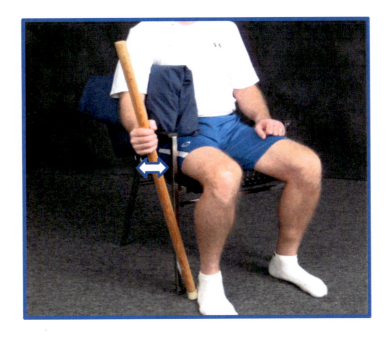

Figure 10-6: Gear Shift Short Arc Shoulder Rotation:

This version of the gear shift exercise applies to the same clinical situations as mentioned in figure 10-3. This version will allow for active assisted shoulder external rotation and active internal rotation. As mentioned previously, the patient should be instructed to relax their shoulder girdle muscles, keep their shoulder girdle depressed, and also have a relaxed grip on the stick. Note how the bottom of the stick is next to the patient's foot. This keeps the stick from slipping. Have the patient move their arm in a pain free arc of shoulder rotation for 30 seconds and then rest for 30 seconds and evaluate their pain status. If there is no increase in shoulder pain continue this exercise for several minutes.

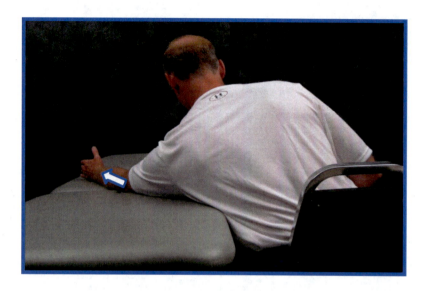

Figure 10-7: Glenohumeral Elevation: Supported Self-Mobilization:

This exercise was historically termed a concave self-mobilization with the idea that if one were to lean his/her trunk forward, the concave portion of the joint moved the most and the head of the humerus moved less. The thought was, that the trunk motion might help make shoulder elevation less painful in the presence of certain orthopedic shoulder conditions. I believe that the support afforded the UE by the table allows us to prescribe a form of active assisted shoulder elevation that is usually less painful for our patients. The table support and spinal/hip motion helps to produce a passive to active assisted shoulder elevation in the plane of the scapula. This exercise procedure provides a gentle way of moving the UE out of the vertical position and away from the body. This is a nice progression from the Gear Shift exercise and can be helpful post injury, post operatively, or in the sub-acute or settled stage of a painful flare up. In these situations, stay within the pain-free boundaries of elevation and make sure that injured shoulder tissues have healed sufficiently before moving the UE too far into elevation. Again, note how the UE is now being moved further away from the body as compared to the Gear Shift exercise. Here is a general rule, the worse the shoulder problem, the more we will have to keep the patient's humerus close to his/her side. This exercise gives us a way to get the humerus away from the body while still providing a degree of support. In addition, this exercise provides a way to maintain motion after a session of manual intervention (mobilization and stretching) for shoulder stiffness impairments.

Therapeutic Exercise

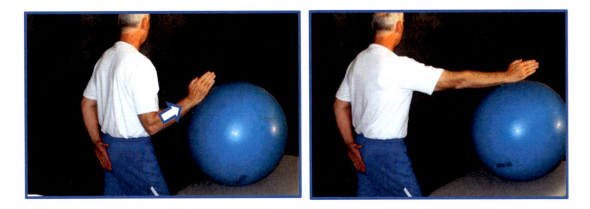

Figure 10-8: Glenohumeral Elevation: Supported Self-Mobilization:

OK, here is a similar exercise procedure which also provides a gentle way of moving the humerus out of vertical position and away from the trunk. The exercise ball will provide a degree of support to the shoulder joint as the patient pushes the ball along a treatment table in your clinic, or a table/counter top at home. The degree of shoulder elevation can easily be changed by raising or lower one of your treatment tables. Think of prescribing this active assisted exercise in cases of arthritic flare ups, tendinopathy management, early on after tendon and labral repair or post injury as shoulder tissues are healing.

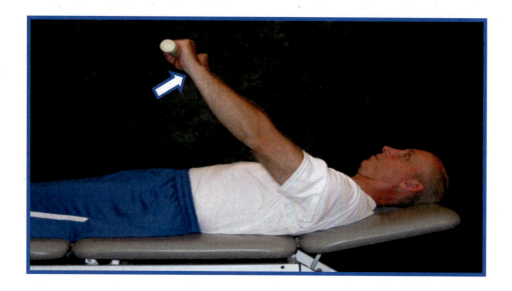

Figure 10-9: Glenohumeral Assisted or Resisted Elevation; Below 90 Degrees – Supine:

Exercise 10-9 has been part of physical therapy for many years. The "cane" or "stick" assisted UE elevation exercise when performed below 90 degrees can take the form of passive motion (PROM), active assisted range of motion (AAROM), Active range of motion (AROM) and resisted range of motion (RROM). This exercise can assist in maintaining capsular extensibility after manual stretching intervention and will assist in maintaining the contractile properties of the UE elevator muscles when performed with AAROM and AROM. It probably goes without saying, but if this exercise is prescribed to assist in maintaining the contractile properties of shoulder elevator muscles, many repetitions would need to be prescribed. To strengthen shoulder elevator muscle such as the Pectorals and the anterior portion of the Deltoids with RROM below 90 degree of elevation, just wrap a cuff weight around the cane-stick. One last note, for post-operative and post injury management, the range of UE movement can be very precisely controlled with this exercise procedure so as to not overstretch soft tissues, and retard or delay healing.

Therapeutic Exercise

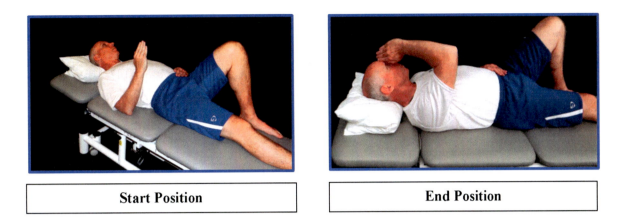

| Start Position | End Position |

Figure 10-10: The Salute Exercise

Let's stay is supine and look at the Salute Exercise. This is an active motion exercise that builds strength in Pectorals and anterior Deltoid (shoulder elevator muscles). Note how load across the shoulder joint and amount of muscle effort to elevate the humerus is reduced by keeping the elbow flexed to 90 degrees. This is a great initial strength building procedure post rotator cuff and labral repair and when dealing with patients who have severely damaged (degenerated and torn) rotator cuffs. Patients who are unable elevate their UE well due to full thickness rotator cuff tears will be able to improve their active elevation by performing many repetitions of this exercise.

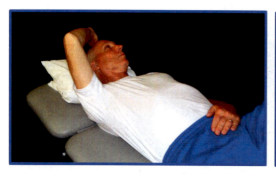 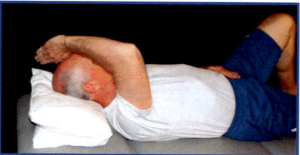

Figure 10-11: The High Salute Exercise

As your patient makes modest gains in elevator muscle strength, increase the arc of motion for this exercise by performing the High Salute. Note how the end position is now at the top of the head. Increase the degree of resistance by wrapping cuff weights around your patient's wrist or have your patient hold onto small hand-held dumbbells. The Salute exercises along with our other shoulder muscle strength building procedures can help to improve our patient's ability to actively elevate his/her UE.

Therapeutic Exercise

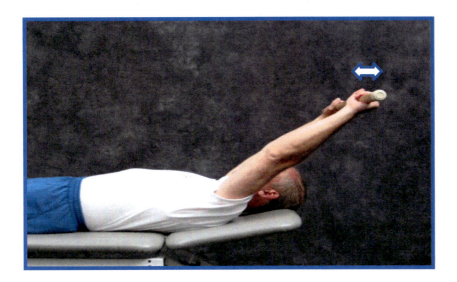

Figure 10-12: Glenohumeral Elevation; Above 90 Degrees –Supine:

Let get our patient's shoulder joints above 90 degrees of elevation and allow the weight of the stick and gravity to provide an additional stretch to shortened soft tissue structures around the shoulder. For the purposes of soft tissue stretching, this procedure should be held at end range elevation for a minimum of 30 seconds up to two minutes or more for both capsular and muscular lengthening purposes. This exercise can assist in maintaining restored motion after a session of manual intervention. If end range is more painful, use gentle oscillations at or close to end range elevation. All shoulder patients performing this motion should be instructed by their therapist to make a self-determination regarding the provocation of impingement symptoms. Sharp or fairly sharp pain in the area of the anterior acromion or pain referred into the upper lateral humeral area are not allowable symptoms, and if elicited the exercise should be discontinued or better yet the arc of movement should be changed by the therapist.

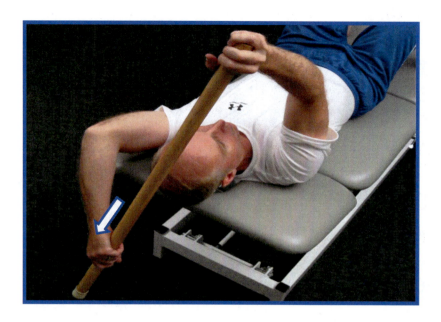

Figure 10-13: Glenohumeral Elevation with External Rotation; Above 90 Degrees-Supine:

Note how this top hand grip on the stick facilitates humeral external rotation along with UE elevation. This will facilitate a greater degree of glenohumeral capsular stretching. This simple self-stretching exercise can be used to maintain motion improvements after treatment with joint mobilization or shoulder muscle stretching. The supine position and UE elevation beyond 90 degrees will incorporate the effect of gravity for additional soft tissue stretching. This is a stretching exercise which will likely affect both capsular and muscular tissues and as such the end range position should be held for at least 30 seconds or up to two minutes or more to facilitate greater elongation of both soft tissue structures. Again, a sharp pain in the area of the anterior acromion is not an allowable symptom and if elicited, the exercise should be discontinued. Further, the patient should be educated by their therapist to not push aggressively past the first stop (end feel) in their available passive motion.

Therapeutic Exercise

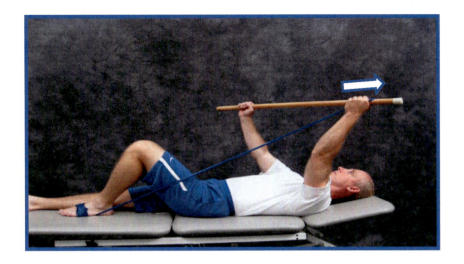

Figure 10-14: Glenohumeral Elevation-Elastic Band Resistance-Supine:

Ok, one more supine elevation exercise that incorporated a cane or stick. There are numerous ways to provide resistance for UE elevation. To this day, manual resisted exercise (MRE), particularly PNF diagonal patterns remain one of the best ways to improve impaired UE elevation secondary to weakness. This version of UE resisted elevation incorporates the patient's opposite UE to facilitate various diagonal patterns of elevation by changing the angle of the cane or stick. Note how the involved UE (hand) has taken an "under grip" on the stick to facilitate humeral external rotation. The elastic band which is looped around the patient's foot will provide an elastic band attachment point and the UE elevation movement pattern let tension the elastic band and provide progressive RROM. Have the patient vary the angle of knee flexion and extension to change the pre-tensioning of the elastic band and as a result the amount of resistance the patient will encounter. Standard multi-set, multi-rep exercise prescription is often used.

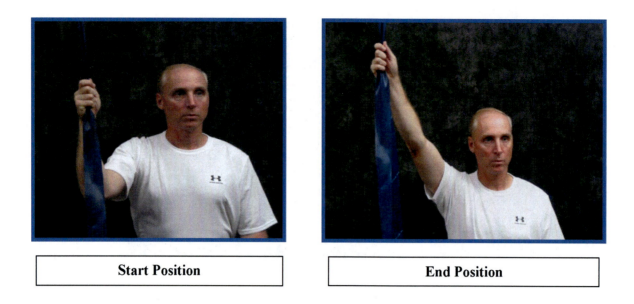

| Start Position | End Position |

Figure 10-15: Assisted UE Elevation-Seated:

Let's get our patient into an upright position and continue to focus on how we can help improve (increase) his/her active shoulder elevation. This Elastic Band assisted elevation exercise can be prescribed if there is impaired UE elevation is due to elevator muscular weakness, cuff tendinopathy, and for post-operative care. Remember, repetitive pain-free assisted motion can increase circulation, promote in tissue healing, and maintain the contractile properties of the UE elevator muscles and while reducing load on the shoulder joint and the tissues that might be painful. I like to prescribe this exercise for 5 minutes at a time. Chose a thickness (color) of elastic band that will help your patient achieve his/her maximum elevation without discomfort. Our goal with this exercise is to lightly stimulate contractile elements without provoking symptoms from them. Lastly, in terms of exercise set up, tie a knot close to the end of the elastic band, toss the end over the top of a door, and then close the door to secure the band. Once the band is secure, assist the patient's shoulder to 90 degrees of elevation with his/her elbow at 90 degrees as well (start position above). Next, pre-tension the elastic band by having the patient sit down. The tension in the band will now assist your patient into UE elevation (end position above).

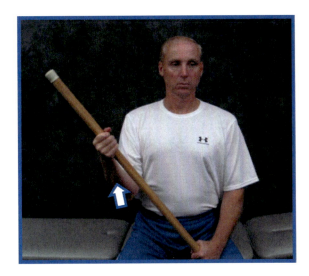 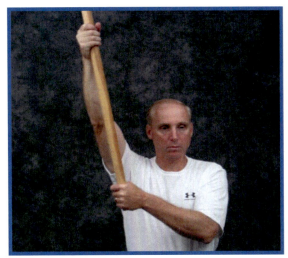

Figure 10-16: Upright Cane Assisted Shoulder Elevation:

OK, let's keep our patient's trunk in an upright position and go back to the stick or a cane to help improve shoulder elevation. The entire spectrum of therapeutic motion (PROM, AAROM, AROM, RROM) can be prescribed here. This exercise may be useful in cases capsular shortening is limiting end range UE elevation. The uninvolved UE is used to provide PROM to stretch the involved (shortened) shoulder tissues. In this case the UE should be held at end range for a minimum of 30 seconds. Remember, the patient should be educated by their therapist to not push aggressively past the first stop, typically a firm (capsular) end feel. Second, if the therapist has determined that there is muscular strength impairment involving shoulder elevation multiple reps of active assisted UE elevation can be prescribed. Also, "place and hold" isometric muscle training can be performed while holding onto the cane. Regarding isometrics, the uninvolved UE places the involved shoulder joint at various spots in the range of UE elevation. The uninvolved hand is released and the patient is asked to maintain the elevated position for a minimum of 6-10 seconds. For strength building will occur if you instruct your patient to lower the cane slowly. Slow controlled lowering is a great way to build eccentric muscle strength.

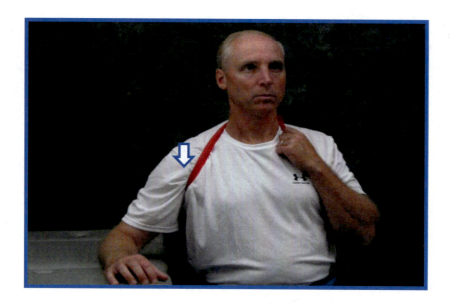

Figure 10-17: Active Caudal Glide Neuromuscular Self-Mobilization–Seated:

As we wrap up this first section on UE elevation, let's take a moment and discuss neuromuscular re-education and an exercise that you may or may not find helpful. If the rotator cuff muscles and other humeral elevator muscles are weak, the axio-scapular and axio-rib muscle (shoulder girdle elevator) muscles may contribute to excessive shoulder girdle elevation during UE elevation. This exercise is a neuromuscular re-education procedure where the patient is taught, against the resistance of elastic band, to feel how to depress their shoulder girdle and is instructed to do so prior to and during UE elevation. This active movement pattern likely inhibits the axio-scapular and axio-rib (shoulder girdle elevator) muscles. Elastic band is looped under the axilla and both ends of the band are brought around the posterior aspect of the cervical spine and anchored with the opposite hand. Numerous repetitions will need to be performed to facilitate neuromuscular re-education and the patient should be instructed to incorporate this movement pattern of active shoulder girdle depression into other daily activities requiring UE elevation and other therapeutic exercises which call for UE elevation.

Therapeutic Exercise

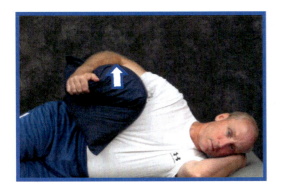 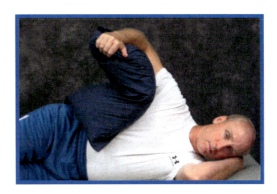

Figure 10-18: Active Short Arc Abduction-Side lying:

Exercise 10-17 concludes our first section on pain management and UE elevation. Now we are going to swing our discussion toward the cranial portion of the rotator cuff. In the exercises that follow, we will discuss tendinopathy management and keep an eye on UE elevation, because it is very difficult to elevate the arm without good function of the rotator cuff. In some circles, the supraspinatus muscle is termed the "cranial portion" of the rotator cuff. This text is part of that circle. The supraspinatus plays a key role in UE elevation and external rotation. Its medially directed line of muscular pull produces humeral head compression, which is a vital dynamic component to UE elevation. This portion of the text will discuss various therapeutic motions (exercises) which stimulate the cranial portion of the cuff and assist in the management of painful supraspinatus tendinopathy and supraspinatus weakness. So, let us look at figure 10-18. This exercise is probably new to most of you but I have used it for many years to help manage symptomatic supraspinatus tendinopathy. his exercise requires a foam filled pillow to be folded in half. The patient is instructed to bend their elbow to 90 degrees (short lever arm), and lightly unload (lift) his/her humerus off the folded foam pillow. As the foam pillow opens just a bit it will provide a small degree of assistance for the short arc, low load abduction motion. This exercise can be used in early post op management of a rotator cuff repair, a painful flare up of glenohumeral arthritis, early motion management of stable humeral head fractures, and painful degenerative supraspinatus tendinosis. Do not force patients to perform painful active abduction of the shoulder, this will only serve to inhibit and irritate the target muscle group.

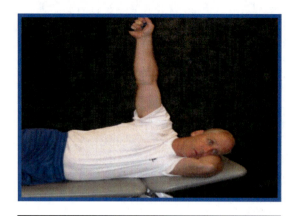
Star position at 90 degrees of abduction

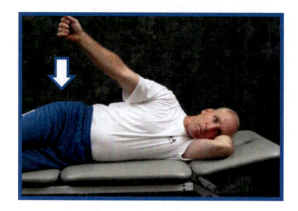
Controlled eccentric lowering of the arm

Figure 10-19: Active UE Abduction Long Lever Arm-Side lying:

Now let's straighten the patient's elbow and lengthen the level arm working over the shoulder joint. This will place more demand on the supraspinatus tendon. The key to this active abduction exercise is finding the right arc of movement and using both concentric and eccentric muscle contractions with stimulate and weakened, degenerated, or partially torn supraspinatus tendon. Instruct the patient to keep his/her elbow straight during the entire movement pattern. Assist the patient's humerus up a 90 degree position (start position) work with the patient to find out what arc of movement in the frontal plane can be used to load the tendon in a way that will make it stronger without further damaging it. Non-symptomatic tendon stimulation can occur from 90 to 75 degrees, 90 to 60 degrees, 90 to 45 degrees, 90 to 30 degrees and so on. Now, let's discuss this last sentence and briefly review tensile loading on the cranial portion of the rotator cuff during exercise training. I believe this is pretty obvious, but if we want to progressive increase tensile load on the supraspinatus tendon, the arc of exercise motion should be short, about 15 degrees, moving the UE from a starting point of 90 degrees of abduction down to the 75 degree position. As the UE is moved more and more in a downward direction toward the patient's side, the cranial portion of the rotator cuff will be subject to a greater amount of tensile load.

Therapeutic Exercise

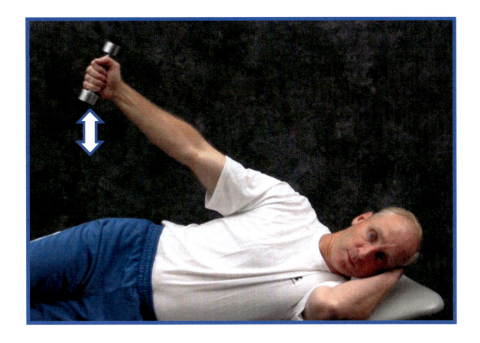

Figure 10-20: Active and Resisted Concentric-Eccentric Abduction-Side lying:

In my opinion the side lying position is often underutilized in the management of both the cranial and dorsal portion of the rotator cuff. Let's stay focused on the cranial portion of the rotator cuff for the time being. Active muscle training for this portion of the cuff incorporating both gravity and free weight resistance (shown above) can be accomplished using a number of different arc of motion similar to exercise 10-19. The therapist should encourage a slow decent of the arm to facilitate eccentric muscle strengthening. Also, MRE concentric and eccentric training for this portion of the cuff is easily accomplished in the side lying position. Pillows or the opposite UE should be used to keep the head and neck in mid-line. Make sure that the shoulder girdle elevator muscles remain relaxed and no excessive cranial migration of the head is seen during this exercise. Remember; not all patients with severe glenohumeral arthritis or full thickness rotator cuff tears will likely not be to accomplish a full arc of motion from 90 to 0 degrees. Lastly, use the patient's pain response and movement quality or lack thereof as part of your clinical decision making with regard to the amount of free weight resistance and number of prescribed of sets and repetitions (Exercise Dosage).

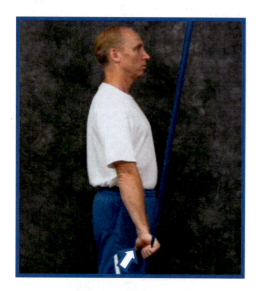 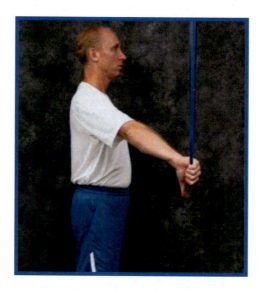

Figure 10-21: Assisted Elevation in the Scapular Plane-Standing:

We are going back to assisted motion with this exercise. UE elevation in the plane of the scapula, cutely called scaption, is a movement that will facilitate contraction of the cranial portion of the rotator cuff (supraspinatus muscle). For early post-surgical repair, after a shoulder injury or after a flare up of a chronic shoulder arthritis or tendinopathy, assisted motion in the scapular plane will prevent atrophy of the supraspinatus and often allow for early pain-free motion training. Adjust the amount of elastic band pre-tension so that assisted scaption motion is pain free, and minimal shoulder girdle elevation and cranial migration of the humeral head is noted. Let's review the basics, elastic band assisted motion modestly builds, lightly stimulates, and likely maintains muscle strength while minimizing pain by reducing joint and soft tissue loading. We need to prescribe a higher number of repetitions for this to happen, so consider prescribing 5 minutes of this assisted motion exercise giving the patient a 10-second rest break every 30 seconds or so. Review point, use of elastic bands and AAROM will reduce the weight of the UE and as a result reduce joint loading and load on irritated or degenerated cartilage and tendons while also modestly improving strength of weakened shoulder muscles.

Therapeutic Exercise

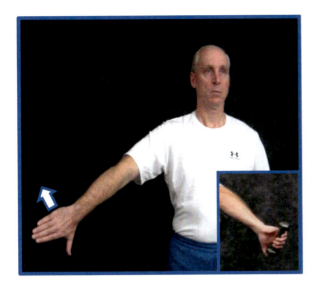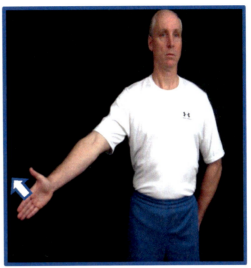

Figure 10-22: Active and Resisted Elevation in the Scapular Plane-Standing:

Utilizing this same patient position, free weight can be added as rotator cuff strength improves. Review chapter 3, Therapeutic Motions and Movements, and Chapter 6 Musculoskeletal Injury and Repair, and the Application of Therapeutic Motion. Remember, use the patient's pain response and movement quality or lack thereof as part of your clinical decision making with regard to increasing free weight resistance and exercise reps. Shoulder girdle elevation and excessive cranial rolling of the humeral head should not be allowed to occur during this therapeutic motion. The amount of free weight and or the arc of movement will need to be reduced if either of these movement abnormalities is seen. Multiple sets and reps can be performed in order to build strength in the cranial portion of the rotator cuff. Note how humeral rotation is varied in the two figures above. The picture on the left demonstrates humeral internal rotation and the one on the right humeral external rotation. Use patient pain response, movement quality, and clinical palpation of supraspinatus muscle contraction to determine how you will position the humerus for this exercise. To better stimulate the supraspinatus tendon in cases of tendinopathy, instruct your patient to perform slow eccentric lower of his or her arm.

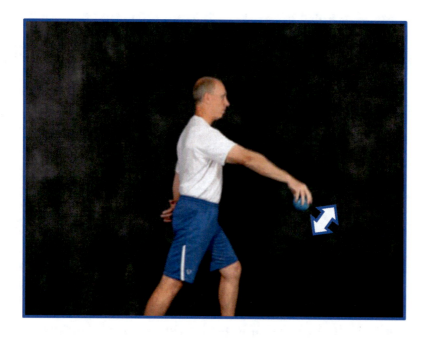

Figure 10-23: Eccentric Strengthening for the Cranial Portion of the Rotator Cuff:

This is the supraspinatus eccentric ball dropping exercise performed in somewhat of an athletic split stance position. For our athletic patients, this exercise can also be performed in the Hip Hinge position, see the Lumbar Chapter. The patient's UE is elevated in the scapular plane to just below 60 degrees. The hand-held weighted exercise ball (1-4 pounds) is released and caught. After the ball is caught, the patient slowly lowers his/her arm downward to about 15 degrees of scaption. If your patient is having difficulty with catching the ball after release, have him/her supinate his/her forearm. This will turn their hand into a palms up position. Now the patient can toss the ball upward, catch it, and slowly control the descent or lowing of the UE. This is an important eccentric muscle-tendon strengthening exercise that can be used by many different patients but is particularly valuable in the rehabilitation of the overhead athlete who is experiencing problems with supra-humeral soft tissue structures.

Therapeutic Exercise

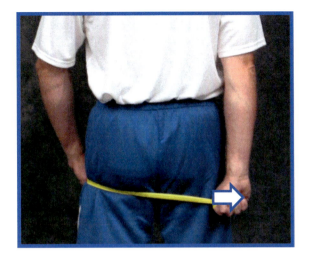 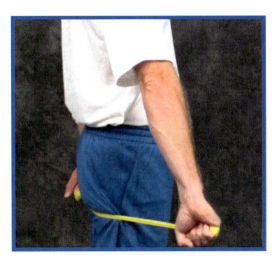

Figure 10-24: Elastic Resistance in the Scapular Plane-Standing:

Note how one hand stabilizes the elastic band while resisted movement in the scapular plane is performed. You may change the pre-tensioning of the elastic band by changing the anchor point of the stabilizing hand to different parts of the trunk such as the sacrum or lateral hip region. Bilateral UE movement (not shown above) can also be performed. Again, shoulder girdle elevation and excessive cranial rolling of the humeral head should not be allowed to occur during the therapeutic motion. The arc of movement will need to be reduced if either of these movement abnormalities is seen. Multiple sets and reps can be performed in order to build strength in the cranial portion of the rotator cuff. This concentric strength building exercise also works very well for overhead throwing athletes as part of an off-season strength building program. Remember, full painful UE elevation and pain free overhead sports function is unlikely if the cranial portion of the cuff is not working well.

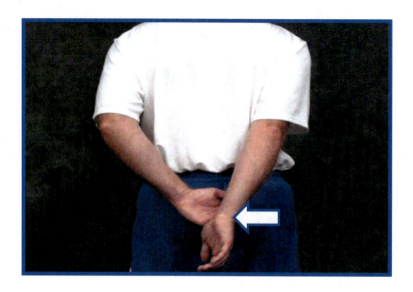

Figure 10-25: Self-Stretching for the Superior Capsular Complex and Cranial Portion of the Rotator Cuff (Supraspinatus):

So, probably an anatomy review is in order. The Superior Capsular Complex (Rotator Interval) is a complicated area of anatomy, but in short it is largely comprised of the Coracohumeral ligament. So, consider the attachment points of these ligaments and you will be able to see how UE adduction can help to elongate a portion of the rotator interval. In this view, the left hand passively adducts the right UE behind the back in order to lengthen the superior capsular complex. But be careful, because will are also elongating a portion of the rotator cuff that commonly thins out and tears. Too much tensile loading of the cranial portion of the cuff is likely not a good idea. Elongation of the rotator interval should be held for at least 30 seconds or up to a minute or more. This stretch may be helpful when applied prior to athletic endeavors, particularly with regard to overhead throwing sports. Do not prescribe this stretch immediately after surgical repair of the supraspinatus.

Therapeutic Exercise

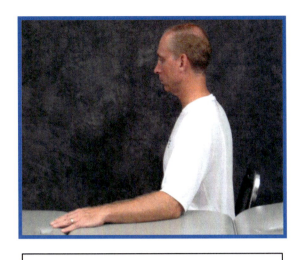
Start Position

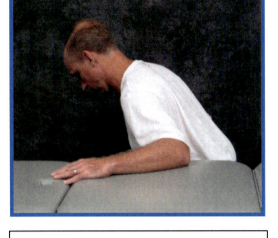
End Position

Figure 10-26: Glenohumeral External Rotation; Passive Concave Self-Mobilization:

This next section of the text will begin discussing the dorsal and ventral portion of the rotator cuff and focus a bit more shoulder rotation verses shoulder elevation. This self-stretching exercise uses a table to support the weight of the upper extremity while the patient's trunk (concave portion of the joint) is moved, facilitating elongation of the anterior (ventral) portion of the rotator cuff (subscapularis) and the anterior aspect of the glenohumeral joint capsule, which is another soft tissues which may limit glenohumeral external rotation. This is a gentle therapeutic motion and useful for stiffness and pain impairments associated with stable humeral head fractures, rotator cuff repairs and adhesive capsulitis particularly the painful and early stiffening phases. The patient is instructed to flex forward at their hip joints and to push backward on a rolling chair if available. This passive self-mobilization can be repeated in a rhythmical fashion without holding the end range position if the condition is more pain dominate or the end position can be held for up to two minutes if stiffness impairment is the principal clinical feature. Note the involved UE should start in the scapular plane and below 60 degrees of abduction. A rolling chair will facilitate keeping the UE in the scapular plane during this passive external rotation self-stretch. Hinging forward on a standard chair will cause the arm to go into extension as well. Humeral extension will facilitate some degree of elongation of the anterior aspect of the rotator interval.

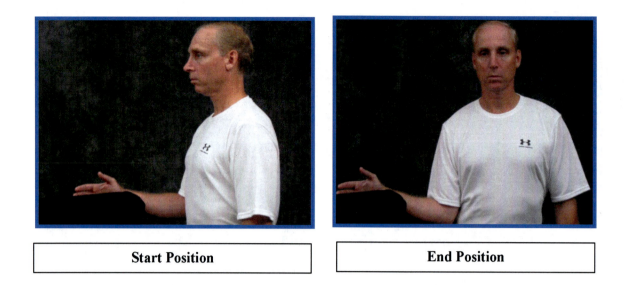

| Start Position | End Position |

Figure 10-27: Glenohumeral Rotation; Subscapularis Self-Stretch-Standing:

Let's have our patient in a standing position and use trunk rotation to give us another option for stretching the anterior shoulder capsule and the ventral portion of the rotator cuff and ventral portion of the capsule. Have your patient adduct his or her humerus down to their side, and place their distal forearm, not hand or wrist, against a door jam or table. The patient is instructed to use their feet in order to rotate their trunk which will produce passive external rotation at the glenohumeral joint. Pressing the distal forearm into the door jam or table will facilitate hold-relax stretching of the subscapularis muscle as external rotation will elongate both this portion of the cuff and the anterior glenohumeral capsule. After several sessions of hold-relax isometric contractions and additional elongation of the target tissue, the final stretching position should be held for at least 30 seconds or up to a minute or more. The humerus should remain in contact with the anterolateral aspect of the rib cage and no shoulder girdle elevation should occur during the performance of this self-stretch.

Therapeutic Exercise

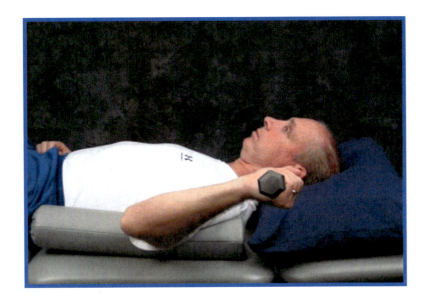

Figure 10-28: Glenohumeral External Rotation Self-Stretch-Supine:

Let's go over one last stretch for restricted shoulder external rotation. Note how the humerus is elevated up off of the table and a free weight is incorporated to increase the load of this stretch. Elevating the humerus into or close to the scapular plane will make this stretch less painful. Also, note how the humerus is also abducted away from the trunk as well to take up some slack in the inferior portion of the capsule. That being said, keep the humerus below 90 degrees as shown above. This stretch is meant for adhesive capsulitis in the frozen or thawing phase. It is an aggressive stretch for stiff shoulders that demonstrates a low level of irritability at the end range of external rotation. The stretch should be held for at least 30 seconds or up to two minutes or more. Note, and this is important, have the patient use their uninvolved UE to move the involved UE out of the stretching position when finished.

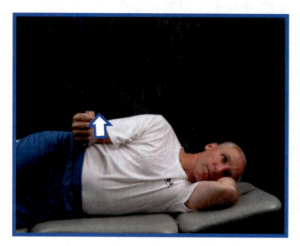
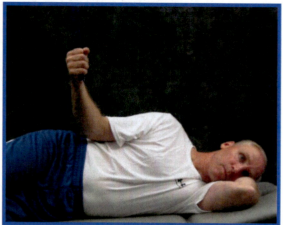

Figure 10-29: Glenohumeral Active-Assisted External Rotation-Side lying:

The last three exercises dealt with tissue elongation with some emphasis on stretching the ventral portion of the capsule and rotator cuff. Now we will turn our attention to training the dorsal portion (Infraspinatus and Teres Minor) of the cuff. Similar to other assisted motions previously discussed, this exercise can be used in early post op management of cuff repairs and debridement procedures and painful flares of glenohumeral arthritis and tendinosis. Note how the elastic band is attached above the patient. In the clinic the band can be attached to a free standing pulley system. At home, it can be attached over the top of a door or to a cane that is set between two chairs. Also the band could be held above the patient by a therapist or family member. Pulling the band down (humeral internal rotation) will pre-tension the band which then allows it to assist the weight of the UE upward into humeral external rotation. The assisted external rotation exercise should be prescribed for 5 minutes giving the patient rest breaks to evaluate his/her pain intensity level. The arc of movement, speed of movement, or amount of elastic assistance is varied as the patient's strength and or pain impairment improves. A pillow or roll can be inserted into the axillary region to slacken the cranial portion of the rotator cuff if irritated.

Therapeutic Exercise

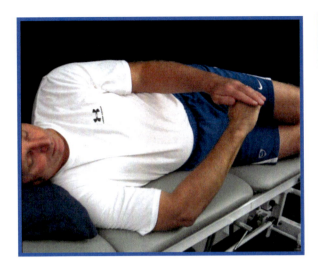 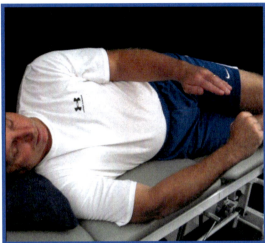

Figure 10-30: Glenohumeral Isometric External Rotation-Side lying:

Exercise 10-30 can be prescribed to improve isometric muscular strength for the dorsal portion of the rotator cuff. This is a therapeutic progression from the active-assisted external rotation exercise (Figure 10-29). The patient may use their uninvolved and undermost UE to place the upper most and involved UE at various points in the range of external rotation. The patient is then instructed to pull their undermost hand away from the uppermost hand in order to isometrically hold the weight of their forearm and distal UE in a mid-position and then in different parts of the range for multiple angle isometric training. Isometric muscle contraction should be held for a minimum of 6-10 seconds and repeated a minimum of 6-10 times. Building a platform of isometric muscular strength is often helpful prior to beginning isotonic muscle training. Regarding orthopedic conditions, this exercise procedure can be prescribed in cases of strength impairment secondary to degenerative thinning of this portion of the rotator cuff, C5, C6 nerve compression resulting in dorsal cuff atrophy, or to assist in post-surgical strength building.

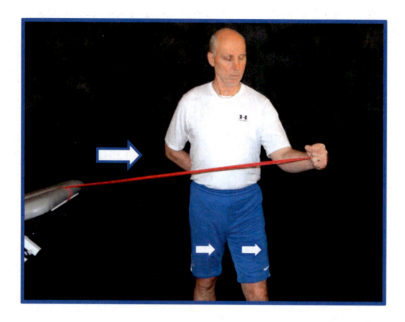

Figure 10-31: Glenohumeral Isometric Training of the External Rotators-Standing:

This therapeutic exercise provides another option for isometric muscle training for the dorsal portion of the rotator cuff. It is often times called the lateral step out exercise. The patient is instructed to place the UE with shoulder external rotator strength impairment in a mid-position with regard to rotation and hold that position as they step outward and away from the point of attachment for the elastic band. Stepping away from the point of attachment will tension the elastic band and force the patient to increase the degree of isometric contraction of their external rotator muscles. The patient should be instructed to not let his/her humerus move in extension or internal rotation. If possible, it is not a bad idea to have your patient's humerus positioned in slight flexion and slight external rotation. Multiple lateral step outs, perhaps as many as several sets of 30 at a time can be performed.

Therapeutic Exercise

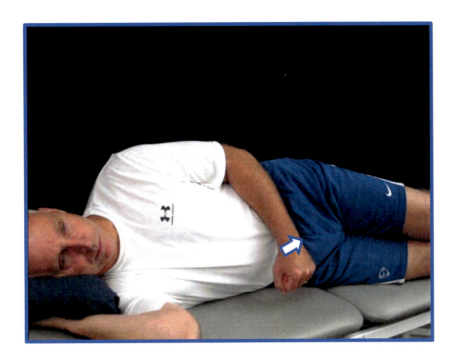

Figure 10-32: Glenohumeral Short Arc Isotonic External Rotation-Side lying:

Once a platform of isometric muscle strength has been built using exercises 10-30 and 10-31, short arc isotonic gravity resisted shoulder external rotation can be performed. In cases of strength impairment affecting this portion of the rotator cuff the short arc motion should initially be performed with the dorsal portion of the rotator cuff close to mid-position where the muscle group will be most efficient. Multiple sets of short arc isotonic muscle contractions can be performed or the therapist could prescribe a rep max program where the target muscle is trained until the quality of the therapeutic movement begins to erode.

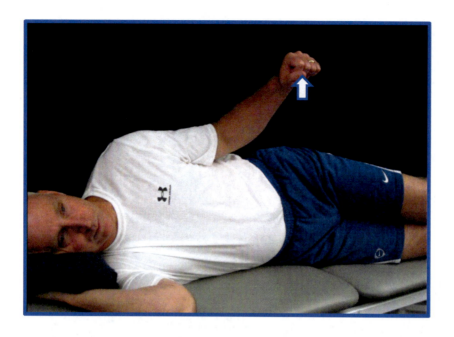

Figure 10-33: Glenohumeral Full Arc Isotonic External Rotation-Side lying:

As external rotator muscle strength improves, the arc of therapeutic motion is increased and the patient is now asked to lift the involved UE above their body. This will shorten the target muscle group more fully and requires a greater degree of strength. The therapist may instruct their patient to perform full arc motions where the start position of the exercise begins with the involved UE in contact with the abdomen, or short arc shoulder external rotation can be performed toward end range as shown above. Free weight is added incrementally with the maximum amount of free weight determined by the therapist as they evaluate the quality of shoulder external rotation as whether symptoms are provoked as weight is added.

Therapeutic Exercise

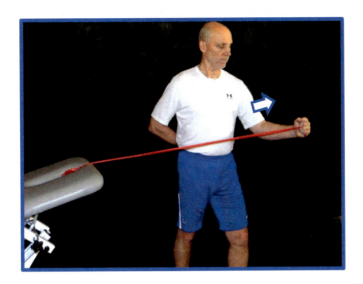

Figure 10-34: Glenohumeral Resisted External Rotation-Standing:

As the strength of the dorsal portion of the rotator cuff improves and keeping post-operative and post injury healing time frames in mind, muscle training with elastic band can be considered. Elastic band thickness (color), single strip or looped as shown above, arc of motion, speed of motion and amount of elastic band pre-tension should be considered. The goal is to achieve a solid palpable muscular contraction of the dorsal portion of the rotator cuff without provoking tendon or joint pain. Joint discomfort, joint noise and movement substitution should not be allowed to occur. Make sure that patients keep their sternum and rib cage up (chest) in an upward and forward position. This will help to keep the head of the humerus centered in the Glenoid fossa. In addition, and particularly in cases of anterior shoulder instability, make sure that your patient can "see" his/her humerus while he/she actively rotates against elastic band resistance. A well-toned dorsal portion (Infraspinatus and Teres minor) will facilitate dynamic caudal gliding of the head of the humerus during UE elevation. Multiple sets of repetitions of isotonic external rotation can be performed to increase strength of these target muscles and tendons. Remember, and this is important, in our patient's with glenohumeral laxity/instability, all rotational strength building motions should be performed with the humerus in the plane of the scapula. Written another way, our patients should always be able to see his/her humerus in their peripheral vision.

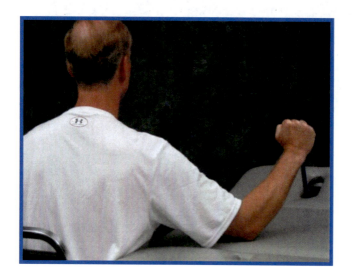

Figure 10-35: Resisted Glenohumeral External Rotation - UE Supported on Treatment Table:

If there is visual evidence of excessive upward rolling of the humeral head (the Deltoid muscle over powering the Cuff) during resisted external rotation or if your patient complains of shoulder pain, support his/her shoulder on a table as seen above. In other words, passively support the patient's humerus close to the shoulder resting position and in the scapular plane. This type of UE positioning can facilitate both concentric and eccentric strength building for the dorsal portion of the rotator cuff. To minimize the chance of subacromial impingement in patients with clinical signs of this condition, keep the humeral abduction below 60 degrees. When first moving the UE away from the side of the body, initially supporting the patient's arm on a table may keep this resisted motion pain-free. Note clinicians will find this to be a good patient position for the application of manual resistive concentric and eccentric dorsal cuff muscle training. As shown above, tie one end of the elastic band to the frame of the table and thread the band through the table cut out. A multi-set, multi-rep exercise dose can be prescribed when dorsal cuff strength impairment is the dominant clinical feature.

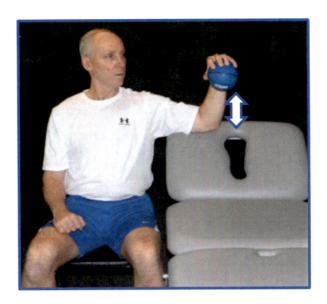 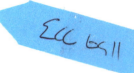

Figure 10-36: Eccentric Posterior Rotator Cuff Strength Building:

This is an eccentric dorsal cuff (Infra and Teres minor) ball dropping (strength building) procedure. The patient's UE is supported on a therapy table with the humerus below 90 degrees and in the plane of the scapula to facilitate a more stable position with the glenoid fossa. Supporting the humerus on the table will minimize deltoid contraction and upward gliding of the head of the humerus. The ball is released, caught, and the forearm, wrist and hand is slowly lowered (internal rotation) toward the table. Supporting the humerus as shown above works well for patients with cuff strength impairment and other load sensitive degenerative changes. Stock up on 1-4 pound hand held plyometric (medicine) balls so you can prescribe the right intensity of therapeutic exercise load.

Therapeutic Exercise

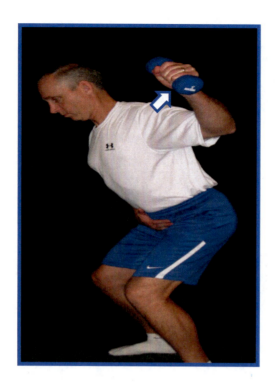

Figure 10-37 UE Elevation with External Rotation – Hip Hinge Position

Now let's take away the table support and also place the patient in a more athletic position. This figure demonstrates the hip hinge position which is discussed in detail in Chapter 18. The patient can be instructed to move their UE up into an elevated position in the plane of the scapula and then perform concentric shoulder external rotation. Clinicians will also find this position useful for the provision of concentric and eccentric MRE for the dorsal portion of the rotator cuff. A multi-set, multi-rep exercise dose can be prescribed when strength impairment is the dominant clinical feature.

Therapeutic Exercise

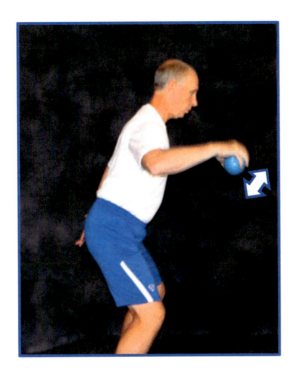

Figure 10-38: Eccentric Posterior Rotator Cuff Strength Building:

This is the ball dropping exercise performed in the hip hinge position as well. Remember, the hip hinge position provides a way to strength a patient's spinal extensor and LE muscles as well. The hand-held medicine ball, typically 1-4 pounds, is released, caught, and the forearm, wrist and hand is slowly lowered. Remember, controlling the descent of the UE will build eccentric posterior cuff strength. The rate of release, catch, and forearm descent can be varied to shift between concentric and eccentric muscle contractions. Be sure to position the humerus below 90 degrees of elevation. For our patients with glenohumeral laxity, the patient should always be able to see his/her humerus in his/her peripheral vision. In other words, train with the humerus slightly forward.

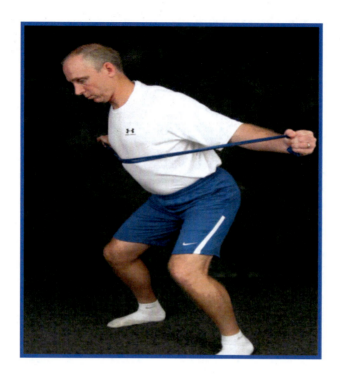

Figure 10-39   Bilateral Scapular Retraction with Bilateral Shoulder External Rotation – Hip Hinge Position

In order to assume the hip hinge position, as seen above and as seen in previous exercises, patients should be instructed to take a wide stance, flex their knees and "push" their buttock in a posterior direction to achieve hip flexion. When in this position bilateral elastic band resisted shoulder external rotation and scapular retraction is performed. A multi-set, multi-rep program should be performed in order to build concentric strength in these muscle groups. Note when incorporating the hip hinge position, lower extremity and spinal extensor muscle strength is also enhanced. Ensure that the patient gently draws their chin down and in toward their Adams Apple in order to elongate the posterior aspect of their cervical spine and to facilitate contraction of cervical flexor muscles during the performance of this exercise. This procedure is an excellent pre-season, in-season and post season athletic strength building exercise for the posterior (dorsal) portion of the rotator cuff and the scapular retractor muscles.

Therapeutic Exercise

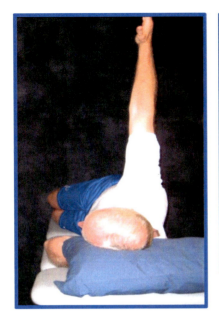 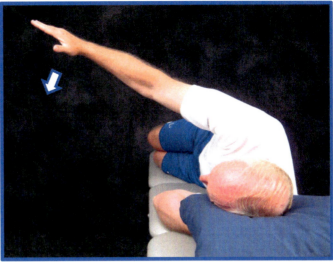

Figure 10-40: Horizontal Abduction and Adduction and the Dorsal Portion of the Rotator Cuff – Side lying:

Horizontal abduction and adduction are important therapeutic motions for developing strength in the dorsal portion of the rotator cuff. Short arc therapeutic motion can be initiated with the patient's finger tips pointing up toward the ceiling (the 90-degree position). After operative repair, shoulder injury, or in the presence of degenerative joint and tendon changes, short arc motion can begin in 15 degree increments away from the vertical position. As healing or the patient's condition improves, the movement arc is expanded eventually reaching a point where the UE is parallel to the floor. Incorporation of scapular protraction adds to this strength building motion as the UE nears a position parallel to the floor. Initially, the patient is asked to control the weight of his UE only. Isometric training can also occur at various points in the range of horizontal adduction. Concentric and eccentric MRE is also easily applied by the therapist as the patient performs this motion in the side lying position.

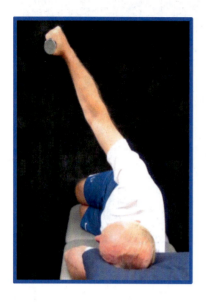
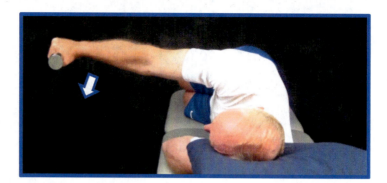

Figure 10-41: Resisted Horizontal Abduction and Adduction and the Dorsal Portion of the Rotator Cuff – Side lying:

As patient strength improves, free weight is added to this horizontal abduction and adduction movement arc. Short arc therapeutic motion can be initiated with the patient holding onto free weight and their UE pointing up toward the ceiling (the 90-degree position). After operative repair, shoulder injury, or in the presence of degenerative joint and tendon changes, short arc motion can begin in 15 degree increments away from the vertical position. As healing or the patient's condition improves, the movement arc is expanded eventually reaching a point where the UE is parallel to the floor. Incorporation of scapular protraction adds to this strength building exercise as the UE nears a position parallel to the floor. Isometric muscle training can also occur at various points into the range of horizontal adduction as the patient is asked to isometrically control the weight of his UE and the prescribed amount of weight. Concentric and eccentric MRE is also easily applied by the therapist as the patient performs this motion in the side lying position.

Therapeutic Exercise

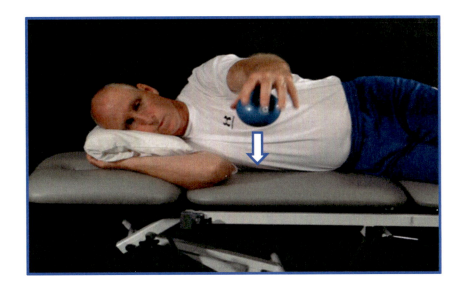

Figure 10-42 Eccentric Strengthening for the Dorsal Portion of the Rotator Cuff – Side lying:

The side lying position and eccentric ball dropping can also be used to build posterior cuff strength. Have the patient "reach forward" and protract his/her scapula in order to recruit scapular stabilized muscles as well. This may improve (reduce) the degree of scapular dyskinesia. The ball is released, caught, and the patient controls the eccentrically controls the descent of his/her arm while holding onto a 1-4-pound hand held medicine ball. The rate of release, catch, and forearm descent can be varied to shift between concentric and eccentric muscle contractions. I like this exercise very much for my over-head athletes.

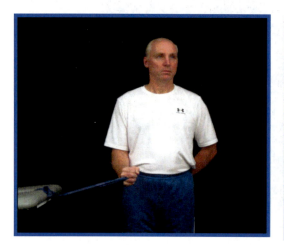 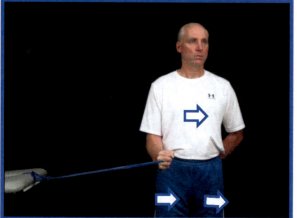

Figure 10:43 Isometric Strengthening of the Glenohumeral Internal Rotators-Standing:

We have discussed previously that if a patient presents with significant strength impairment affecting a muscle group, that it may be beneficial to first build a platform of isometric strength before beginning with short arc or full arc isotonic motions. Similar to the external rotation lateral step out exercise the internal rotation step out exercise provides a good option for isometric muscle training the ventral portion of the for rotator cuff. The patient is instructed to place the UE with shoulder internal rotator strength impairment in a mid-position with regard to rotation and hold that position as they step outward and away from the point of attachment for the elastic band. Multiple lateral step outs, perhaps as many as 30, should be performed. As your patient's ventral cuff strength improves, increase the thickness of elastic band resistance.

Therapeutic Exercise

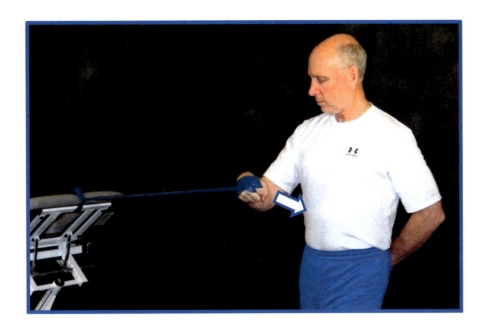

Figure 10-44: Resisted Internal Rotation – Standing:

Unlike the cranial and dorsal portion of the rotator cuff, the ventral portion of the rotator cuff is less commonly involved in degenerative thinning and tearing, but it can be subject to weakness impairment secondary to chronic arthritis, or tearing secondary to repeated micro and macro trauma. Similar to the dorsal portion of the rotator cuff, the ventral portion of the cuff (subscapularis) exerts an important biomechanical effect on the head of the humerus. The dorsal and ventral portion of the rotator cuff exerts a medial and caudal pull on the head of the humerus during elevation of the UE. Without this biomechanical effect, full UE elevation would not be possible. A multi-set, multi-rep isotonic exercise dose can be prescribed incorporating plate weights on a pulley system or the correct thickness of elastic band when strength impairment of this important internal rotator is present. Once again, in cases of anterior capsuloligamentous laxity, make sure your patient performs isotonic resisted internal rotation with his/her humerus in the plane of the scapula. As mentioned before, and as shown above, our patients with shoulder instability should be able to "see" their humerus in their peripheral vision while performing their repetitions.

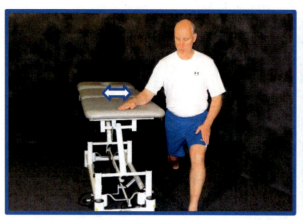 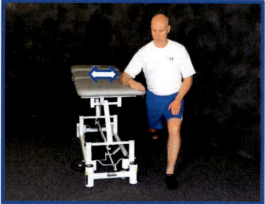

Figure 10-45: Glenohumeral Stabilization- Active Towel Slide for the Dorsal and Ventral Portions of the Rotator Cuff:

This is one of our most important glenohumeral stabilization and cuff strength building exercises. This is an advanced therapeutic exercise that will strengthen both the dorsal and ventral portion of the rotator cuff. As such, the patient will gain improved dynamic (muscular based) stability. Rotator cuff strength impairments and glenohumeral capsular laxity (hypermobility) are the two primary orthopedic conditions that will benefit from this exercise. Short arc shoulder external rotation and internal rotation movements are performed at a high rate of speed. Fast, short movement is the goal! Note, the patient's chest should be kept in an upward and forward position to assist in centering the humeral head in the Glenoid fossa. Have your patient perform multiple 10-second reps. Three sets of six to ten, 10-second table slides is about right for many patients. For the more athletic patients, perform the exercise in a lunge position as shown. Perform this exercise for 30 seconds with a 30 second rest cycle and repeat for 2-5 minutes.

Therapeutic Exercise

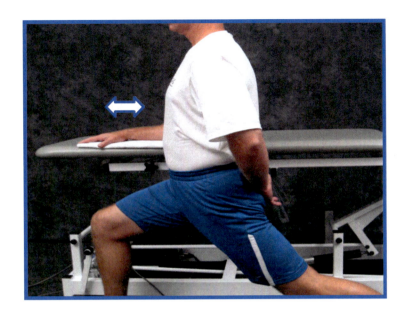

Figure 10-46: Glenohumeral Stabilization- Resisted Towel Sliding-Flexion-Extension:

Glenohumeral stabilization muscle training can also be performed using short arc shoulder flexion and extension at a high rate of speed. Again, fast and short movement is the goal and fast means as fast as the patient/athlete possibly can! Also, short means short, the humerus should not be advanced front or behind the patient's trunk. Remember to have your client keep their sternum and rib cage in an up and forward position to assist in centering the humeral head in the Glenoid fossa. To add a component of LE strength building, prescribe this exercise in the lunge position as shown above. Regarding exercise dosage, prescribe this procedure for 2- 5 minutes with a 30 second work cycle and a 30 second rest cycle. Note, 30 seconds of sustained high rate speed is very challenging.

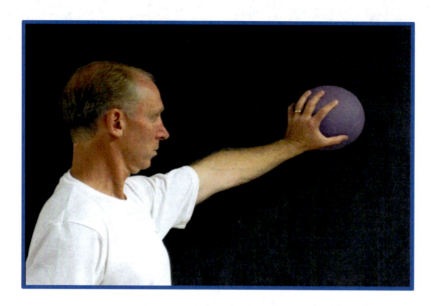

Figure 10-47: Glenohumeral Stabilization- Ball Rolling:

This glenohumeral and scapulothoracic stabilization exercise is performed at a much slower rate of speed as compared to the towel slide exercise but does offer the advantage of rotator cuff and serratus anterior muscle training with the UE in an elevated position. The scapula needs to function as a stable base for the humerus during UE elevation and also needs to rotate in rhythm with the humerus during all planes of UE elevation. This closed kinetic chain exercise promotes isometric muscular contraction of the serratus anterior and light contraction of the shoulder elevator and rotator cuff as the ball is moved in an upward, backward, and forward direction. Therapists can be creative regarding arcs and patterns of motion as long as those patterns are pain free.

Therapeutic Exercise

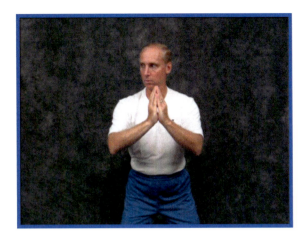 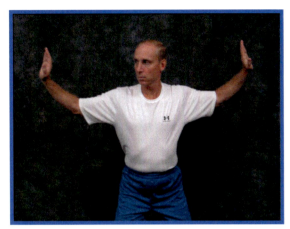

Figure 10-48: The Palms Together-Palms Away Exercise – Standing:

A good portion of Chapter 10 has dealt with management of the rotator cuff. I would like to end this section of the chapter by demonstrating two simple therapeutic throwing drills that clinicians can prescribe for an overhead throwing athlete who has reached the point in his intervention where light short toss throwing is about to start. A full throwing program including long toss likely exceeds what most orthopedic clinicians are able to provide an athlete. This drill will assist the clinician who does not have a strong handle on the overhead throwing motion and it will provide the patient with a biomechanically correct way to initiate his or her throwing motion again. The exercise movement begins with both palms together; the hands break apart and move downward with the lateral aspect of both thumbs "swiping" past the anterior proximal aspect of each thigh. This is the beginning of a full arm circle. The patient is then instructed to move both elbows high such that the "glove side" arm/elbow is parallel to the ground and symmetric with the throwing side (left in the case of the figure above). Note how the palm on the throwing hand (left) is facing away from the intended target. In the cocked position, if your patient were standing in stretch position on a pitching mound, his/her palm should face backward and toward short stop for a right-handed thrower and backward and toward where a 2nd basemen would play for a left-handed thrower. This movement pattern can be performed repetitively with or without a ball in the hand.

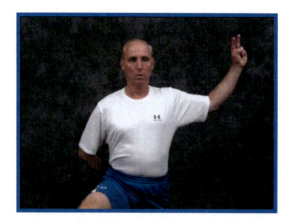 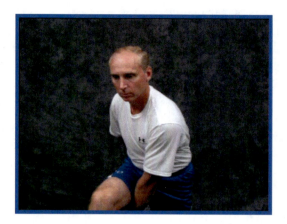

Figure 10-49: The Full Finish Exercise – Half Kneeling:

In this stage of cuff rehabilitation where throwing is about to start, this throwing drill will give a clinician another biomechanically sound procedure for the overhead throwing athlete. The start position is one where the patient's arm has rotated out of the fully cocked position, the ball is now facing forward, and the body is no longer closed off to the intended target as shown in exercise 10-48. Many rotator cuff problems begin due to lack of a full finish during the throwing motion. Lack of a full finish does not allow for enough deceleration time for the arm. Lack of full arm deceleration places a great deal of extra load on the rotator cuff tendons. Regarding the end position for this throwing drill, notice how the lateral aspect of the upper end of the humerus is fully facing the target which would be directly in front of the patient. Inexperienced throwers often stop their arm motion with the lateral aspect of the upper end of the humerus facing laterally at the conclusion of a throw. Over time, this will irritate and could very well damage the cuff tendons. Have your patient practice this throwing motion to a full finish with or without a ball in their hand. It is best to play catch with the patient at approximately 10-15 feet when first starting out.

Therapeutic Exercise

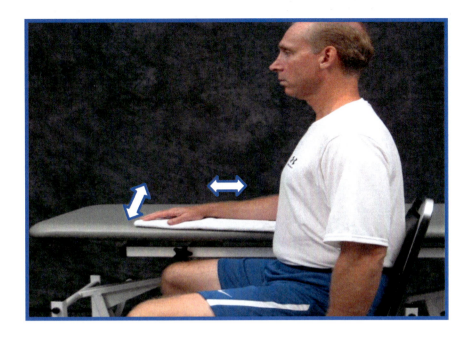

Figure 10-50: Glenohumeral Stabilization- Resisted Towel-Table Slide Exercise-Seated:

Let's go back to the towel slide exercise and slow it down quite a bit and I do mean slow. The previous two towel slide exercises were advanced high-speed procedures. But the towel slide exercises can also be applied to significant weakness and pain impairments associated with acute post op, post injury and in relation to flare ups of chronic conditions such as osteoarthritis. This seated version can be prescribed for patients who do not tolerate the more athletic lunge position. The arc of movement and amount of frictional resistance should be varied so that the ER/IR or the flexion/extension movement is non-painful. Remember, rotator cuff muscle training that provokes joint or soft tissue pain will ultimately inhibit the same muscles that you hope to make stronger for the patient. The arc and speed of movement and amount of frictional resistance (pressing down onto the towel) should be varied so that this therapeutic motion is non-painful. For exercise dosage, prescribe this procedure for 2- 5 minutes with a 30 second work cycle and a 30 second rest cycle

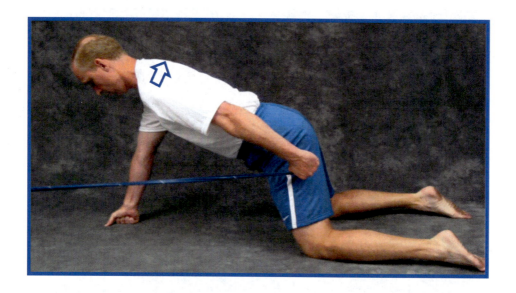

Figure 10-51: Scapular Muscle Isometric Protraction Closed Kinetic Chain – Four Point Position:

The next four exercises in this chapter essentially deal with the various forms of scapular protraction and improving strength in the Serratus Anterior muscle. In this first exercise, scapular muscle stabilization (strengthening) is achieved by reducing the B of S from four points of reference in contact with the ground to three points on the ground as the uninvolved UE pulls against the resistance of an elastic band. Isometric closed chain protraction of the scapula is performed on the right side in the figure above to strengthen the Serratus Anterior muscle. For patients with good joint cartilage and no subacromial impingement isometric protraction could be held for 30 seconds or more. Again, if the suprahumeral soft tissue structures are healthy, UE elevation should be greater than 90 degrees for optimal training of the Serratus muscle.

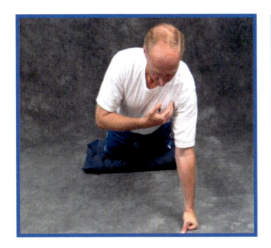 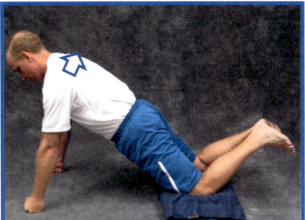

Figure 10-52: Alternating Isometric Scapular Muscle Protraction- Prone on Knees
Abdominal Drawing:

This is an alternating UE closed kinetic chain Serratus Anterior strength building exercise. I like to call it the "shoulder slapper" exercise. Isometric scapular protraction is maintained throughout the exercise as the patient's hands alternately slap the top of the opposite shoulder. Three sets of 6-10 repetitions is often a good starting point. To repeat, the emphasis of this procedure is to maintain a unilateral isometric scapular protraction as the patient alternately moves from both UE's in contact with the floor to one UE in contact with the floor. Note, have your patient keep the back of the cervical spine in a nicely elongated position by gently drawing their chin down and in towards their Adams Apple. Abdominal drawing (Chapter 18) should also be performed during the course of this exercise.

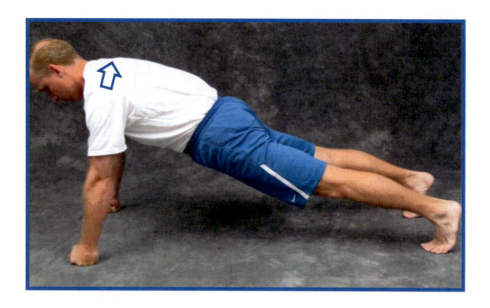

Figure 10-53: Scapular Muscle Isometric/Isotonic Protraction Closed Kinetic Chain – Prone Plank Position

For your more advanced patients with impaired UE elevation and deficits in protractor muscle strength, the prone plank position with abdominal drawing can be used to facilitate both isometric scapular protraction and isotonic scapular protraction. Isotonic muscle training can be performed with a minimum of three sets of 6-10 repetitions and isometric training should be held for a minimum of 6 to 10 seconds with a similar number of repetitions. During the rest phase, the patient should relax their glut squeeze and abdominal muscle drawing, let their knees flex to the ground, and lightly "shake out" their upper extremities. Let's talk a little bit about risk verse reward. I am all for improving scapulohumeral rhythm, serratus anterior muscle strength and possibly reducing the degree of scapular dyskinesia in our patients. I also mentioned previously that the scapula is an important mobile base, which needs to rotate in rhythm with the humerus during all planes of UE elevation. But let's make one point perfectly clear, isometric and isotonic scapular protraction muscle training is not worth the cost of glenohumeral cartilage damage or damage to the cuff tendons. These two structures are by far the most important in terms of overall function of the shoulder and too much closed chain scapular protraction training could eventually damage both structures.

Therapeutic Exercise

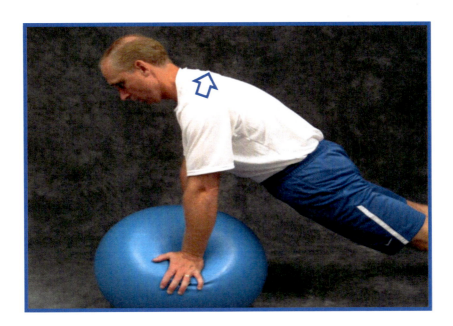

Figure 10-54: Scapular Muscle Isometric/Isotonic Protraction Closed Kinetic Chain with Swiss Ball– Prone Plank Position

Lastly, for your more advanced patients with impaired UE elevation and deficits in protractor strength, the prone plank position with abdominal drawing can be used to facilitate both isometric scapular protraction and isotonic scapular protraction. Incorporation of the Swiss exercise ball will further elevate the patient's C of G, add an unstable exercise platform, and as a result increase muscular demand. Isotonic muscle training can be performed with a minimum of three sets of 6-10 repetitions and isometric training should be held for a minimum of 6 to 10 seconds with a similar number of repetitions. During the rest phase, the patient should relax their glut squeeze, abdominal muscle drawing, let their knees flex to the ground, and "shake out" their upper extremities. Don't forget my comments regarding cartilage, cuff tendons and closed chain scapular protraction. If shoulder pain is provoked during the course of this exercise, it should be discontinued.

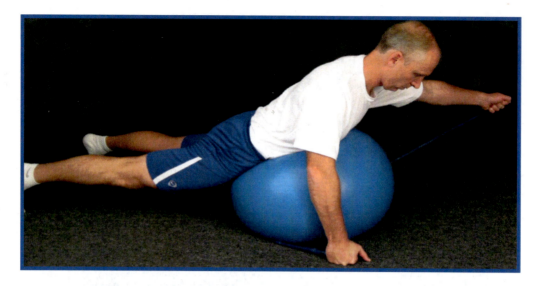

Figure 10-55: Swiss Ball Supported Elastic Band Resisted Lower Trap Muscle Training, Unilateral and Bilateral:

In terms of common muscular imbalances that appear with some degree of frequency at the shoulder girdle, it is not uncommon to find weakness impairment affecting the lower trapezius muscle. There are a number of ways to train this superficial spinal/ shoulder muscle and here is one of the better ones. Have the patient get into a level 1 Swiss ball supported position (Chapter 18) and perform isotonic elastic band resisted UE elevation up the 10 o clock or 2 o clock position depending on which UE is performing the motion. The patient's head would be considered at the 12-o clock position. Perform a minimum of three sets of 6-10 reps. Note how the elastic band is wrapped around the lower aspect of the Swiss ball in order to secure it. UE elevation is performed with the humerus in an externally rotated position. Elongation of the posterior aspect of the neck is essential during the performance of this exercise.

Therapeutic Exercise

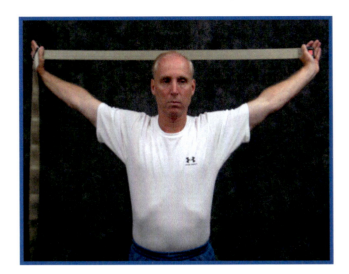 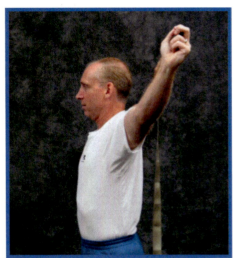

Figure 10-56: Glenohumeral Self-Stretching Pectoralis Major - All Three Portions

This self-stretch exercise is placed at the end of this chapter for two reasons. First it is an excellent way to stretch all three portions of the Pectoralis Major muscle. Second, stretching this muscle provides us an opportunity to review a common pattern of muscle imbalance that often affects the shoulder girdle secondary to aging, degenerative change, and common postural impairments. In brief, it is not uncommon to find shortening of the glenohumeral internal rotator muscles and weakening of the external rotators. This stretch provides a good way to lengthen some of these commonly shortened internal rotator muscles. Hold this muscular self-stretching for a minimum of 30 seconds or up to one minute. To isolate different portions of the muscle, stretching can occur at different points in the range of UE elevation.

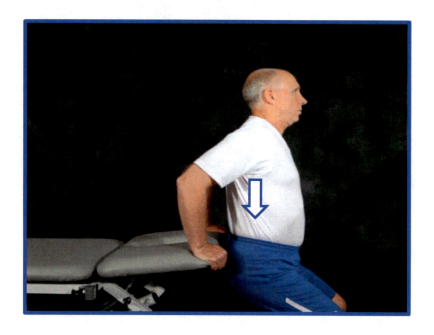

Figure 10-57 Self-Stretching for the Rotator Interval:

I would like to end the shoulder capture by discussing two more capsular self-stretches for the shoulder joint. The first, and shown above, is Glenohumeral extension self-stretching. Your patient can simply place his/her palms on the edge of a table or counter-top and just bend his/her knees. As the patient bends at his/her knees, both glenohumeral joints will be passively pressed into extension. I believe that this motion will elongate and therapeutically stretch the anterior capsule and the anterior aspect of the rotator interval. Like all forms of self-stretching, for a tensile load to produce a plastic change in soft tissue, stretching for up to a minute or more is likely necessary. Cyclic loading with progressive oscillations is another route to plastic elongation.

Therapeutic Exercise

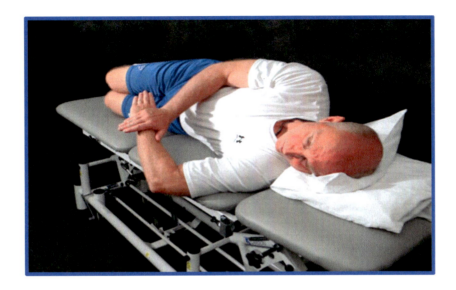

Figure 10-58: Self-Stretching for the posterior Capsule:

One last exercise here in the shoulder chapter. This as you can probably see is a passive internal rotation self-stretch which some folks like to call the sleeper stretch. I think that is a silly name, but you should know it anyways. Note how the patient is not directly lying on his shoulder and how one hand presses the under-most shoulder into internal rotation. This self-stretch will assist in elongating the posterior portion of the shoulder capsule. Like all self-stretches for the extremity joints, and here comes your end of the chapter review, it is prescribed for end feels that are firm (capsular) and early (tight). Same deal, stretching for up to a minute or more is likely necessary for permanent (plastic) changes and cyclic loading with progressive oscillations is another route to the same.

Chapter 11

Therapeutic Exercise for the Elbow

Chapter 11 will look at exercises for the patient with various elbow impairments. Here is a bulleted list of some of the more important topic areas that will be covered in this chapter.

- Managing Elbow and Forearm Motion Impairment
- Improving UE strength Without Eliciting UE Pain
- Managing Elbow Muscle and Tendon Pain

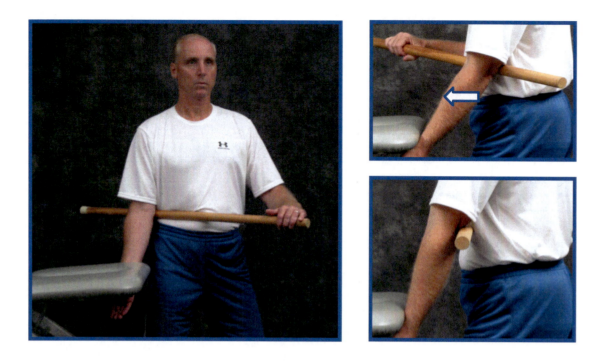

Figure 11-1: Elbow Extension Self-Mobilization-Humerus Ventral; Version 1:

This self-mobilization will assist in maintaining elbow extension after manual intervention such as joint mobilization, joint manipulation or hold-relax muscle stretching. This exercise will place a tensile load on the anterior capsule and improve elbow extension impairment following a distal humerus or proximal forearm fracture as well as certain arthritic changes limiting full elbow extension assuming calcific hypertrophy is not limiting full extension. The patient is instructed to pull the dowel rod posteriorly with one hand, which will force the anterior distal humerus in an anterior direction. The self-mobilization should be held for a minimum of 30 seconds or up to two minutes or more.

Therapeutic Exercise

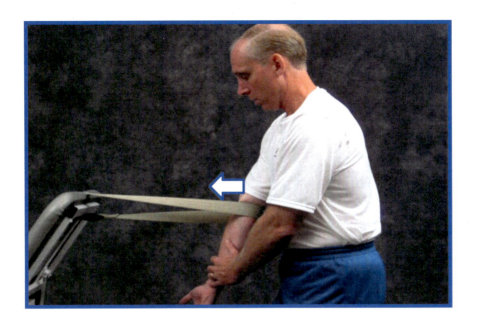

Figure 11-2: Elbow Extension Self-Mobilization-Humerus Ventral; Version 2:

This version of humerus ventral self-mobilization is best applied in the clinic using a mobilization belt and table as shown. The patient is to step backward holding their arm and forearm stable. The belt will pull (glide) the distal humerus in a ventral direction in relation to the ulna and radius. Similar to exercise 11-1, this therapeutic exercise will stretch the anterior elbow capsule and assist in maintaining and in some cases of less severe capsular restriction, improve elbow extension. The self-mobilization should be held for a minimum of 30 seconds or up to two minutes or more.

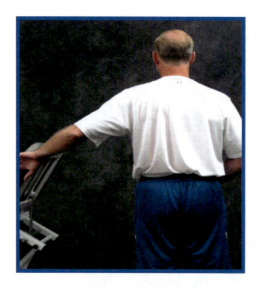 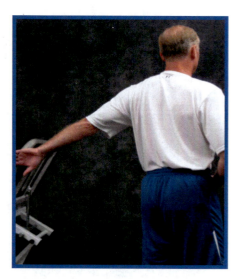

Figure 11-3: Biceps Self -Stretch:

This is a muscular self-stretch and as such should not be applied to the elbow in cases of capsular restriction. For joint limitation due to capsular shortening see figures 11-1 and 11-2. Use this exercise for general flexibility purposes, shortening of the biceps, before and after muscle strength training and before sports competition. Use your feet and turn your trunk allowing your elbow to straighten with your forearm in a pronated position. Hold-relax stretching can be incorporated by gently tensing the elbow flexor muscles, relaxing them, and turning the trunk further in order to promote a greater degree of elbow and UE extension. Hold the fully elongated muscle position for a minimum of 30 seconds or up to a minute or more. Unfortunately, this stretching position also places a great deal of tensile load on the brachial plexus and if a tension sensitive radiculitis is present; this stretch should not be performed.

Therapeutic Exercise

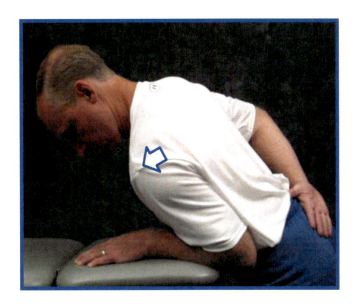

Figure 11-4: Elbow Flexion Self -Mobilization:

This exercise can be applied in cases of impaired elbow flexion. This exercise is commonly applied post immobilization secondary to an elbow fracture. The forearm is placed on a table top and the patient is instructed to advance their trunk forward between their upper extremities. Hold–relax muscle stretching can be incorporated by pressing the palms into the table and intermittently tensing the elbow extensor muscles. Greater degrees of elbow flexion are attained as the patient continues to advance their trunk forward. The chest should be held in an upward and forward position and the back of the cervical region should be elongated. Hold end range elbow flexion for a minimum of 30 seconds or up to two minutes or more.

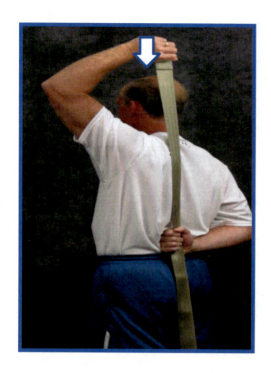 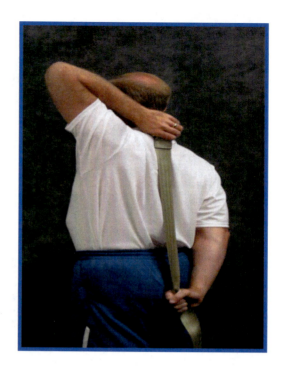

Figure 11-5: Triceps Self -Stretch:

This exercise is termed the triceps self-stretch and really does a great job at fully elongating the long head portion of this muscle. The patient is to fully elevate and fully adduct their UE before their elbow is passively flexed. Passive elbow flexion is obtained by pulling downward on the belt as shown in figure 11-5. Hold-relax muscle stretching can be achieved by intermittently tensing the elbow extensor muscles. As noted elsewhere in this text, muscle stretching procedures should be held for a minimum of 30 seconds or up to a minute or more after at least three hold-relax isometric contractions and joint re-positioning have been performed. Here is a point to remember regarding Hold-Relax stretching. At the conclusion of the isometric contraction, if additional range of motion is achieved then neuromuscular relaxation has been accomplished, not muscle stretching. When no further range of movement can be achieved after the Hold-Relax method and this final position is now held for a minimum of 30 seconds or up to a minute or more, then the process of muscle stretching has started.

Therapeutic Exercise

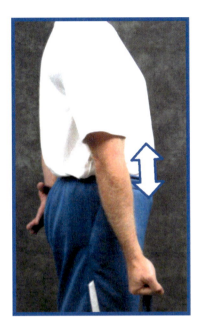 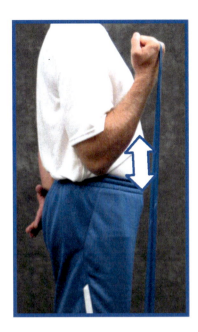

Figure 11-6: Elbow Self-Mobilization/Strengthening-Option 1:

Next we will begin a short series of four elastic band exercises which provide both assisted and resisted motions. These next four exercises, 11-6 through 11-9 provide light movement therapy for conditions such as symptomatic elbow arthritis and the associated muscular atrophy often seen with painful arthritic conditions. The prescribed thickness of band or the number of plates on a pulley system should be based upon muscle strength, symptom intensity and movement quality during the exercise. In cases of painful elbow arthritis, we do not want the patient to struggle to perform a motion nor do we want the movement to produce pain. So, choose the thickness of elastic band carefully and don't overdue the resistance training in these cases. In option 1, the patient simply steps on the elastic band to anchor it distally. Again, chose a thickness and amount of pre-tensioning that will allow for full (if possible) and pain free resisted elbow flexion and elastic band assisted elbow extension. Perform repetitions until elbow flexor muscles become slightly fatigued and the movement quality begins to decline. This exercise procedure along with exercises 11-1 and 11-2 will assist patients with weakness impairments and stiffness impairments affecting elbow extension.

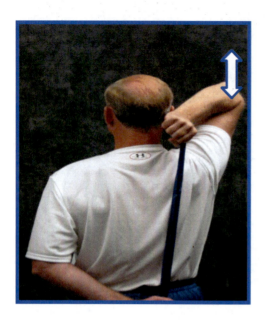 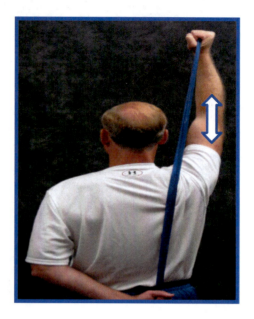

Figure 11-7: Elbow Self-Mobilization/Strengthening-Option 2:

In option 2 the patient anchors the elastic band with one hand behind the sacrum or buttock region and performs light repetitive elastic band resisted elbow extension and elastic band assisted elbow flexion. Choose a thickness and amount of pre-tensioning that will allow for full and pain free elbow motion. This statement may be obvious, but the choice of assisted verses resisted elastic band motion is primarily based on whether the impaired motion is predominately caused by stiffness, weakness, or pain. When motion is impaired due to pain, the best choice for therapeutic motion is assisted movement. When motion is impaired due to weakness, the best choice for therapeutic motion is resisted movement. Regarding resisted motion, perform repetitions until the target muscles become slightly fatigued and the movement quality begins to decline. Lastly, when motion is impaired by stiffness, often assisted movement is initially the best form of therapeutic movement when used in conjunction with muscular self-stretching and capsular self-mobilization exercise (Figures 11-4 and 11-5). Elastic band resistance training for the elbow flexors and extensors also provides a very good way to build muscular endurance for patients (low load-high rep training) and athletes wishing to train theses muscle groups.

Therapeutic Exercise

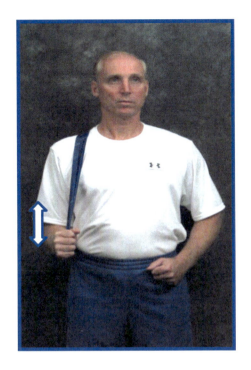 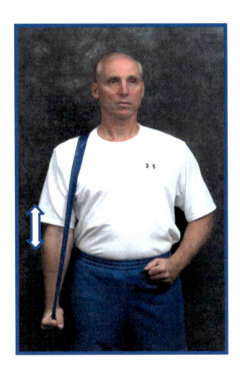

Figure 11-8: Elbow Self-Mobilization-Strengthening-Option 3:

In option 3 the patient anchors the elastic band with one hand along their side, wraps the band around their back, and drapes the remaining portion over the front of their chest. Option 3 will provide elastic resisted elbow extension and elastic band assisted elbow flexion. Chose a thickness and amount of pre-tensioning that will allow for full and pain free elbow extension with light resistance and elastic band assisted elbow flexion. This exercise option along with option 4 allows the humerus to remain at the patient's side during the therapeutic motion. In some cases, where shoulder injury or pathology is involved, the patient will find this to be a comfortable exercise training position. Perform repetitions until the target muscles become slightly fatigued and the movement quality begins to decline. When treating a patient with impaired elbow flexion secondary to stiffness, assisted elbow flexion prescribed along with exercises 11-4 and 11-5 will assist your patient in improving this restricted motion.

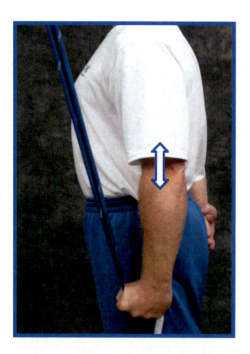 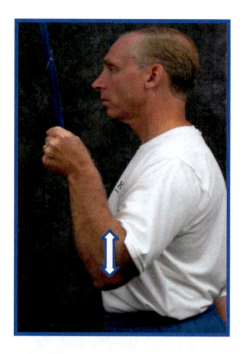

Figure 11-9: Elbow Self-Mobilization-Strengthening-Option 4:

In option 4 the patient knots one end of the elastic band, drapes the band over the top of a door and secures it by closing the door. Option 4 will provide elastic resisted elbow extension and elastic band assisted elbow flexion. Chose a thickness and amount of pre-tensioning that will allow for full and pain free elbow extension with light resistance and elastic band assisted flexion. This exercise option along with option 3 allows the humerus to remain at the patient's side during the therapeutic motion. In some cases, where shoulder pathology such as impingement tendonitis is involved, the patient will find this to be a comfortable exercise training position. In addition to impaired motion due to elbow arthritis, these elastic band movements prescribed along with self-mobilization and self-stretching exercises are also helpful after a period of immobilization post fracture. To repeat, perform resisted elastic band muscle training until the target muscles become slightly fatigued and the movement quality begins to decline.

Therapeutic Exercise

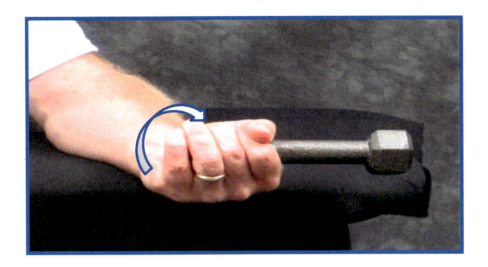

Figure 11-10: Forearm Self-Stretching-Supination:

Let's move a little more distally now and discuss the forearm joints and soft tissues. This is a classic exercise often performed in the clinic with an asymmetric weight device (weight placed on one end of a bar) at home; a hammer could also be used. This is a self-stretch used in cases of stiffness impairment. Most often, this exercise is prescribed after a course of immobilization due to distal humerus, proximal, mid or distal forearm fracture. Examination findings need to demonstrate active and passive motion restriction in the same direction, in this case restricted active and passive forearm supination. Hold this self-stretch for a minimum of 30 seconds or up to 2 minutes or more. Your patient should feel a stretching sensation in the forearm only and not in the ulnar aspect of the wrist. At the conclusion of this stretch, have the patient use their opposite hand to remove the asymmetric weight out of the involved hand (UE). There is nothing real fancy about this stretch, but it is often necessary to prescribe due to stiffness impairment after a number of different orthopedic fractures.

Therapeutic Exercise

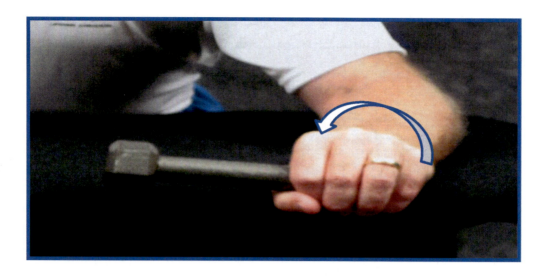

Figure 11-11: Forearm Self-Stretching-Pronation:

Now let's stretch the forearm joints and soft tissue in the opposite direction. Again, this is a sustained self-stretch used for cases of stiffness impairment. Most often, this exercise is prescribed after a course of immobilization due to distal humerus, proximal, mid or distal forearm fracture. Examination findings need to demonstrate active and passive motion restriction in the same direction, in this case, restricted active and passive forearm pronation. Similar to exercise 11-10, have the patient keep their UE supported on a table and hold this self-stretch for a minimum of 30 seconds or up to 2 minutes or more. Note, in addition to sustained self-stretching, repetitive arcs of forearm supination and pronation can be performed with an asymmetric weight in order to improve forearm muscle strength. After an injury, the arc of these two forearm motions should be pain free. Also monitor that no joint noise is elicited at the forearm or intercarpal articulations.

Therapeutic Exercise

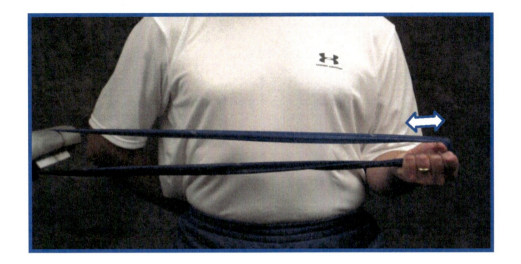

Figure 11-12: Forearm Self-Mobilization/Strengthening-Resisted Supination with Assisted Pronation:

Somewhat similar to exercises 11-6 through 11-9, elastic band assisted and resisted movement therapy for forearm supination and pronation can be applied in cases of painful arthritic movement impairment and post elbow or forearm fracture management. Remember, in cases of painful movement associated with arthritis, keep the resisted motion at a level where all repetitions are pain free. In cases of non-symptomatic motion restriction, make sure there is enough tension on the elastic band to pull the joints and soft tissues (assisted movement) into the entire available range of motion. In cases of weakness impairment, the amount of elastic band resistance should not exceed the strength of the weakened muscular tissue. In other words, the quality of movement should always be good and the patient should not have to struggle against the resistance provided by the band.

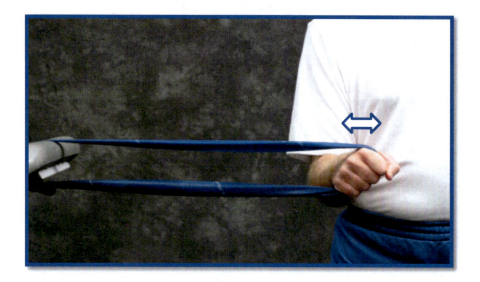

Figure 11-13: Forearm Self-Mobilization/Strengthening-Resisted Pronation with Assisted Supination:

The legend associated with Figure 11-12 discussed and reviewed some of the orthopedic conditions associated with prescription of this type of therapeutic exercise. Let's briefly discuss another use for elastic band strength training and a couple more clinical conditions (figure 11- 14 and 11-15). Elastic muscle resisted training can be used to build strength in the forearm supinator/wrist extensor muscle group and the forearm pronator/wrist flexor muscle group in athletes and others. In the case of healthy athletes with sound cartilage and tendons, rep max programs with elastic resistance can be very helpful to improve sports performance. Note: make sure that self-stretching of the same muscle groups is performed before and after rep max strength training.

Therapeutic Exercise

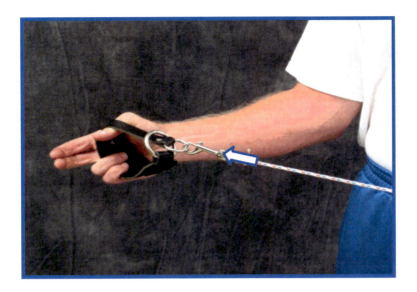

Figure 11-14: Resisted Forearm Supination with Lateral Epicondylitis:

The legend associated with Figure 11-13 brought athletic strength training into the discussion when utilizing these therapeutic motions. Let's go back to common orthopedic conditions and briefly discuss epicondylitis-losis and strength training. In an acute flare up and for first time occurrence epicondylitis in the younger patient (less than 35 years), controlled use, immobilization and supportive bracing is a key aspect of epicondylitis management. As the condition improves therapeutic strength training may be incorporated. Initial attempts at muscle training must be pain free and minimizing grip pressure as shown above is a key aspect of non-symptom provoking resisted training. This figure demonstrates how fingers can be released during resisted supination training for the forearm supinator/wrist extensor muscle groups. This will minimize the extent of muscle contraction and may allow for pain free training. In cases of epicondylitis-losis and strength building, make sure your patient really understands the importance of rest breaks in between each set of 10-30 reps, whatever you prescribe. For example, during a 30 second rest break the patient should be evaluating his/her pain intensity level If pain starts to increase, make a change in the exercise speed, resistance or movement arc.

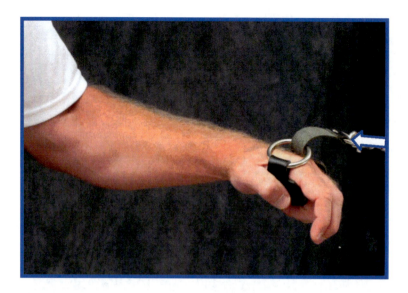

Figure 11-15: Resisted Forearm Pronation with Medial Epicondylitis:

Let's stay with our discussion of epicondylitis, strength training and focus on the medial aspect of the elbow. Again, in an acute flare up and for first time occurrence epicondylitis in the younger patient (less than age 35 years), controlled use, immobilization and supportive bracing is a key aspect of management. Upon resolution of some or all of the inflammation, strength training should be applied. Regarding medial epicondylitis-losis, resisted forearm pronation is a key therapeutic movement. Similar to our discussion of lateral epicondylitis in the previous figure, muscle training should be pain free and grip pressure should be minimized. Regarding that, figures 11-14 and 11-15 demonstrate how a pulley system strap can be positioned and how the fingers can be released during resisted pronation for the forearm pronator/wrist flexor muscle groups. In cases of painful degenerative tendinosis research has shown that resisted training is helpful for pain reduction and strength restoration.

Chapter 12
Therapeutic Exercise for the Wrist-Hand

Chapter 12 will look at exercises for patients with various wrist-hand impairments. Here is a bulleted list of some of the more important topic areas that will be covered in this chapter.

- Managing Motion Stiffness Impairments at the Wrist
- Managing Motion Stiffness Impairments at the Fingers
- Increasing Forearm, Wrist, and Hand Strength
- Managing Epicondylitis with Wrist Flexion and Extension

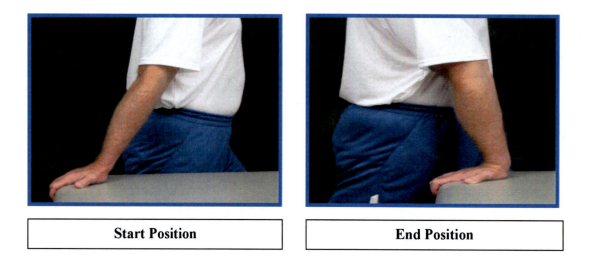

| Start Position | End Position |

Figure 12-1: Self-Stretching Wrist Flexors:

This exercise promotes passive wrist extension and can be prescribed for capsular restriction and muscle shortening. Unlike the Biceps self-stretch exercise which is not to be prescribed for elbow capsular restriction, movement substitution at other joints is not likely with this self-stretching procedure. Have your patient place the palmar surface of their hand at the end of a table with their fingers flexed over the edge. Their body must be "in front" of their UE. This will initially keep the wrist in a more neutral position. The patient is then instructed to step backward and bring their UE with them. This movement will passively extend the wrist joint. Hold this stretch for at least 30 seconds or up to a minute or more. A pulling or stretching sensation should be felt somewhere along the anatomical course of the muscles and tendons. Discomfort, particularly discomfort that seems to be intercarpal discomfort within the wrist should not be allowed to occur.

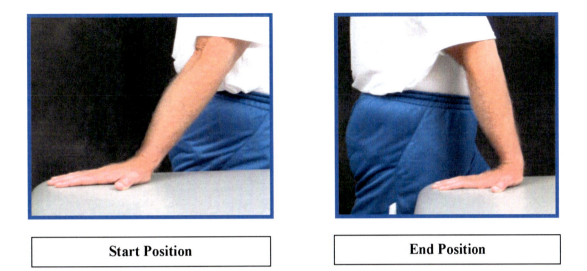

| Start Position | End Position |

Figure 12-2: Self-Stretching Finger Flexors Version 1:

This exercise promotes passive wrist and finger extension and should be prescribed primarily for muscle shortening of the long finger flexor muscles. Shortening of these muscles can occur due to overuse (gripping activities) and orthopedic injuries requiring a period of immobilization involving the wrist/hand area. Have your patient place the palmar surface of their hand and fingers at the end of a table with their fingers flattened against the table. Their body must be "in front" of their UE. This will initially provide for a start position where the muscles are slackened and the wrist is not fully extended. The patient is then instructed to step backward and bring their UE with them. This movement will passively extend the wrist which will in turn begin to lengthen the target muscle groups. Hold this stretch for at least 30 seconds or up to a minute or more. A pulling or stretching sensation should be felt somewhere along the anatomical course of the muscles and tendons. Discomfort, particularly discomfort that seems to be intercarpal discomfort within the wrist should not be allowed to occur.

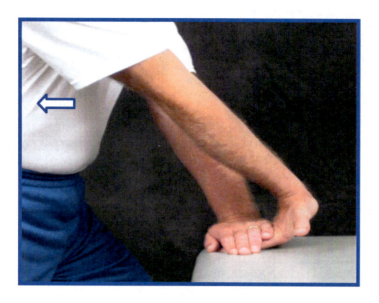

Note the end position for the heel of the hand

Figure 12-3: Self-Stretching Finger Flexors-Version 2:

Note, in this figure the fingers have been more securely stabilized onto the table and the palm of the hand is now "lifted" off the table. The patient is taught to use their opposite hand to hold the IP joints in full extension and allow the MCP joints to be extended more fully for greater lengthening of the long finger flexor muscles. Hold this stretch for at least 30 seconds or up to a minute or more.

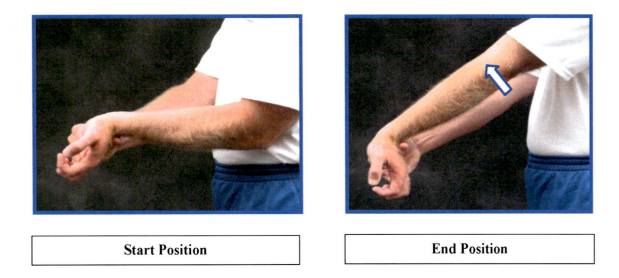

| Start Position | End Position |

Figure 12-4: Self-Stretching Wrist Flexors-Off the Table and on the Field:

The first version of this exercise was demonstrated with figure 12-1. This version is essentially the same, but now the wrist-hand area is not placed on a table. This version is great for pre sport participation (on the field), during various forms of upper body weight training which requires an element of gripping, when taking a break from typing on a computer or many different forms of material handling work that requires repetitive gripping. In terms of movement sequence, carefully pull the wrist into extension. Do not force end range wrist extension. After the wrist has been placed in extension, the patient should actively and fully extend their elbow joint to completely lengthen this muscle group. Hold this stretch for at least 30 seconds or up to a minute or more.

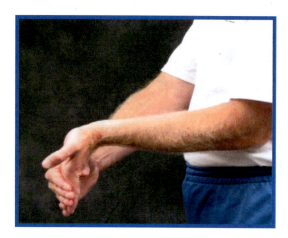 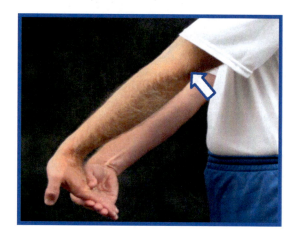

Figure 12-5: Self-Stretching Finger Flexors-Off the Table and on the Field:

The first version of this exercise was demonstrated with figure 12-2. This version is essentially the same, but now the wrist-hand and fingers are not placed on a table. This version is great for pre sport participation (on the field), during various forms of upper body weight training that requires an element of sustained gripping, when taking a break from typing on a computer, or many different forms of material handling work that requires gripping. In terms of movement sequence, carefully pull the wrist and all finger joints into extension. Do not force end range wrist or finger extension particularly if these movements are painful. After the wrist and fingers have been placed in extension, the patient should actively extend their elbow joint to fully lengthen these muscle groups. Hold this stretch for at least 30 seconds or up to a minute or more.

Therapeutic Exercise

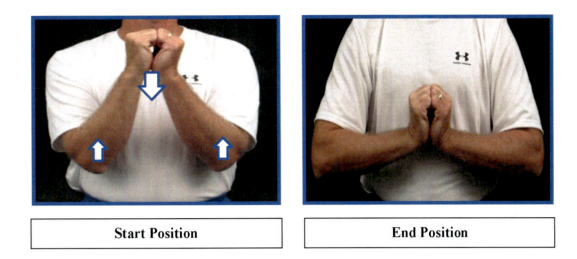

Figure 12-6: Self-Mobilization-Wrist Extension:

This is a very basic but also very useful self-mobilization exercise used for impaired (restricted) wrist flexion. The patient is initially instructed to gently, not fully, flex their fingers in order to slacken the long finger flexor muscles. Then instruct your patient to place their hands close to their chin and their elbows pointing downward. Next, the patient is instructed to move their hands in a caudal direction toward their belly button and to lift their elbows upward. When the first stop in passive wrist extension is felt, the patient is to stop the downward movement of their hands. This exercise should be performed lightly and rhythmically with multiple repetitions when a painful wrist extension impairment is present. The end position is held for a more sustained period of time if the orthopedic condition is less painful and more stiffness dominate.

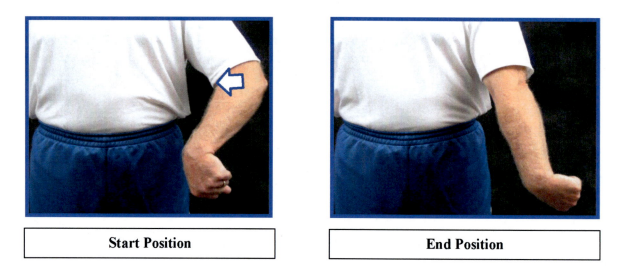

| Start Position | End Position |

Figure 12-7: Self-Stretching Finger Extensors:

Instruct the patient to hold their involved hand (fingers) at their side in a comfortable position with their shoulder girdle relaxed. Next the patient is instructed to make a fist. After the patient makes a fist, they are to flex their wrist while maintaining finger flexion. Then the patient is taught to fully pronate their forearm while maintaining wrist and finger flexion. Lastly, have the patient fully extend their elbow. This movement sequence will fully elongate the lateral elbow muscle group. The patient should experience a stretching sensation in the anatomically correct area only. In Chapter 11, we briefly brought up the subject of epicondylitis. If a patient is experiencing symptoms associated with the lateral version of this condition and muscle flexibility impairment is present, this exercise should be prescribed. Medial epicondylitis and muscular flexibility impairment can be addressed with exercises 12-1 — 12-5.

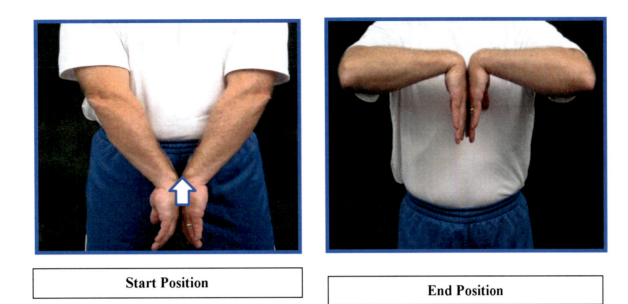

| Start Position | End Position |

Figure 12-8: Self-Mobilization-Wrist Flexion:

This is a very basic, but also very useful self-mobilization exercise used for impaired (restricted) wrist flexion. This movement intervention begins by having the dorsal aspects of both hands next to one another and placing them in front of the lower abdominal region (below the belly button). The patient is then instructed to lift their hands up toward their chin and stop this motion when the finger tips are just above the belly button. As this occurs, the wrists will passively flex. This exercise should be performed lightly and rhythmically with multiple repetitions when painful wrist flexion impairment is present and the end position can also be held for a more sustained period of time if the orthopedic condition is less painful and more stiffness dominate in its clinical presentation.

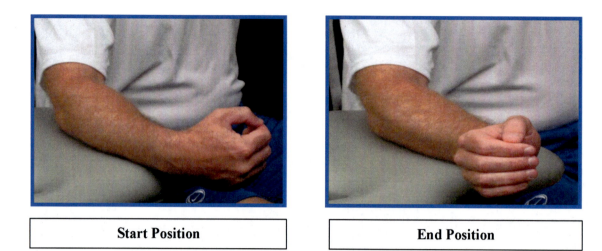

| Start Position | End Position |

Figure 12-9: Active Wrist Extensor and Flexor Muscle Training with Reduced Effect from Gravity:

In cases of acute flare ups of elbow tendonitis and in cases of painful degenerative tendinosis, this exercise may provide a way for patients to begin pain free therapeutic motion. Note how the patient's elbow is flexed, forearm is in a neutral position, and how the fist is open and fingers are relaxed. All of these conditions must be met to initially minimize loading on inflamed or painful musculotendinous tissues. The patient is instructed to perform short arc pain free wrist flexion and extension. Gravity resisted motion is minimized when the forearm is in a neutral position and the UE is supported on a table. Perform this initial tendonitis/tendinosis exercise for 5 minutes strictly following a 30 second work phase and 30 second rest phase protocol. Light self-massage and pain free self-stretching as demonstrated by the therapist can also be incorporated during some of the rest periods. This short arc isotonic movement must be pain free for the entire duration of the exercise. If the isotonic motion provokes any discomfort, the speed and or the amplitude of motion will likely need to be reduced. Total work time can be progressed as tolerated.

Therapeutic Exercise

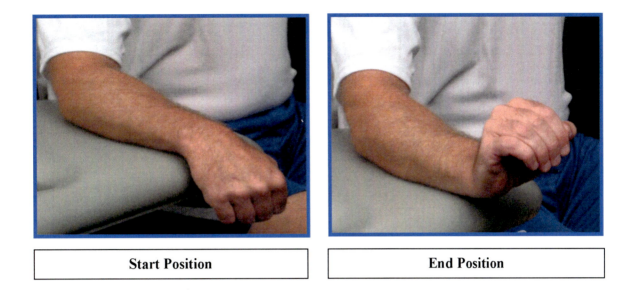

| Start Position | End Position |

Figure 12-10: Active Wrist Extensor or Flexor-Gravity Resisted, Elbow Flexed:

Changing muscle length and the effect of gravity make for the next advancement from the exercise shown in figure 12-9. The painful muscle tendon unit can be lengthened slightly by either pronating or supinating the forearm. Resistance can be increased by lifting the weight of the hand against gravity. The forearm is pronated for gravity resisted wrist extensor training in cases of lateral epicondylitis or lateral tendinosis and the forearm is supinated for gravity resisted wrist flexor training in cases of medial epicondylitis or medial elbow pain due to tendinosis. Isotonic wrist motions are performed in the pain-free range. The involved muscle-tendon unit is still not fully lengthened with the elbow positioned in flexion. For this first phase of gravity resisted training the patient's fist is to remain open and the fingers relaxed. Perform this second level tendonitis/tendinosis exercise for 5 minutes strictly following a 30 second work and 30 second rest protocol. Light self-massage and pain free self-stretching as demonstrated by the therapist can also be incorporated during some of the rest periods. Movement must be pain free for the entire duration of the exercise. If the isotonic motion provokes any discomfort, the speed and or the amplitude of motion will likely need to be reduced. Total work time can be progressed as tolerated.

Therapeutic Exercise

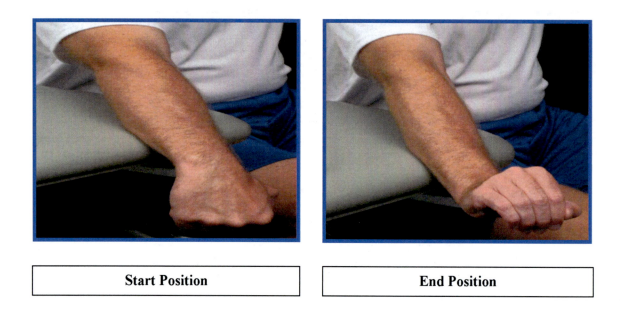

Start Position — End Position

Figure 12-11: Active Wrist Extensor or Flexor-Gravity Resisted, Elbow Extended:
The next advancement in this muscle training series is to have the patient fully extend their elbow. Short arc isotonic wrist motions are performed in the pronated position (shown above) or supinated position with the involved (painful) muscle-tendon units in a more fully lengthened position. As the patient's condition improves, the muscle-tendon unit should be more fully challenged by performing an expanded range of wrist flexion or extension and varying the degree of grip pressure by making a fist. Clenching the hand or opening the hand will change the length-tension relationship of the involved muscle-tendons. This should be incorporated to assist in keeping the exercise movement pain free or to further challenge the muscle-tendon units. Perform this third level tendonitis/tendinosis exercise for 5 minutes making sure that the patient takes a rest break every 30 seconds to evaluate his/her pain level. Light self-massage and pain free self-stretching as demonstrated by the therapist can also be incorporated during some of the rest periods. Movement must be pain free for the entire duration of the exercise. If the isotonic motion provokes any discomfort, the speed and or the amplitude of motion will likely need to be reduced. Total work time can be progressed as tolerated.

Therapeutic Exercise

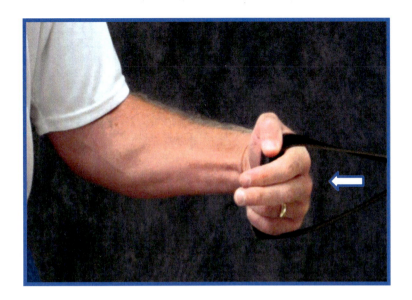

12-12: Resisted Wrist Flexion with Reduced Grip Pressure:

If resistance greater than the effect of gravity is required in order to progress strength training, a pulley system (above) or an elastic band can be incorporated as shown here. This discussion was first brought up in Chapter 11 during resisted forearm motions. Resisted training for medial elbow pain or wrist flexor strength impairment should be challenging, but should not provoke the patient's primary symptoms. If elastic band or pulley system resistance is incorporated, grip pressure and grip adjustment may need to occur for higher level resistance training. Note how two fingers have been released from the pulley system strap in order to reduce grip pressure and control pain during this therapeutic motion. Perform this therapeutic procedure when treating tendonitis/tendinosis for 5 minutes making sure that the patient takes a rest break every 30 seconds to evaluate his/her pain level. To repeat, vary the arc and speed of movement as well as the grip pressure and pulley strap or elastic band placement on the patient's distal UE such that their primary symptoms are not reproduced during muscle training. Total work time can be progressed as tolerated.

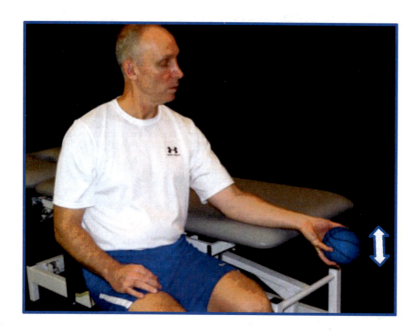

Figure 12-13: Eccentric Strengthening for the Flexor-Pronator Muscles:

This intervention is known as the eccentric ball dropping exercise for the wrist flexors. This version of flexor-pronator (medial elbow) muscle strength building works very well for the more athletic medial elbow pain patient. It is an excellent way to shift between concentric and eccentric muscle training. The patient actively flexes his/her wrist, to release the ball, catches it, and slowly carries the weight of the ball downward (eccentric loading of muscles and tendons) into wrist extension. All of the eccentric ball dropping-catching exercise require some practice. Your patients with better hand-eye coordination will do well this them.

Therapeutic Exercise

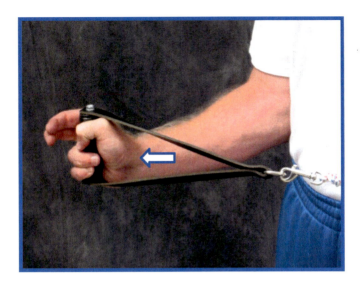

Figure 12-14: Resisted Wrist Extension with Reduced Grip Pressure:

This figure demonstrates the incorporation of a pulley system for lateral elbow pain or wrist extensor strength impairment. Speed changes and continual grip adjustment (taking finger(s) off) of the elastic band, or pulley system handle or strap is a key to minimizing the chance of a painful flare up during therapeutic tendon reloading (strength building). Note how two fingers have been released from the pulley system strap in order to reduce grip pressure and control pain during this therapeutic motion. Have your patients perform this tendonitis/tendinosis exercise for 5 minutes making sure that he/she takes a rest break every 30 seconds to evaluate his/her pain intensity level. If tendon pain is noted, vary the arc and speed of movement as well as the grip pressure and pulley strap or elastic band placement on the patient's distal UE such that their pain symptoms are controlled. Light self-massage as demonstrated by the therapist can also be incorporated during some of the rest periods.

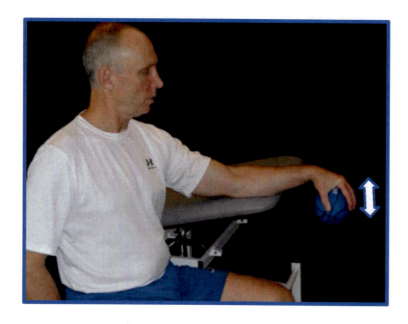

Figure 12-15: Eccentric Strengthening for the Extensor-Supinator Muscles:

This intervention is known as the eccentric ball dropping-catching exercise for the wrist extensors. It version of extensor-supinator (lateral elbow) muscle strength building works very well for the more athletic lateral elbow pain patient. It is an excellent way to shift between concentric and eccentric muscle training. The patient actively extends his/her wrist, releases the ball, catches it, and slowly carries the weight of the ball downward (eccentric phase) into wrist flexion.

Therapeutic Exercise

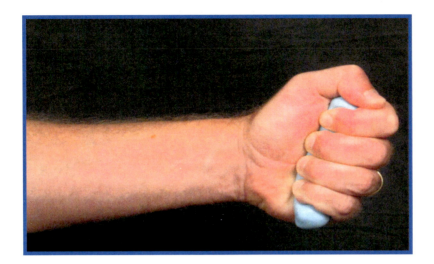

Figure 12-16: Wrist-Hand Isotonic and Isometric Muscle Training with Exercise Putty:

Yes, this picture above is showing exercise putty. We need to look at this basic strength building exercise in order to reinforce some key points made earlier regarding medial and lateral elbow pain and to underscore the importance of this cute little piece of therapeutic equipment. Regarding elbow pain, epicondylitis is often caused by activities that require a great deal of repetitive gripping. So, don't over use putty squeezing activities when managing this type of elbow condition. Make sure the patient does not over grip and squeeze too hard. Squeezing should not provoke pain. Also, I would prescribe a 30 second work and 30 second rest protocol by passing the putty back and forth between hands. Remember, the patient should be evaluating whether or not any discomfort has been provoked during the 30 second rest phase as the putty is squeezed in the opposite hand. If so, adjust the intensity of muscle contraction. The therapist can demonstrate a light gripping pressure by gripping the patient's distal forearm at different intensities.

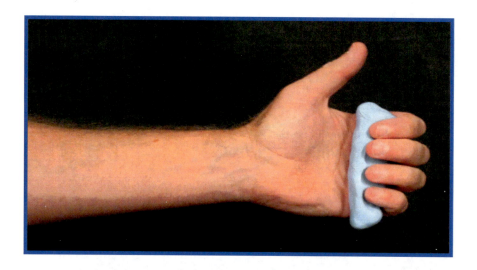

Figure 12-17: Wrist-Hand Isotonic and Isometric Muscle Training with Exercise Putty:

There is a host of orthopedic elbow, forearm, wrist and finger fractures which require a course of immobilization. When the cast comes off, the hand, wrist and forearm muscles will be weak. Grip strengthening with exercise putty is one of the things to prescribe if strength impairment is found post immobilization. Again, I would follow the 30 second work and 30 second rest protocol by passing the putty back and forth between hands at the 30 second mark. Remember, during the 30 second rest break the patient should evaluate whether any pain has developed in the involved wrist-hand. If so, have the patient reduce the intensity of the gripping pressure. Total work time can range from 5 up to 15 minutes.

Therapeutic Exercise

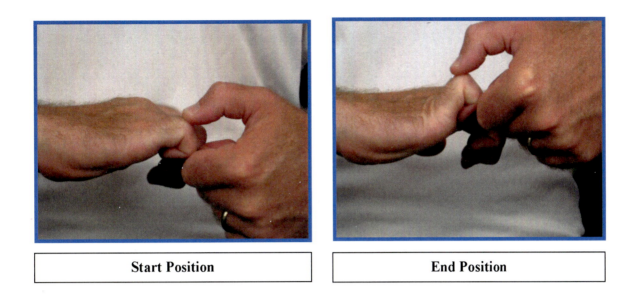

| Start Position | End Position |

Figure 12-18: Self-Stretching Dorsal Interossei:

This is an often forgotten, but very effective self-stretching procedure. Shortening of the intrinsic muscles of the hand can adversely affect hand and finger function as well as cause hand and finger discomfort. Wrist and hand injury, overuse, or degenerative changes can cause shortening of these muscles. Instruct your patient to pronate their forearm, passive flex their two IP joints, and then passively extend through their MCP joint. Once positioned in extension, passive adduction can also be added through the MCP joints. Note, do not over flex the IP joints prior to extending through the MCP joints. Protect the small amount of cartilage found at the IP joints by not flexing them too forcibly. Muscular self-stretching should be held for a minimum of 30 seconds or up to a minute or more.

Therapeutic Exercise

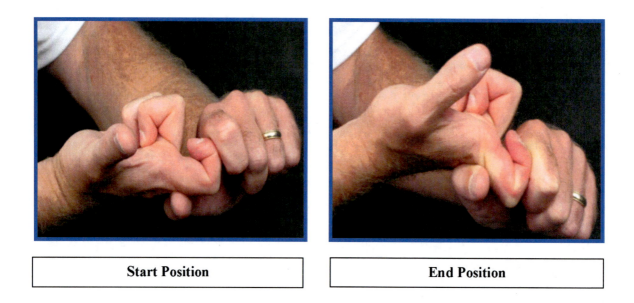

| Start Position | End Position |

Figure 12-19: Self-Stretching Palmar Interossei:

This too is an often forgotten, but very effective self-stretching procedure. Shortening of the intrinsic muscles of the hand can adversely affect hand and finger function as well as cause hand and finger discomfort. Wrist and hand injury, overuse, or degenerative changes can cause shortening of these muscles. Instruct your patient to supinate their forearm, passive flex their two IP joints, and then passively extend through their MCP joint. Passive abduction through the MCP joints can also be added. Note, do not over flex the IP joints prior to extending through the MCP joints. Protect the small amount of cartilage found at the IP joints by not flexing them too forcibly. Muscular self-stretching should be held for a minimum of 30 seconds or up to a minute or more.

Therapeutic Exercise

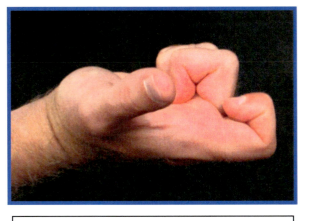
Start Position

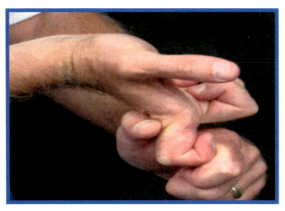
End Position

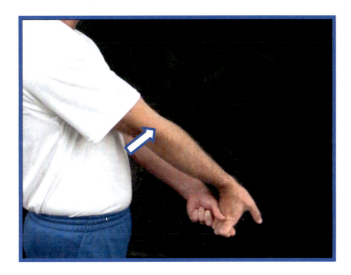

Figure 12-20: Self-Stretching-The Lumbrical Muscles:

To completely stretch the intrinsic muscles of the hand, instruct your patient to supinate their forearm, passively flex their two IP joints, and then passive extend through the MCP joint. Note, do not over flex the IP joints prior to extending through the MCP joints. In order to stabilize the proximal attachment point of this intrinsic muscle and fully stretch the lumbrical muscles, once the IPs are flexed and the MCP joint is extended, instruct the patient to passively extend their wrist and elbow. Muscular self-stretching should be held for a minimum of 30 seconds or up to a minute or more.

Chapter 13

Therapeutic Exercise for the Hip

Chapter 13 will look at exercises for patients with various hip impairments. Here is a bulleted list of some of the important topics covered in this chapter.

- Building strength in the proximal hip joint muscles.
- Protecting the lumbar spine during proximal hip muscle strength training.
- Using Closed Kinetic Chain wisely
    - Building lower extremity strength without provoking pain.
    - Protecting the hip joint cartilage.

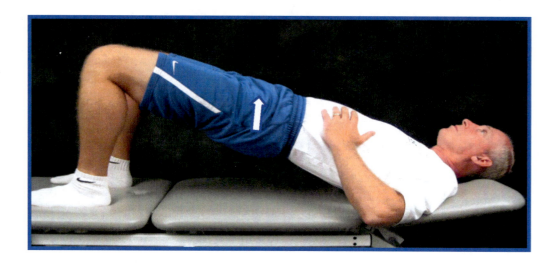

Figure 13-1: Proximal Hip Muscle Training-Bridging:

Bridging is an exercise that is helpful for improving LE strength including the proximal hip muscles and the spinal extensor muscles. Typically, this exercise motion does not provoke symptoms when arthritic changes are present in the hip. This exercise position has a low C of G and large B of S, so this strength building procedure can be useful in a number of different practice environments and bridging is helpful for strength impairments associated with lumbar disc disease, stenosis, and orthopedic hip conditions such as hip joint arthritis, total hip replacement, and after a hip fracture has healed or been surgically stabilized. In the older client, multiple sets of 6-10 repetitions are a good place to start with this basic exercise. To further build muscular endurance, sustained isometric contractions can also be incorporated along with isotonic training. Occasional clinical palpation of the buttock muscles during the performance of a bridge is necessary to ensure your patient is making a large enough arc of movement for an efficient contraction of the target muscles. If hamstring muscle cramping occurs or if discomfort in the patellofemoral joint(s) is provoked, change the angle of knee flexion during the exercise. For younger clients, incorporate a Swiss Exercise Ball placed under the lower extremities when prescribing bridge exercises.

Therapeutic Exercise

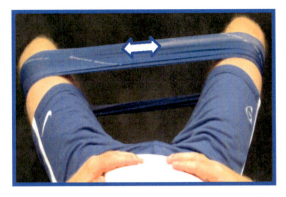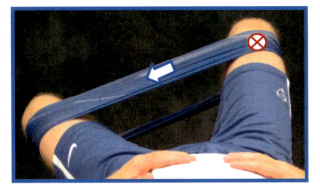

Figure 13-2: Resisted Hip Abduction-External Rotation- Hook lying Butterfly Exercise:

Resisted hip abduction-external rotation exercise performed in hook lying, sometimes called the "Butterfly" is a therapeutic exercise that is helpful for improving strength in the proximal hip abductors and external rotator muscles. Typically, this exercise motion does not provoke symptoms when arthritic changes are present in the hip. The exercise position has a low C of G and large B of S, so this procedure can be useful in a number of different practice environments. Multiple sets of 6-10 repetitions are a good place to start and choice of elastic band thickness relates to both strength and pain impairment. This movement pattern should not be a struggle and should not produce pain. As seen above, both bilateral and unilateral lower extremity movement patterns can be performed. In the older client, multiple sets of 6-10 repetitions followed by a rest break is a good place to start with this basic exercise. To further build muscular endurance, sustained isometric contractions can also be incorporated along with isotonic training. If hamstring muscle cramping occurs or if discomfort in the patellofemoral joint(s) is provoked, change the angle of knee flexion during the exercise. Lastly don't let your patient's knee "slap" back together. The knees should slowly return to the mid-line to facilitate a degree of eccentric muscle training.

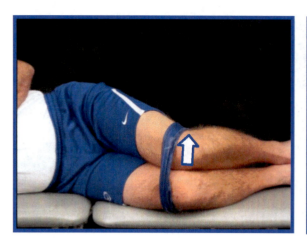 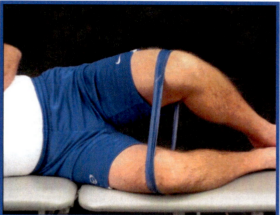

Figure 13-3: Resisted Hip Abduction-External Rotation-Side lying The Clam Shell Exercise:

Once your patient's hip abductor/external rotator muscle have shown improved strength with the resisted Butterfly exercise, transition the patient into side lying for the gravity resisted Clam Shell exercise. Again, this therapeutic exercise is helpful for improving strength in the proximal hip abductors and external rotator muscles. Usually this exercise motion does not provoke symptoms when arthritic changes are present in the hip particularly if the arc movement and amount of resistance is controlled. Similar to hook lying, this exercise position has a low C of G and a fairly large B of S if when hips and knees are flexed. This exercise can be useful in a number of different practice environments. Multiple sets of 6-10 repetitions are a good place to start and choice of elastic band color (thickness) relates to both strength and pain impairment. This movement pattern should not be a struggle and should not produce pain. To further build muscular endurance, sustained isometric contractions can also be incorporated along with isotonic training.

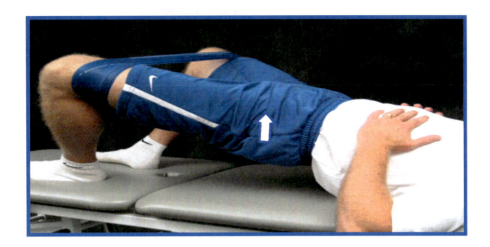

Figure 13-4: Resisted Hip Abduction-External Rotation (Butterfly) with Isometric Hip Extension (Bridging):

This OKC exercise is performed in the hook lying position and combines the bridging motion followed by hip abduction and external rotation. Older clients with lumbar spine and hip arthritis and associated strength impairments affecting their spinal extensors and proximal hip extensors will likely benefit the most from this exercise. The arc of movement should be pain free and clinicians should monitor that patients are not holding their breath as this exercise is a little more difficult than 13-1 and 13-2. A multi-set, multi-rep isotonic exercise dose can be prescribed and the position can be held for isometric muscular endurance training as well. If hamstring muscle cramping occurs or if discomfort in the patellofemoral joint(s) is provoked, change the angle of knee flexion during the exercise.

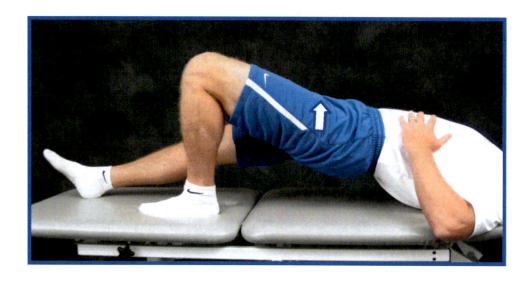

Figure 13-5: Proximal Hip Muscle Training- Single Leg Bridging:

Single leg bridging is more challenging and patients with more significant proximal hip muscle weakness or more advanced grades of hip arthritis may not be able to perform this exercise without provocation of symptoms. When prescribed for patients with proximal hip muscle weakness I like to have the patient switch back and forth between legs every 6-10 repetitions. Note, for more advanced patients or for individuals simply seeking a general lower extremity strength building procedure, the opposite LE can be held off the table for isometric training of the hip flexor muscles as single leg bridging is performed. A multi-set, multi-rep isotonic exercise dose can be prescribed and the position can be held for isometric muscular endurance training. If hamstring muscle cramping occurs or if discomfort in the patellofemoral joint(s) is provoked, change the angle of knee flexion during the exercise.

Therapeutic Exercise

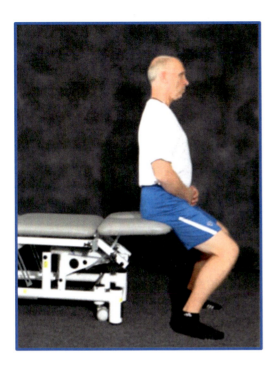 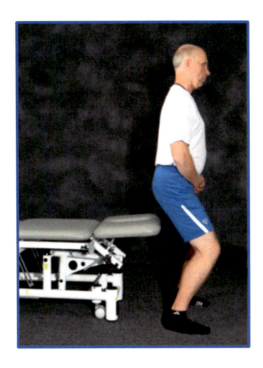

Figure 13-6: Sit to Stand LE Strength Building:

Figures 13-1 – 13-5 looked at some very important LE, proximal hip, and spinal extensor muscle strength building exercises. Now let's transition into closed kinetic chain and discuss one of the most important and powerful exercises we can prescribe for our patients. This is the elevated sit to stand LE strength building exercise. There are many patients who can benefit from this exercise motion including patients with orthopedic conditions affecting their LE strength such as hip and knee arthrosis, lumbar stenosis, and other debilitated patients who have generally become weakened. This exercise works very well in a clinical setting where the patient is initially placed on the edge of an elevated Hi-Lo table and the clinician determines the correct number of repetitions. As the patient's strength improves, and if his/her LE joints tolerate, the table can be progressively lowered. Creative physical therapists working in many different practice settings will find this exercise very helpful and perhaps one of the key exercises to be prescribed to keep some of our patients walking.

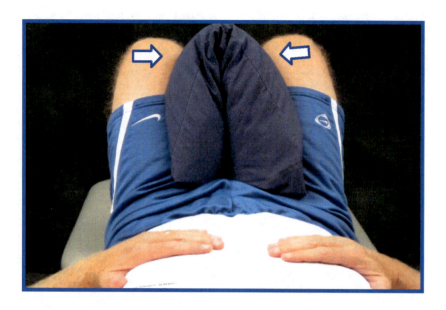

Figure 13-7: Isometric Hip Adductor Muscle Training-Hook lying, (The Pillow Squeeze):

This exercise is also performed in the hook lying position and can be viewed as a short arc isotonic and or isometric adductor muscle training exercise otherwise known as the pillow squeeze exercise. Hip adductor weakness is fairly common in our elderly patient and in association with various common orthopedic hip conditions. In addition, after an adductor muscle tear, the strength of the adductor muscles will need to be addressed and this fairly easy exercise can be a good place to start. Multiple sets of 6-10 short arc isotonic reps can be prescribed with additional incorporation of isometric muscle contraction if deemed appropriated by the therapist.

Therapeutic Exercise

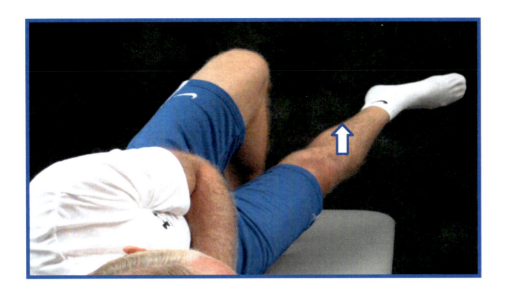

Figure 13-8: Isotonic Hip Adductor Muscle Training- Side lying, Open Kinetic Chain:

Non-weight bearing open kinetic chain (OKC) isotonic muscle strength training for the adductors is often the next logical strength building progression after a platform of isometric strength has been built with the pillow squeeze exercise. Free weight (cuff weight) attachment is easily applied either above or below the knee for additional resistance and therapists should also consider the application of concentric and eccentric MRE for additional strength training. MRE for the adductor muscles is easily applied in this position and in the hook lying position. To expand on a comment made on the previous page, research has demonstrated that for athletes who have suffered an adductor muscle tear, successful performance of both concentric and eccentric adductor muscle training is needed before return to sport.

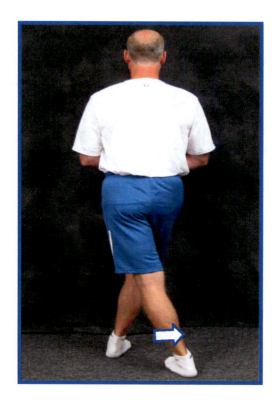

Figure 13-9: Isotonic Hip Adductor Muscle Training-Cover- Over Stepping, Closed Kinetic Chain:

Closed chain cross over stepping is an important CKC exercise that assists many different patients with strength, balance, and lower extremity coordination impairments. Patients must adapt to a changing B of S as hip adductor muscles pull the one lower extremity across the other. Therapist supervision for patients with balance difficulties is needed as the base of support is reduced during this movement pattern. High speed front and back cross-over karaoke stepping is an excellent speed, balance, and coordination exercise that provides isotonic training of the hip adductor muscles. Foam balance beams may be added to increase the difficulty of the movement pattern.

Therapeutic Exercise

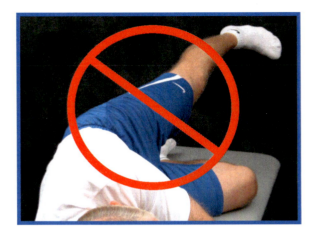 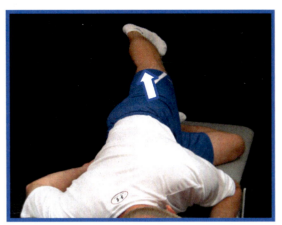

13-10: Isotonic Hip Abductor Muscle Training- Partial-Prone Position, Open Kinetic Chain:

We turn our attention back to the hip abductors with exercise 13-10. The movement pattern for the LE is a combination of hip abduction and extension. Incorporating hip extension will reduce the hip abduction contribution from the TFL and increase the muscular contribution from the target (gluteal) muscles. The position shown on the right hand figure is termed partial prone. Note the position of the under most UE and the pelvis. If hip abductor muscle weakness is present, the standard side lying position usually does not facilitate a solid contraction of the target muscle group and the TFL and quad muscle produces a LE abduction/flexion movement pattern. Note, if pain is provoked during this exercise movement pattern, clinicians should change the hip position in terms of rotation. Often pre-positioning the hip toward external rotation will reduce hip mediated discomfort. A multi-set, multi-rep program isotonic exercise dose should be prescribed.

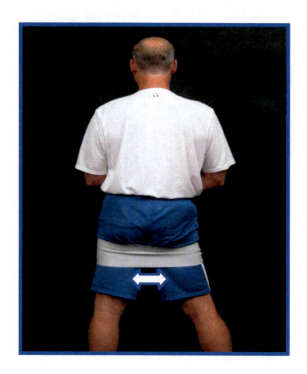

Figure 13-11: Isotonic Hip Abductor Muscle Training- Side Stepping, Closed Kinetic Chain:

Closed chain side stepping is an important exercise that assists many different patients with various levels of strength, balance, and lower extremity coordination impairments. For some patients, balance training without resistance requires therapist supervision as the patient must constantly adjust to a changing B of S. For more athletic patients, high speed elastic band resisted side stepping builds hip abductor strength, balance and coordination. When training athletes, have them flex at the hips and knee into an "athletic ready position" during the performance of this exercise. Two additional points of review; the further the elastic band is from the hip joints the greater the resistance for the proximal hip muscles. In this first version of the side stepping exercise the elastic band is close to the hip joint and this will assist us in reducing load on the joint and may keep this exercise pain free for our patients with hip arthritis.

Therapeutic Exercise

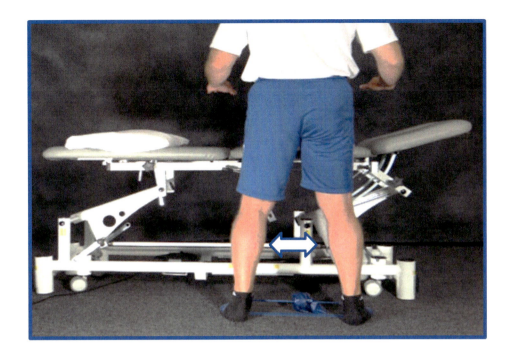

Figure 13-12: Isotonic Hip Abductor Muscle Training- Side Stepping:

Now note the placement of the elastic band in the picture above. Wrapping the elastic band around the patient's forefeet will increase the length of the lever arm over which the elastic band resistance occurs. If your patient is able to perform the side stepping exercise successfully and without symptom increase with the elastic band placed around the feet, strengthening of the proximal hip muscles will occur much more quickly. One additional point, to increase the degree of safety and prevent a fall from occurring, have your patient perform this exercise in front of an elevated treatment table or counter top so he/she can grab hold if necessary.

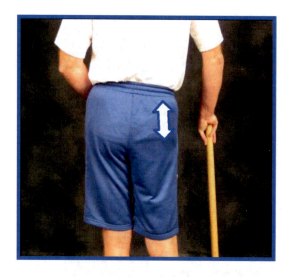 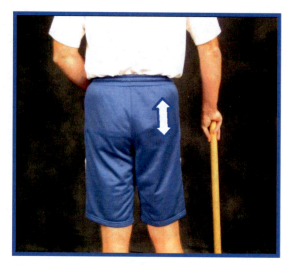

Figure 13-13: Isotonic Hip Abduction,

Closed Kinetic Chain:

The two figures above demonstrate closed kinetic chain left hip abductor muscle training. A cane or dowel is given to the patient and placed on the ground to increase the base of support and to shift weight (load) away from the left hip in this case. Next, while standing on an aerobic step (not seen above), the patient is instructed to drop and then elevate the right side of their pelvis. Concentric muscular contraction of the proximal hip abductors on the left side will elevate the right side of the pelvis. This is a great therapeutic exercise for healthy hips with sound articular cartilage. Patient with hip joint osteoarthrosis may not be able to tolerate the compressive loading associated with the single leg stance position, left in this case, despite shifting the C of G to the right with a cane or stich in the patient's right hand (above). After performing a set of repetitions have your patient self-traction the LE that has been weight bearing.

Therapeutic Exercise

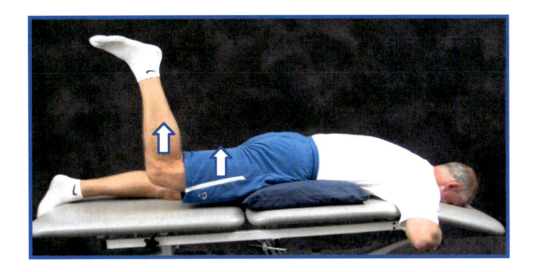

13-14: Isotonic Hip Extensor Muscle Training- Prone over a Pillow, Open Kinetic Chain:

Figure 13-14 swings the discussion back to the hip extensor muscles and demonstrates one of the positioning options for short arc isotonic hip extensor muscle training. Support is provided to the lumbar spine by placing a pillow across the abdomen. Flattening of the lumbar lordosis will prevent lumbar hyperextension and reduce the compressive loads on the lumbar spine during this lower extremity movement. Note how the back of the cervical spine is lengthened and also kept in a mid-position throughout the exercise. Given the start position for the hip joint, choice of this exercise position works well when the patient has enough strength to perform end range hip extensor muscle training. Multiple sets of short arc isotonic motion can be prescribed based on the patient's level of strength.

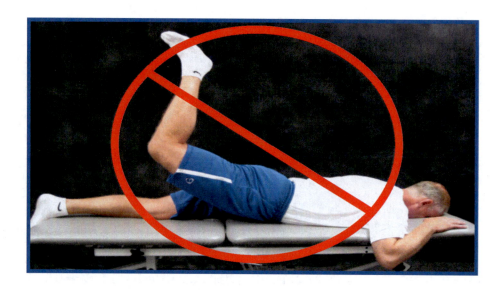

Figure 13-15: Isotonic Hip Extensor Muscle Training – Incorrect Position, Open Kinetic Chain:

The lower extremity movement performed in this position will also facilitate hip and spinal extensor muscle contraction and as such this exercise can be used to improve strength impairments affecting these two muscle groups. That said, repetitive muscle contraction superimposed upon the close pack position of a joint or lower lumbar motion segment in this case may have a deleterious effect on facet joint cartilage and posterior disc space if performed over a long time period. Therefore, I do not recommend this exercise position for our patients.

Therapeutic Exercise

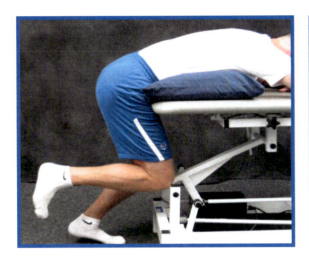 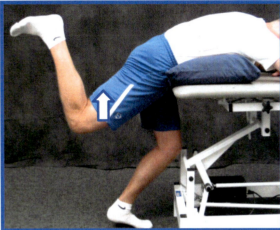

Figure 13-16: Isotonic Hip Extensor Muscle Training – Prone over the Edge, Open Kinetic Chain:

The two figures shown on this page demonstrate the start and the end position for what I feel is the best way to provide patients with a larger arc of open kinetic chain hip extensor muscle training. The excursion of movement from a more fully flexed to fully extended position affords the patient a much greater range of gravity resisted movement. Note how the back of the cervical spine is lengthened and kept in a mid-position. Also, note how the lumbar spine is also supported through the abdomen by both the treatment table and pillow. Add a second pillow for additional comfort and support. Similar to exercise 13-14, prescribe multiple sets of 10 repetitions or a rep max program may also be prescribed. Remember, when the quality of movement performance begins to erode in a multi-set program or a rep max program, the exercise should be stopped for that session.

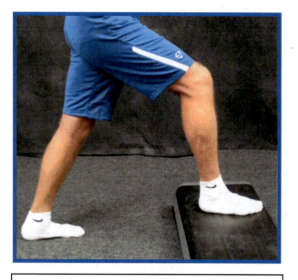
Start Position

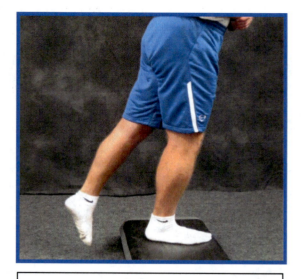
End Position

Figure 13-17: Isotonic Hip Extensor Muscle Training– Split Stance Step Up, Closed Kinetic Chain:

There are many different ways to improve proximal hip extensor and quad muscle strength in a CKC environment. The split stance step up exercise is one possible way to initiate CKC muscle training. The Quadriceps and the proximal hip extensor muscles are trained during this exercise, but if the start position for this procedure incorporates a split stance (hip flexion), contraction of the proximal hip extensor muscles are favored. This exercise may provide functional carry over in terms of balance training and stair climbing. Athletic patients can be asked to perform this movement with greater amounts of speed and use a step that is higher than the one seen in this figure. Multi-set and rep max programs can be assigned depending on the age, physical condition, strength and status of hip and knee joint cartilage.

Therapeutic Exercise

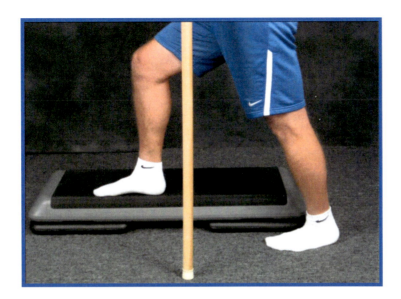

Figure 13-18: Isotonic Hip Extensor Muscle Training– Split Stance Step Up, Reduced Loading, Closed Kinetic Chain:

In cases of hip pain due to arthritis or injury, a cane or dowel can be provided to the patient and placed in the opposite hand in order to shift weight away from and partially unload the involved hip. If this eliminates pain during this CKC therapeutic motion, the exercise is allowed to continue. If not, the height of the step is reduced and the speed of movement is changed in an attempt to provide pain free CKC exercise training. Two canes or two dowel rods may also be used to further reduce load on the involved lower extremity. If there is significant cartilage degeneration at the hip or knee joints, a 30 second work and 30 second rest program beginning with two to five minutes of total exercise time is often a good way to start this exercise when both pain and strength impairment is present. During the rest phase the patient is encouraged to let their involved LE hang over the edge of the step for additional unloading (traction) of intra-articular structures.

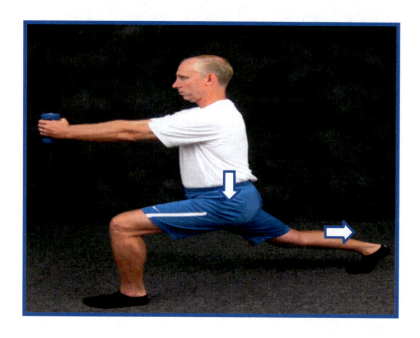

Figure 13-19: Advanced Hip Extensor Muscle Training-The Glut Slide, Close Kinetic Chain:

This is a higher level exercise where the end position as shown in figure 13-17 resembles a lunge or split stance squat position. The movement pattern by which the patient achieves this position is different than a typical lunge. The more athletic patient wishing a sports training procedure or a patient who is rehabbing their lower extremity muscles after a surgical procedure or injury is asked to slide one foot in a posterior direction. The front lower extremity will flex at the hip and knee joints. The quadriceps and proximal hip extensors will eccentrically control flexion at both joints. To increase the demand placed upon the target muscle groups, a weight can be held with the UEs as shown above. Placement of the hand held weight closer to or further away from the patient's trunk will vary the level of resistance. Further discussion regarding the numerous benefits of the lunge exercise will occur in Chapter 14. For our younger or more athletic patients consider the prescription of a rep max program where the movement pattern is performed until significant fatigue in the lower extremity muscles is perceived.

Therapeutic Exercise

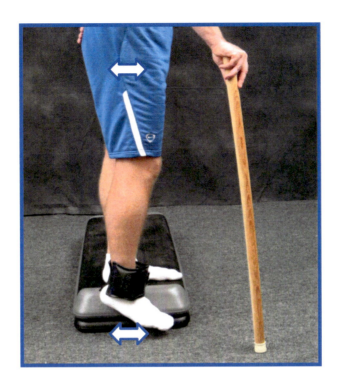

Figure 13-20: Hip Self Traction- Pendulum Swings, Standing, Open Kinetic Chain:

We are going to swing the discussion back to open kinetic chain motion and patients with symptomatic and load sensitive arthritic changes in the hip joint. Weighted pendular swings can be performed in the clinical setting and easily applied as part of a home-based exercise program. The key is to minimize muscular contraction around the hip joint and let the LE "dangle" as relaxed short pendular motions are performed. If a patient is able to do this, a light traction load will be provided to the hip joint. The addition of cuff weight will typically improve the effect of this exercise. Five to ten pounds is usually about right. Perform short pendular swings for at least 30 seconds or let the LE hang (traction without movement). Treatment for up to five minutes or more can be prescribed. This exercise can also be prescribed as a warm up or cool down procedure when performing other hip strength training exercises and it can also be interspersed between the same.

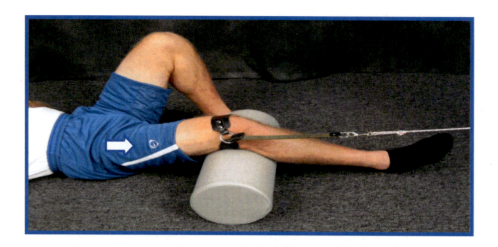

Figure 13-21: Sustained Hip Joint Traction –Supine with LE Supported, Open Kinetic Chain:

Let's stay on the subject of providing a traction load to load sensitive (degenerated) articular cartilage. This unloading exercise incorporates the attachment of a leather strap and cable attached to a weight stack on a pulley system. This is a very good way to unload hip cartilage and reduce hip pain by providing traction to the superior weight-bearing surface of the hip. Apply 20-40 pounds of traction for 10-20 minutes. Use a therapeutic roll and or pillows to support the involved hip is close to the resting position in slight flexion and external rotation. Therapists should encourage patients to let their LE fully relax on the therapeutic roll or pillow(s). In addition, therapists should clinically palpate the muscles around the patient's hip to ensure that they remain relaxed during the course of treatment.

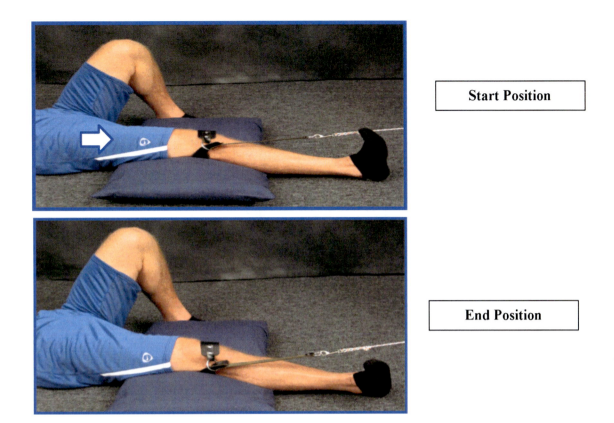

Figure 13-22: Active Hip External Rotation with Traction – Supine, Open Kinetic Chain:

The next exercise is set up in the same way as exercise 13-21. Provide the patient with sustained traction for 10-20 minutes and instruct him/her to perform intermittent active external rotation of the hip. Support the involved hip joint in the resting position and deliver 20-40 pounds of traction. Have the patient perform active hip external rotation under traction with a speed and arc of movement that reduces hip discomfort.

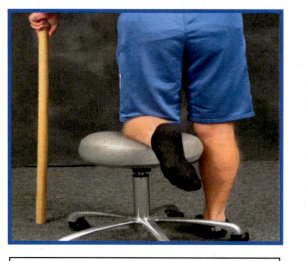
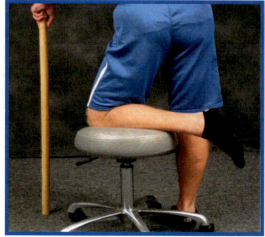

| Start Position | End Position |

Figure 13-23: Hip Active External Rotation-Standing, Open Kinetic Chain:

This exercise does not incorporate a traction load, but it does attempt to reduce load through the hip. When performing this short oscillatory therapeutic motion a stool with a rotating padded top in needed. Make sure that the patient does not place much compressive loading through the LE (hip joint) that is in contact with the stool. Note how a cane or dowel is used to shift load away from the LE in CKC. Injured and arthritic hips often like or at least better tolerate light non-loaded oscillatory motion toward external rotation. The main idea behind this active therapeutic motion is to reduce hip pain and provide for very light muscular activation for the hip rotator muscles. Movement arc and speed need to be controlled, so that reported hip pain intensity is less after the exercise is performed. In some cases of arthritic hip pain, the arc of motion needs to be quite small. Follow the 30 second work and 30 second rest or some variation such as 15 second work/ 45 second rest for at least five minutes. In cases of severe arthritic hip pain exercise 13-18 can be interspersed.

Therapeutic Exercise

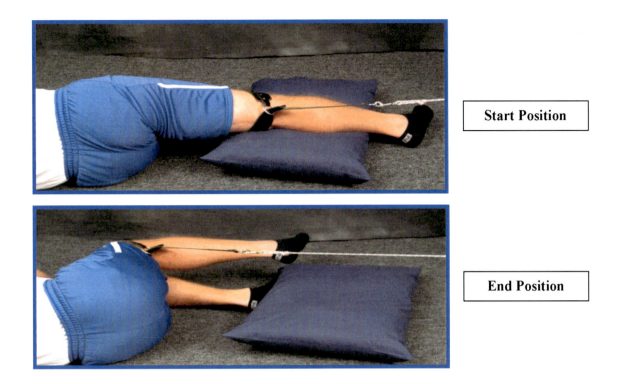

Figure 13-24: Resisted Hip Flexion- Side lying Open Kinetic Chain:

This exercise attempts to manage compressive load through the hip and seeks to generate a greater degree of muscle activation for the hip flexors. So, if a degenerated or injured hip is painful during weight bearing and hip flexor strength impairment is found during clinical examination, exercise 13-24 may be indicated. The therapist may first attempt to reduce load dependent hip pain with exercises 13-20 and 13-23 and then instruct the patient to move into the side lying position, on a table adjacent to a pulley system, in order to perform resisted OKC short arc isotonic hip flexion. Keep the painful hip well supported with pillows during this exercise motion. Follow the 30 second work and 30 second rest exercise cycle for at least 5 minutes progressing the total training time as hip flexion strength improves.

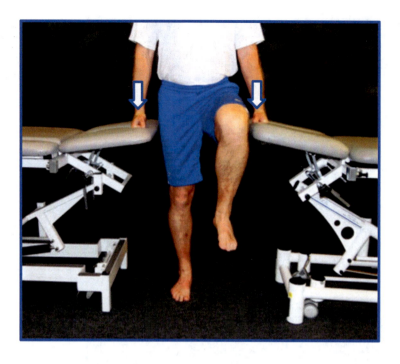

Figure 13-25: Resisted Hip Flexion- Standing, Closed Kinetic Chain:

This is a standing version of exercise 13-24. The goals are the same here. We are attempting to control (reduce) compressive load through the articular cartilage and subchondral bone of our patient's hip (s) and provide a strength build motion for our patient's hip flexor muscles. So, if your patient demonstrates load intolerance, have him or her stand between two tables, or a counter top and the back of a chair, press down with both hands. This will significantly reduce the compressive loading on both hip joints and both tibiofemoral joints and allow our patients to build hip flexor strength without provoking LE joint pain.

Therapeutic Exercise

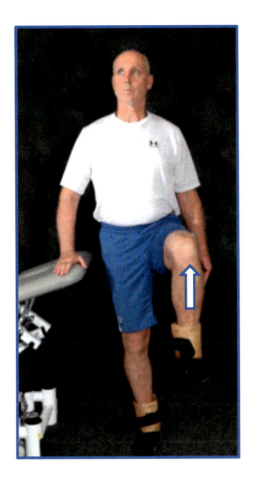 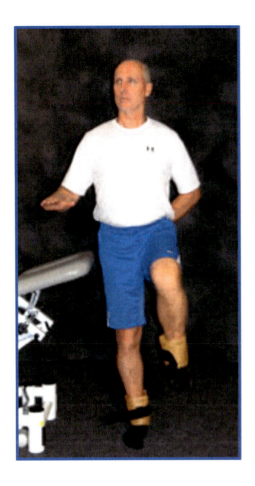

Figure 13-26: Resisted Hip Flexion- Standing, Closed Kinetic Chain:

Now let's take away some of the support and discuss hip flexor strength training and balance impairment. If your patient's hip joints are tolerant of the compressive loading that occurs while in standing, this exercise is easy to set up and instruct. In essence, this is the stationary marching exercise. Isotonic hip flexion can occur in an alternating fashion, at various speeds, and at various amplitudes. Cuff weights, as shown above, can be added for additional resistance. If your patient needs stationary balance training, have him or her remove a hand from an adjacent table as shown above.

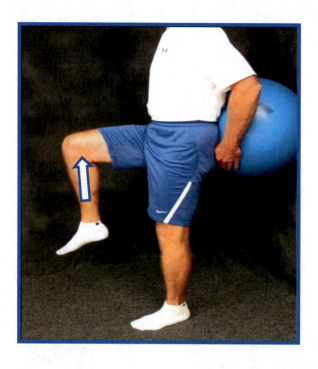

Figure 13-27: Hip Flexion- Open Kinetic Chain with Wall-Swiss Ball Support

Before we start with a short section on hip joint soft tissue self-stretching let's look a one more stationary balance exercise. This is a simple, but important exercise for our senior patients and others having some difficulty with gait, balance during single limb support, and hip flexor strength impairment. The patient is instructed to lean back against a wall or wall and a Swiss Exercise Ball and perform isotonic hip flexion. Isometric hip flexion can be interspersed for additional single leg balance training. For other more athletic patients recovering from a LE injury or surgical repair, this stationary single leg stance exercise can lead to more advanced plyometric training including single leg hopping, jumping, and skipping once sufficient tissue healing has occurred.

Therapeutic Exercise

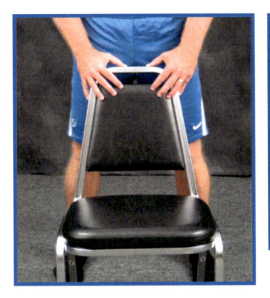
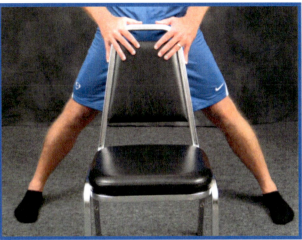

Figure 13-28: Hip Adductor Self- Stretching – Standing:

This final portion of Chapter 13 begins a segment on hip muscle self-stretching. It is not uncommon to find adductor muscle shortening secondary to injury and arthritic hip disease. With this first procedure the patient is to reduce a portion of the weight bearing load through the hips by leaning forward onto a table or chair. The patient is then asked to abduct both lower extremities until a mild pulling sensation is felt in the target area. At that point a strong isometric posterior pelvic tilt is performed in order to elevate the proximal pelvic attachment point of the adductor muscles. This will further separate attachment points and provide for additional muscle stretching. This stretch should be held for at least 30 seconds or up to a minute or more.

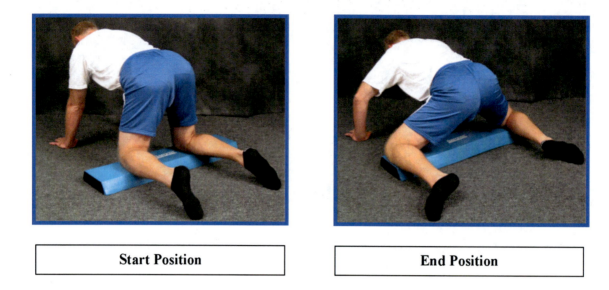

| Start Position | End Position |

Figure 13-29: Hip Adductor Self - Stretching – Four Point:

Perform this stretch in conjunction with 13-28 and should be performed prior to sports competition. The hips are now pre-positioned in flexion prior to the execution of bilateral hip abduction. Hip flexion will allow for the more posteriorly positioned adductor muscles to receive the majority of stretching. Once the LE's are positioned in bilateral hip abduction, a strong isometric posterior pelvic tilt that emphasizes abdominal drawing is performed in order to elevate the proximal attachment point of the adductor muscles. This will further separate muscular attachment points and provide for additional muscle stretching. This stretch should be held for at least 30 seconds or up to a minute or more.

Therapeutic Exercise

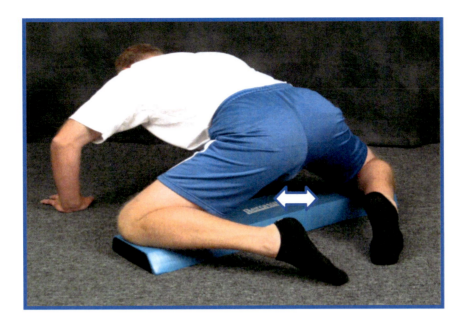

Figure 13-30: Hip Adductor Self - Stretching in External Rotation- Four Point:

The hips are now pre-positioned in flexion and external rotation prior to the execution of bilateral hip abduction. This version of the exercise will promote stretching of different adductor muscle fibers. Once the LE's are positioned in bilateral hip abduction and external rotation, a strong isometric posterior pelvic tilt that emphasizes abdominal drawing is performed in order to elevate the proximal pelvic attachment point of the adductor muscles. This will further separate muscular attachment points and provide for additional muscle stretching. This stretch should be held for at least 30 seconds or up to a minute or more.

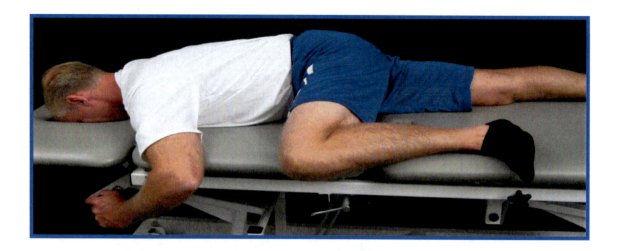

Figure 13-31: Hip Adductor Self -Stretching- Prone:

This prone lying version of adductor muscle stretch is somewhat similar to exercise 13-28 in terms of LE positioning. Patients with adductor shortening, particularly shortening after an adductor muscle tear, can be shown how to elongate various portions of this muscle group in the prone lying position. This position allows a patient to easily change the angle of hip flexion to the spot where stretching is best perceived. Evjenth, in his Muscle Stretching in Manual Therapy text describes an excellent adductor manual stretching procedure in this same position. All muscular self-stretch procedures should be held for at least 30 seconds or up to a minute or more.

Therapeutic Exercise

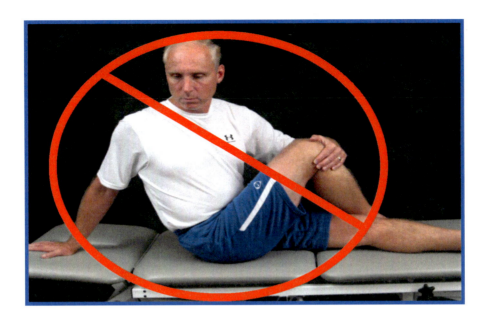

Figure 13-32: Piriformis Muscle Self-Stretching - Seated:

I am sorry to say that this exercise is still an often performed procedure used to affect stretching of the deep buttock muscles including the famous piriformis muscle. Clinicians who prescribe this exercise are forgetting some simple rules. Those rules relate to joint protection and body mechanics. Most PTs would agree that flexing and twisting the lumbar spine in an upright (loaded) position is a bad idea. Well, that is what happens with this stretch. Stretching buttock muscles is not worth placing the lumbar spine in this position. Instead, place the patient in supine where the lumbar discs are unloaded and flex the hip beyond 90 degrees after pre-positioning the joint in external rotation. Or better yet, teach your patient exercise 13-33.

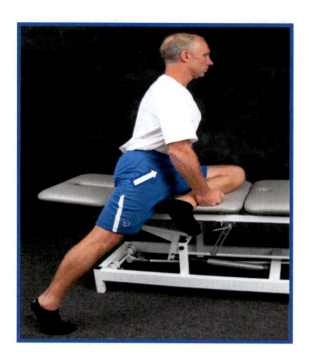

Figure 13-33: Piriformis Muscle Self-Stretching - Hip Hinge Position:

This figure demonstrates self-stretching of the piriformis and other deep rotator muscles of the hip with the entire spine is in good alignment. The LE is positioned on the table by flexing and externally rotating the hip joint. Additional hip flexion is obtained by keeping the lumbar spine straight (chest upward and forward) and hinging forward at the left hip joint in this case while sliding the right foot backward. This hip hinging movement will activate spinal stabilizer (extensor) muscles while slack is taken up in the deep hip rotator group. Note how we were able to lengthen the lower extremity tissues without compromising the spinal position. This deep buttock muscle stretch can be helpful in temporarily relieving sciatic discomfort. All muscular self-stretch procedures should be held for at least 30 seconds or up to a minute or more.

Therapeutic Exercise

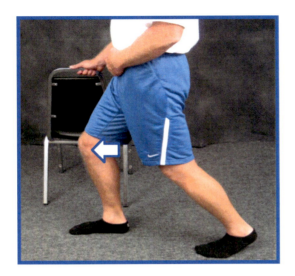 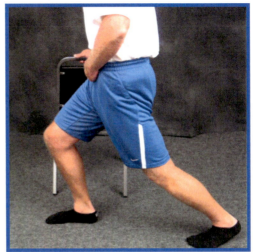

Figure 13-34: Hip Flexor Muscle Self-Stretching- Standing:

This is a very useful version of hip flexor muscle stretching. The patient is asked to hold onto a chair, table or countertop and position their lower extremities in a split stance. Next, the patient is instructed to perform a posterior pelvic tilt by squeezing their buttock muscles together and pulling their lower tummy upward and inward. Their hand may be used to reinforce the abdominal positioning. Posterior rotation of the pelvis will begin taking up slack in the hip flexor muscles. Once the patient has assumed a posterior pelvic tilt, the patient is then instructed to flex their front knee (figure on the right) and in so doing "drag" their back LE into hip extension. This position along with slight lumbar side bending to the opposite side will fully elongate the hip flexor muscle. All muscular self-stretch procedures should be held for at least 30 seconds or up to a minute or more.

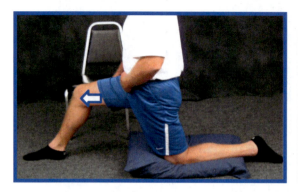 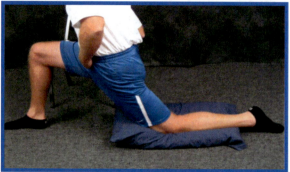

Figure 13-35: Self-Stretching for the Hip Flexor Muscles- Half Kneeling:

This next version of hip flexor muscle stretching will, in addition to stretching the Psoas muscle, also begin to elongate the Rectus Femoris muscle. The patient is asked to hold onto a chair, or some other low surface and position one knee onto the ground. Next, the patient is instructed to perform a posterior pelvic tilt by squeezing their buttock muscles together and pulling their lower tummy upward. Their hand may be used to reinforce the upward and inward positioning of the lower abdomen. The posterior rotation of the pelvis will begin taking up slack in the hip flexor muscles. Then the patient is instructed to flex their front knee and in so doing "drag" their back LE into hip extension (See figure on the right). The patient is also encouraged to not "leave their trunk behind" and end up in a lordosis. In other words, the patient should hinge (flex) forward at the hip as the knee on the same side flexes. When viewed from the side the trunk, pelvis and thigh should all appear to be in a straight line. This position along with slight lumbar side bending to the opposite side will fully elongate the hip flexor muscle. All muscular self-stretch procedures should be held for at least 30 seconds or up to a minute or more.

Therapeutic Exercise

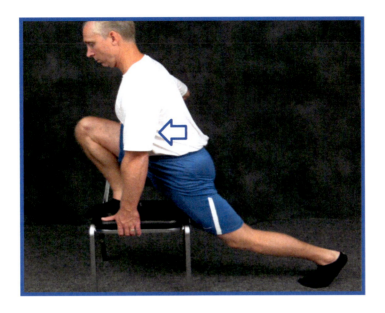

Figure 13-36: Self-Stretching for the Hip Extensor Muscles- Standing:

Shortening of the proximal hip extensor muscles is not a common impairment but this stretch will promote improved hip flexion which is necessary, among other things, for donning certain lower body garments. Also there are times when buttock pain from sciatica can be temporarily relieved with this stretch and piriformis self-stretching (figure 13-33). Lastly, to teach a person the (feel) of hip hinging, (Chapter 18, The Lumbar Spine) this movement pattern is quite helpful. A chair without arms or a low table is needed for this procedure. The patient is instructed to place one foot onto a chair or a table making sure the knee is initially pre-positioned around 60-75 degrees of flexion. Active hip flexion with trunk hinging is performed over the involved leg which will flex the knee on the side of stretching to greater than 90 degrees. The patient's chest is to stay in an upward and forward position and the heel of the back foot may come off the ground. The spine is to remain straight and without lumbar hyperextension. All muscular self-stretch procedures should be held for at least 30 seconds or up to a minute or more.

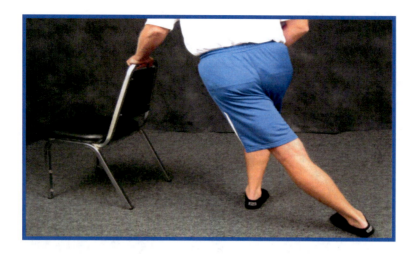

Figure 13-37: Self-Stretching TFL-ITB- Standing:

This self-stretching procedure for the lateral hip and thigh soft tissues begins with the patient in standing within arm's length of a wall chair or table top. The LE closest to the wall is crossed behind the other LE. This places the involved LE into hip adduction, extension, and preferably slight external rotation. The UE is then flexed slightly allowing the pelvis to translate toward the wall which will increase the amount of hip adduction. A light pulling sensation should be felt in the lateral hip and thigh of the LE that is crossed behind. Note, do not allow excessive lumbar side bending to occur, it is not necessary for effective stretching of shortened lateral hip tissues. Also, the LE where tissue stretching is to occur should only be partially weight bearing. Often, and this is important, too much weight is placed on the LE that is crossed behind. All self-stretch procedures should be held for at least 30 seconds or up to a minute or more.

Chapter 14

Therapeutic Exercise for the Knee

Chapter 14 will look at exercises for patients with impairments affecting knee flexion and extension. Here is a bulleted list of some of the more important topic covered in this chapter.

- Exercises to facilitate knee extension
    - Protecting the patellofemoral cartilage.
    - Managing acute arthritic flare ups and knee extension
    - Dealing with acute post-surgical and post-injury and knee extension
- Non-loaded to loaded strengthening exercises for the knee extensors
    - Transitioning from open kinetic chain (OKC) to partial weight-bearing closed kinetic chain (CKC) and finally full weight-bearing quad strengthening exercises.
        - Protecting the Tibiofemoral meniscus and other load sensitive tissues during lower extremity strength building.
- Exercises that facilitate knee flexion
    - Knee flexion stiffness impairment
    - Knee flexion weakness impairment

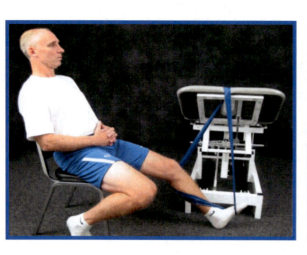 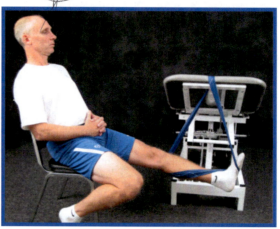

Start Position — **End Position**

Figure 14-1: Assisted Quadriceps Muscle Training–Seated, Open Kinetic Chain:

Assisted quad training performed as shown here may be one of the most useful therapeutic movements for the knee joint. This exercise is valuable for many different knee conditions. First, this exercise works very well for patients with swelling impairments post surgically and post injury. Second, use this procedure for individuals with load sensitive tibiofemoral osteoarthritis. Third, patients with symptomatic patellofemoral arthritis who experience discomfort due to muscular based patellar compression will find that this exercise often reduces anterior knee pain and provides light quad muscle activation.[33] Assisted quad training allows our patients to train for longer periods of time without provoking knee discomfort which can ultimately inhibit the very muscle we are attempting to strengthen. Typically, the exercise is performed for 10 minutes with intermittent rest breaks as needed. Exercise time can be increased to 20 minutes in some cases. This exercise is easily adapted for home use by placing the elastic band over a doorknob and having the patient sit alongside a closed door.

Therapeutic Exercise

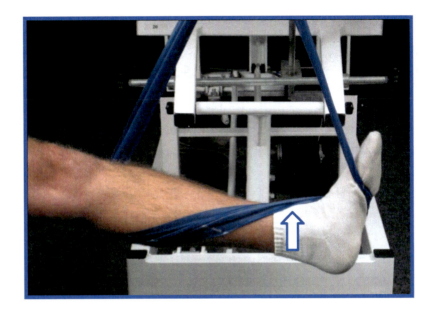

Figure 14-2: Assisted Quadriceps Muscle Training-Seated, Close Up View of Elastic Band Attachment:

This picture demonstrates the elastic band attachment to the lower leg. In the clinic a looped piece of elastic band can be secured to a hook on a pulley system, or a cut out section of a mobilization table. At home the band is wrapped around a door knob. After securing the band, the patient or therapist places the loop around the popliteal fossa. Next, the inside portion of the band, (the portion between the patient's legs) is wrapped around the lateral aspect of the ankle. This forms a simple sling for the lower extremity. The patient is instructed to flex their knee actively against the resistance of the band and then allow the band to assist their knee joint into full extension. Band thickness and initial pre-tension determines how much motion assistance the patient will receive. If using an electric mobilization table, raise or lower the table and or change the angle of the head section to change the tension in the elastic band. In figure 14-1, note how the patient has moved his bottom forward on the chair, this will slacken the hamstring muscles and assist in preventing dorsal translation of the tibia as the knee is extended to an end range. This becomes very important during the performance of exercise 14-3. Remember, the arc of assisted knee extension is to be pain-free so shorten the arc of motion if necessary.

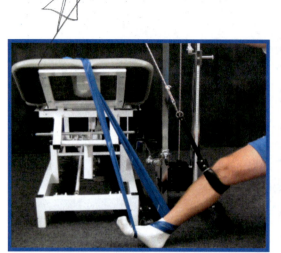 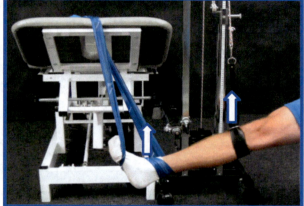

Figure 14-3: Assisted Quadriceps Muscle Training with Anterior Tibial Translation – Seated, Open Kinetic Chain:

I use this version of assisted knee extension in more severe cases of patellofemoral chondrosis. We can produce a millimeter or two of anterior tibial translation with the leather strap wrapped around the proximal tibia. The strap is part of a pulley system and weight is added in 5 pound increments until enough anterior tibial translation is produced to unload the posterior surface of the patella away from the trochlear groove of the femur. In most cases we can alleviate patellar crepitation and discomfort. Similar to the previous exercise, the elastic band will promote assisted knee extension and light activation of the quad muscle. Prescribe this exercise for 10-20 minutes with rest breaks as needed. Remember, if anterior knee pain is experienced, additional weight is added in 5-pound increments to promote increased anterior tibial translation.[33] To review, the elastic band LE sling is wrapped around the leg in the following way. Once attached to the table head section or a pulley system hook, place the "looped" band around the popliteal region. Next, take the inner part of the looped band (the portion between the legs) and wrap it around the outside aspect of the ankle.

Therapeutic Exercise

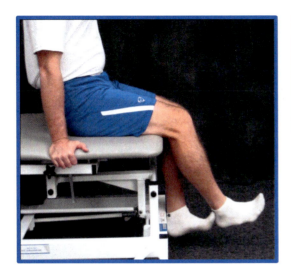 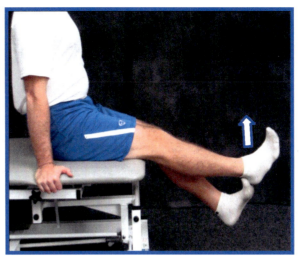

Figure 14-4: Assisted Knee Extension with Opposite LE– Seated:

Ok, we just discussed the various benefits of the pulley system and elastic band assisted knee extension exercises. In my opinion, those two exercises are the best way to perform OKC knee extension when an orthopedic condition is resulting in a pain or swelling impairment affecting knee extension. If elastic band and a pulley system is not available and we want to facilitate light quad muscle activation, then self-assisted knee extension can be a good exercise choice. The figures above demonstrate this classic therapeutic exercise. Therapists treating patients with knee pain, weakness, and swelling impairments including post-surgery, post injury or a flare up of a chronic condition, should not forget this therapeutic exercise if elastic band is not available. The arc of passive or assisted motion should be within the pain free range and for a patient whose tissues are healing after an injury; they should be less painful and less swollen at the conclusion of this exercise. Given the clinical situation, if full knee extension is desired or available remember to have the patient lean backward so that the hamstring muscles do not prohibit full range of movement.

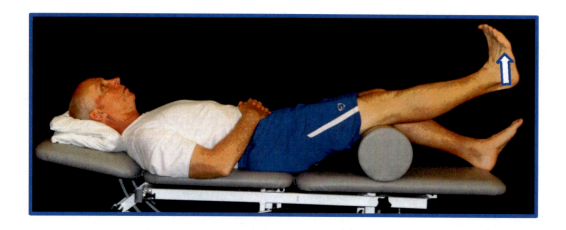

Figure 14-5: Short Arc Quadriceps Muscle Training:

This exercise that is as old as the profession of Physical Therapy. The quadriceps muscle seems to respond to most all painful knee conditions and advancing age by atrophying. If our patients have suffered an injury or have had surgery on some aspect of their LE, the quad muscle will likely weaken and this exercise can be a good starting point in a progressive strength building program. In addition, this exercise is used in many different PT practice arenas to assist patients with generalized weakness. You will likely find yourself prescribing this exercise a great deal of the time.

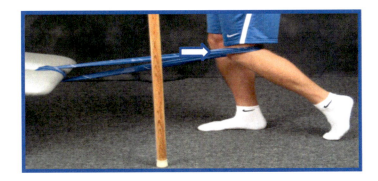

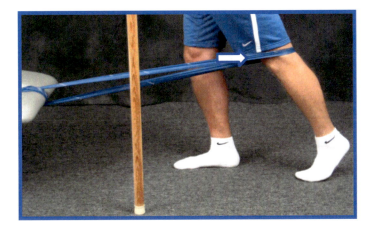

Figure 14-6: Resisted Quadriceps Muscle Training, Terminal Knee Extension(TKE) – Toe Touch Weight Bearing (TTWB):

This and the next two exercises provide a nice way to transition patients from OKC exercise to CKC exercise. I use exercises 14-6 and 14-7 with cases of quadriceps strength deficit both with and without posterior knee joint capsular shortening limiting full passive knee extension. If there is load sensitive tibiofemoral pain or weight bearing restriction this resisted quad training procedure is performed with TTWB only. The knee is moved from a slightly flexed to an extended position by essentially moving from the tip toe to the ball of the foot. Reduced weight bearing can also be achieved by the use of a walker, cane, or the back of a chair. The involved LE is placed behind the uninvolved in a position that more closely mirrors a normal gait pattern. This exercise is an excellent quad muscle training procedure that also lightly stretches the posterior knee capsule. This exercise can be useful for many different knee conditions demonstrating weakness, stiffness, and swelling impairments. Exercise dosage is typically for 5-10 minutes with rest breaks as needed.

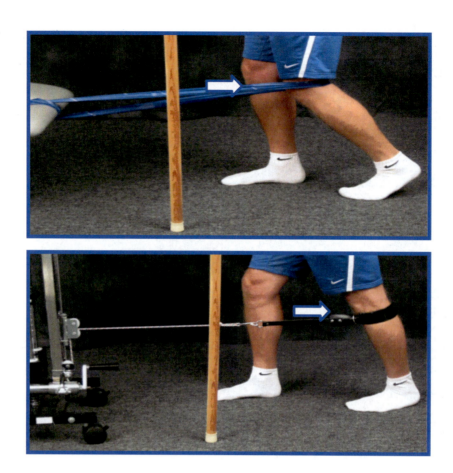

Figure 14-7: Resisted Quad Muscle Training, Terminal Knee Extension – Partial Weight Bearing (PWB):

As a patient's tolerance to weight bearing improves, the start and end position of the foot can change. This exercise will increase the compressive loading through the tibiofemoral joint progressing from TTWB (14-6) to PWB by having the patient start the exercise on the ball of their foot and move their knee into extension by placing their foot flat on the ground. Again, a cane (shown above), walker, or the back of a chair can be used to reduce weight bearing through the involved knee/lower extremity. Resisted quadriceps training is provided by a leather strap attached to a plate weight pulley system. Elastic band attached to a table or pulley system frame also works well. Exercise dosage is typically for 5 -10 minutes giving the patient rest breaks as needed. The leather strap placed around the proximal tibia will assist in reducing a small amount of patellofemoral compression. Consider prescribing this exercise in cases of quad weakness and passive knee joint extension restriction.

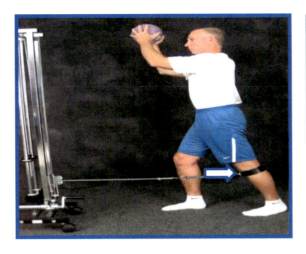
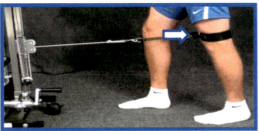

Figure 14-8: Resisted Quad Muscle Training, Terminal Knee Extension – Full Weight Bearing (FWB):

Exercise 14-11 places the patient in a split stance without the assistance of a cane or walker to reduce loading through the knee. Resisted quadriceps training is provided by attaching a leather strap to the LE and attaching the strap to a pulley system with plate weights. An elastic band attached to a table or pulley system frame also works well. The knee is moved from flexion into full extension. For the more athletic patient, UE elevation against some form of resistance can also be prescribed as short arc resisted knee extension is being performed. Exercise dosage is typically for 5-10 minutes with rest breaks as needed. For symptomatic patellofemoral chondrosis the band or leather strap should be placed around the proximal tibia as this may slightly reduce compressive loading at the PF joint by translating the tibia forward. For patients with anterior knee instability, the band or leather strap should be placed around the distal femur as shown in the top photo. Consider prescribing this exercise in cases of quad weakness and passive knee joint extension restriction.

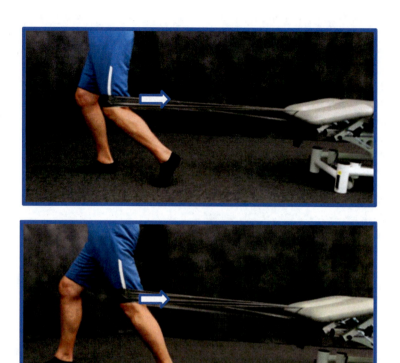

Figure 14-9: Assisted Terminal Knee Extension for Stiffness Impairment:

Look at the placement of the elastic band now. Visualize a pulley system with a rope (cable) and strap placed around the anterior distal femur as well. Note how the placement of the elastic band in the picture above, will pull the patient's knee into extension. This is very valuable exercise that you can prescribe any time your patient presents with a knee extension limitation (stiffness impairment). Instruct your patient to flex his/her knee against the resistance offered by an elastic band or weighted pulley system. The tension in the elastic band or pulley system with plate weights will passively pull (assist or stretch) the patient's knee into extension. I like to have patients perform this exercise at a walking pace so their knee is repetitively pulled into extension for 5 to 10 minutes. If balance is an issue, place a walker or the back of a chair in front of your patient. Next, we finish up this section of the knee chapter with two versions of hamstring stretching.

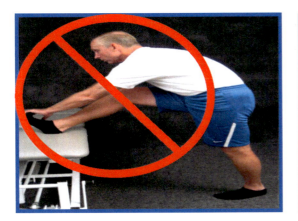 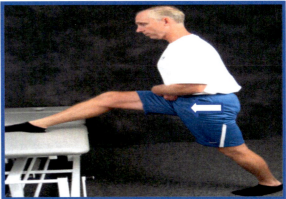

Figure 14-10: Hamstring Self-Stretching in Standing: Correct and Incorrect Position:

Exercises 14-1 – 14-9 all related in some way to knee extension impairment. Shortened hamstrings can relate to limited knee extension as well. The figure on the left shows everything that can go wrong with the standing hamstring self-stretch. The cervical, thoracic and lumbar regions are in a poor position and the sciatic nerve is on stretch. The figure on the right is a much better attempt. This figure shows the correct components to the standing hamstring self-stretch. The key to correct stretching is transverse plane rotation of the pelvis and lumbar spine as a unit toward the same side as the lower extremity where stretching is to occur. This pelvic rotation will move the ischial tuberosity in a dorsal direction separating the muscular attachment points. No rotation is to occur between the lumbar spine and pelvis. Other keys include plantar flexion of the ankle, slight knee flexion, and slight cervical and thoracic extension. Muscle stretching can be a good thing. Unnecessary nerve stretching is not. If a patient's sciatic nerve is irritated, it is questionable whether or not we should even prescribe hamstring self-stretching. All muscular self-stretch procedures should be held for a minimum of 30 seconds or up to a minute or more.

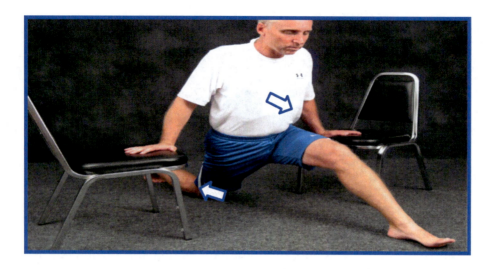

Figure 14-11: Hamstring Self-Stretching in a Half-Kneel Position:

This is a more advanced version of hamstring self-stretching where the patient first places himself in the half kneeling position. The LE where stretching is to occur is extended out in front of the patient with the knee slightly flexed and the heel of the foot touching the ground. Next, the pelvis is positioned at a right angle to the LE where hamstring stretching is to occur (the opposite side of the pelvis is brought forward). The pelvis must remain orientated in this way during the stretch. Now the patient is to press down lightly onto the chairs, unloading their knee and they must slide that knee backward while hinging forward at the hip on the side where stretching is to occur. To repeat, as the knee slides back the patient must hinge forward at the opposite hip and keep their pelvis from rotating backward as the knee moves backward. Once stretching is felt in the target area, continue to press down onto both chairs. This will deliver a light self-traction to the lumbar spine. The ankle on the stretch side should be plantar flexed and the cervical and thoracic spine should be slightly extended. Again, don't stretch nerves; stretch the target tissue which is muscle in this case. Hold this muscular self-stretch for 30 seconds or up to a minute or more. Next, our knee chapter transitions over to progressive LE strength building exercises.

Therapeutic Exercise

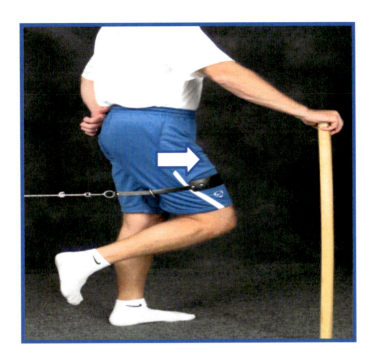

Figure 14-12: Resisted Hip Flexion with the Knee Positioned or Immobilized Close to the Resting Position (Hip Swings) - Open Kinetic Chain:

This portion of the knee chapter swings our discussion toward prescription of LE strength building exercises.

If your patient's knee joint is unable to tolerate weight bearing such as after an acute flare of arthritic pain or right after an injury or surgical intervention, therapists may wish to prescribe an OKC hip swing exercise. The arc of hip flexion motion is typically small, but the speed can vary greatly depending on the patient. Additional balance support and unloading of the opposite (uninvolved) LE is easily provided with a walker or cane if needed. A timed program with a work: rest cycle works very well for the therapeutic exercise. This exercise will assist in building strength in the hip extensor and hip flexor muscles and provide light activation of the quad muscle. This exercise can be adapted for home use with a long knotted circle of elastic band with the knotted end attached and stabilized by closed door.

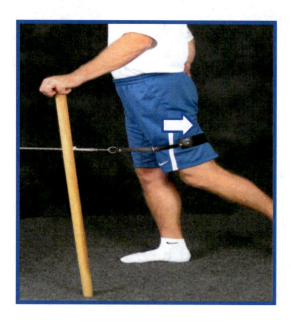

Figure 14-13: Resisted Hip Extension with Knee Positioned Close to the Resting Position – Open Kinetic Chain:

When your patient's knee joint is unable to tolerate weight bearing through his or her hip or more to the point of this chapter tibiofemoral joint, such as after an acute flare of arthritic pain or right after an injury or surgical intervention, therapists may wish to prescribe an OKC hip swing exercise. The arc of hip extension motion is typically small but the speed can vary greatly depending on the patient. Additional balance support and unloading of the opposite (uninvolved) LE is easily provided with a walker or cane if needed. Five to 10 minutes with rest breaks as needed works well for this exercise. Exercise 14-13 will build strength in the proximal hip flexor and extensor muscles and provide light activation of the hamstring muscles.

Therapeutic Exercise

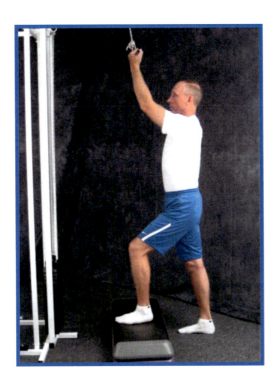

Figure 14-14: Assisted Step Ups – Pulley System and the Pull Down Bar, PWB:

The Step-Up exercises, and in particular assisted step ups allow our post-surgical and post injury patients with swelling and load intolerance and our older arthritic patients with load sensitivity perhaps due to meniscal degeneration, and some symptomatic patellofemoral chondrosis patients a way to perform a PWB CKC motion early in their rehab process. Using a pulley system, a pull down bar, and the entire weight stack, the patient is instructed to use their UE's to assist as much as necessary, so the step up maneuver is pain free. Again, I believe that if a strength building exercise becomes painful, the target muscle will become inhibited and strength improvement will be negated. Exercise dosage can vary from a typical multi-set, multi-rep program or a timed program using rest breaks as needed.

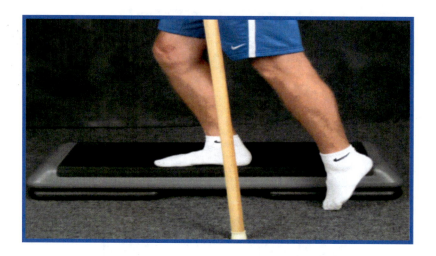

Figure 14-15: Assisted Step Ups- Canes, Dowels, Chairs or Walkers, PWB:

If a pulley system and pull-down bar are not available or to provide a home based procedure for exercise 14-14, the patient is instructed to press down on one or two canes, dowel sticks, the backs of two chairs or a walker in order to reduce loading on the involved and symptomatic knee. Exercise dosage can vary from a typical multi-set, multi-rep program or a timed program with rest breaks. Remember; adjust the speed, arc and amount of UE assistance, so the exercise motion is pain free. Pain free active assisted motion will promote increased circulation, tissue healing, and light stimulation of contractile tissues.

Therapeutic Exercise

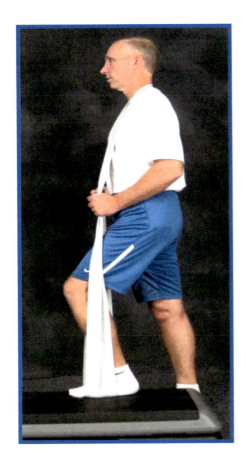
Start Position

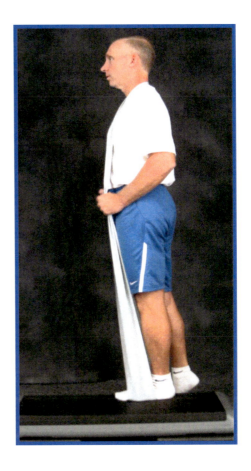
End Position

Figure 14-16: Resisted Step Ups, FWB:

If the knee joint(s) are able to handle a greater amount of load, a large loop of elastic band can be easily incorporated to provide additional RROM both in the clinic and as part of a home based exercise program. As the patient's strength and load tolerance improves, the intensity of the exercise dosage can increase in terms of total training time and number of repetitions. Athletic clients, young patients who are about to return to normal activities, and patients with no degenerative change affecting their tibiofemoral and patellofemoral joint can perform this therapeutic exercise at a high rate of speed.

Therapeutic Exercise

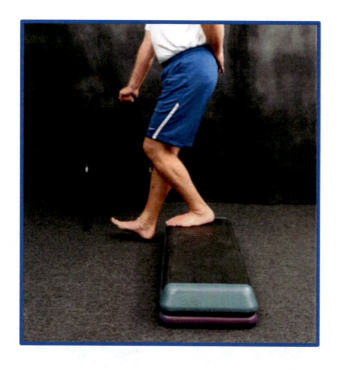

Eccentric training for the L LE

Figure 14-17: Eccentric Step Down, FWB:

Eccentric quad muscle training is next on our agenda. Eccentric muscle contraction is a great way to build muscle-tendon strength. Eccentric quad strength is vital for many daily activities. Our patients will not be able to descend stairs safely without good eccentric quad muscle control. If you find eccentric strength impairment, start with a small step and give your patient something to hold onto. As your patient's eccentric muscle strength is improves, he/she will be able to control the rate of knee flexion and lightly touch his/her foot to the ground. Note, symptomatic patellofemoral chondrosis may hold some patients back from being able to tolerate this exercise. Chronic quad and patellar tendinopathy may benefit from this eccentric strength building procedure.

Therapeutic Exercise

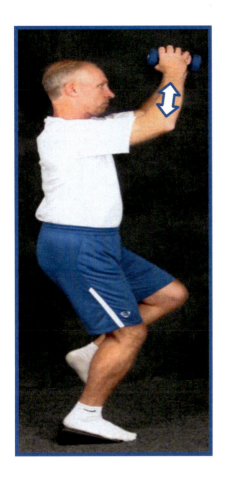

Figure 14-18: Isometric Lower Extremity Strength and Balance Training - Rapid UE Elevation:

The active assisted and resisted exercises 14-14 – 14-17 provide a level of strength building for the quad muscle in the last 20 some odd degrees of knee extension. The isometric LE strength building which occurs in this exercise is similar. In the figure above, the patient's C of G is raised and the B of S is made quite small by standing on a Thoracic Mobilization Wedge or foam pad. This will increase the demand of the exercise and resultant muscular effort. CKC single leg balance and isometric strength training is achieved as the patient is asked to rapidly elevate and depress their UE's while holding onto a free weight, pulley system cable-handle, or elastic band. Typically, the patient is asked to balance on one leg and perform this rapid UE movement for 10-15 seconds. After each exercise period the patient "shakes out their leg" with a small oscillatory OKC motion that will temporarily reduce compressive loading through the knee joint.

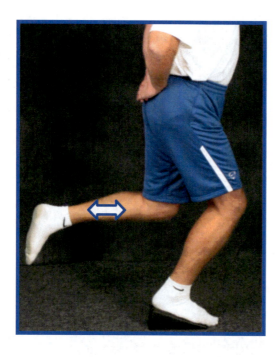

Figure 14-19: Isometric Lower Extremity Strength and Balance Training – Rapid LE Short Arc Flexion and Extension:

In this figure the patient's C of G is raised and the B of S is made quite small by standing on a Thoracic Mobilization Wedge or a foam pad. CKC single leg balance and isometric strength building toward end range knee extension is achieved as the patient is asked to rapidly flex and extend his/her opposite hip. LE strength building will occur as the involved LE reacts to the changes in the C of G. Typically, the patient is asked to balance out on one leg and perform this rapid LE movement for 10-15 seconds. After each exercise period the patient shakes out their leg and repeats the procedure as deemed appropriate by the therapist.

Therapeutic Exercise

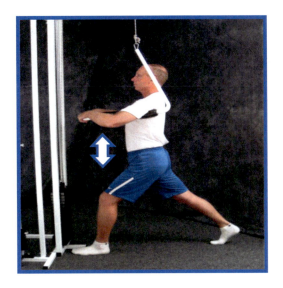 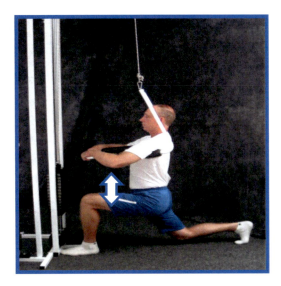

Figure 14-20: Assisted Lunge/Split Stance Squat Training in the Unloading Frame- PWB:

OK, let's build LE strength with our patient's knee joint(s) closer to 90 degrees of flexion. Sorry to say that most clinics do not have this piece of equipment and it is a shame. Not only can we get our post-surgical knee patients up and moving more quickly in a CKC exercise environment, but the unloading frame also has great use for patients with balance impairments. An unloading frame simply attaches to a standard pulley system where a Latissimus pull down bar would typically be attached. Using a standard plate weight system, the patient is given assisted knee extension training during the upswing of the motion (left) and resisted motion as he/she lowers his/her body and against the resistance of the plate weights. The frame and plate weights can assist in unloading pain sensitive LE joints. Squatting motions, step ups, marching and other single leg balance activities can also be performed in the unloading frame. Exercise dosage can vary from a multi-set, multi-rep program or 5-10 minutes exercise session using rest breaks as needed The split stance positioning of the LE's can be alternated after each set.

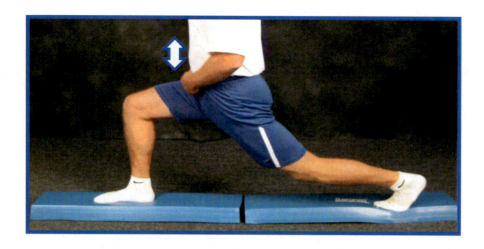

Figure 14-21: Lunge/Split Stance Squat Training on Unstable Surface- FWB:

As knee joint loading tolerance improves and to challenge our more athletic patients and other without balance impairment, take the unloading frame away and prescribe this split stance squat/lunge exercise. This exercise is made more challenging by using a less stable surface as seen above. This procedure is ideal for latter phase rehabilitation of ACL reconstruction, rehabilitation of minor knee injuries, generalized tibiofemoral hypermobility, and injury prevention exercise training. Exercise dosage for the more athletic client can vary from the standard multi-set and multi-rep program to a timed program using a 45 second work and 15 second rest program for 5-10 minutes. The split stance positioning of the LE's can be alternated after each set. When alternating lead leg position in the athletic client, have that individual perform a lunge jump. One additional note on foam balance beams which provide an unstable surface. These balance beams are ideal for other forms of plyometric jump training exercises such as "bottom kick" jumps, hip flexion or "tuck" jumps, jump turns and single leg jumps.

Therapeutic Exercise

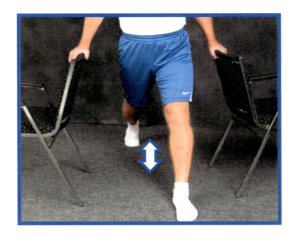 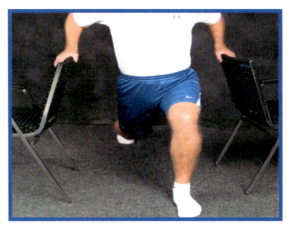

Figure 14-22: Assisted Lunge Training – PWB:

The lunge/split stance squat may be one of the greatest LE strength building movement patterns there is, and it is not just for athletic performance improvement or final phase surgical rehabilitation of the knee. Figure 14-22 demonstrates a clinic and home based version of this exercise. This version may be used as a transition from OKC muscle training to CKC muscle training in the post-surgical and post injury patient once the right amount of tissue healing has occurred (Chapter 6). Further our patients with load sensitive osteoarthritic changes in their hips and knees along with an element of strength impairment will find this exercise very useful. Exercise dosage can vary from the standard multi-set and multi-reps program to a timed program with rest breaks as needed. The split stance positioning of the LE's can be alternated after each set of reps or after each 30 second training phase. Let's review some lunge basics. First, and with regard to the back leg, the patient is to remain on the ball of their foot as the back knee flexes and then fully extends. Second, and regarding the front leg, the patient should lower his/her trunk to drop straight down while keeping the front tibia vertical. See Figures 14-20 and 21.

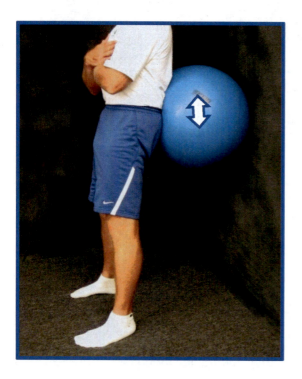 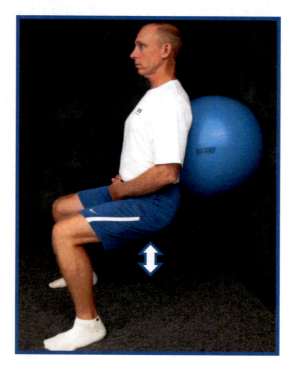

Figure 14-23: Swiss Ball Wall Slides

To this day, the wall slide exercise is still an important LE strength building procedure for many of our patients. The initial positioning of the feet in relation to the wall is a key point if load sensitive knee joint arthritis is present. The patient's feet must be away from the wall to minimize the loading of trunk weight on the knees and to prevent advancement of the tibia over the toes during knee flexion. The end position of the tibia should be vertical, similar to the positioning of the front leg during the downward movement of a lunge. Both isotonic and isometric training routines can be prescribed for this exercise. Incorporation of this exercise into a home based exercise program is very simple. For isometric training, hold each repetition a minimum of 6-10 seconds and repeat a minimum of 6-10 times for patients with strength impairment. The degree of knee flexion should be stopped short of any pain provoking position and short of any osteoarthritic tibiofemoral or patellofemoral noise or crepitation. When tolerated, this exercise allows for LE muscle strength building deeper in the range of knee flexion.

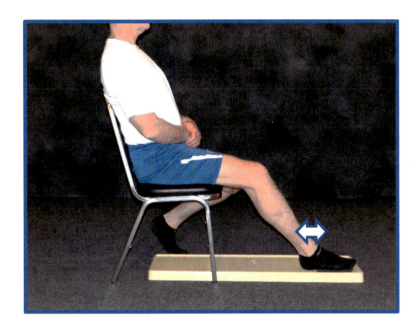

Figure 14-24: The Furniture Slider Exercise – Short Arc Near the Resting Position:

In the figure above, a furniture slider pad has been placed under the patient's knee. This pad greatly reduces friction and allows our patients to easily slide their feet (short arc knee flexion and extension) back and forth. Immediately after a surgery, an injury, or immediately after a flare up of a chronic arthritic condition, this non-loaded, reduced friction, short arc motion can assist in reducing pain and swelling. Shown above, are short arc knee flexion and extension movement that keep the patient's knee close to the resting position. Prescribe this exercise for 5-10 minutes at a time taking rest breaks as needed.

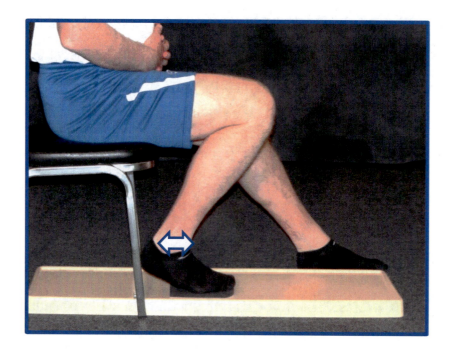

Figure 14-25: The Furniture Slider Exercise – Short Arc Oscillations Focusing on Flexion:

In the figure above, the patient has flexed his knee close to end range and is now performing a short oscillatory (very small) flexion-extension motion. To repeat, this pad greatly reduces friction and allows our patients to easily slide their feet (short arc knee flexion and extension) back and forth. Immediately after a surgery, an injury, or immediately after a flare up of a chronic arthritic condition, this non-loaded, reduced friction, short arc motion can assist in reducing pain, swelling, and as shown above assist with flexion stiffness impairment. Shown above, short arc flexion and extension movements performed further into the range of flexion as the patient's pain, swelling, or stiffness allows. Prescribe this exercise for 5-10 minutes at a time taking rest breaks as needed.

Therapeutic Exercise

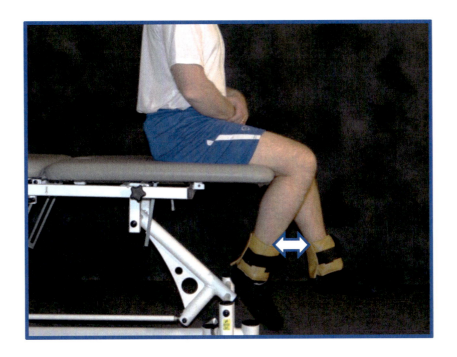

Figure 14-26: The Knee Joint Pendulum Exercise:

Joint traction and oscillatory motion provide two of the most powerful pain relieving modalities we can provide to our patients. This exercise, the knee joint pendulum exercise, provides both. Choose an amount of weight (cuff/ankle weight), typically in the neighbor of 2-8 pounds that provides a degree of knee joint pain relief for your patient. Next, find an arc and speed of pendular motion that also makes the patient's knee less painful. This exercise is useful as a warm up procedure applied prior to other exercises and manual intervention and for both pain and swelling impairments.

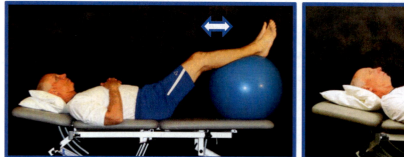 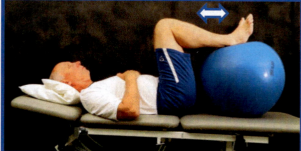

Figure 14-27: Swiss Ball Assisted Knee Flexion:

Let's continue to focus on knee flexion or lack thereof. If your patient's knee demonstrates stiffness or pain impairment limiting his/her ability to bend their knee, use a Swiss Ball and their uninvolved LE to "pull" the involved knee into flexion. Instruct your patient to stay just short of pain provocation is pain is the dominate feature or instruct your patient to lightly move into the first stop if flexion is limited by capsular shortening or arthritic changes. As your patient reaches the first flexion stop (end feel) you can choose to have him or her perform short quick oscillatory flexion and extension motion. For swelling impairments use slower larger amplitude flexion and extension motions in order to achieve more of a muscle pumping effect.

Therapeutic Exercise

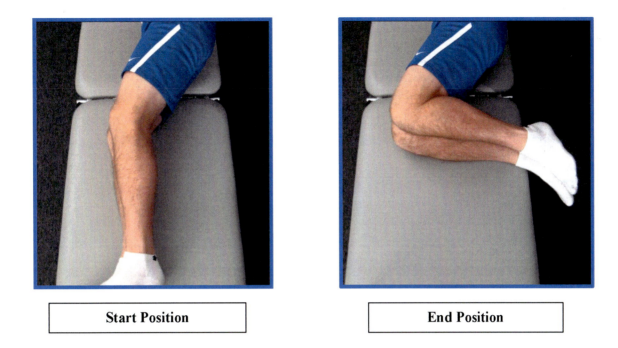

| Start Position | End Position |

Figure 14-28: Assisted Knee Flexion with Opposite LE- Side lying:

Let's stay on the subject of knee flexion. Having worked with many injured athletes, I found this exercise helpful for acute (PROM) and sub-acute (AAROM) hamstring muscle tears. The hamstring muscles have the dubious honor of being the most frequently torn LE muscle. The LE with the muscle tear is placed in the uppermost position and passive or active assisted knee flexion is performed with the lower most (uninvolved) side. I like to "buddy tie" the two ankles together during passive and active assisted motions in the early phases of muscle healing. The length/tension on the hamstring muscle can be increased or decreased by flexing or extending at the hip joints. Intermittent (throughout the day) light, slow pain free reps will improve circulation and assist healing of a torn hamstring muscle. A timed program of 30 seconds of movement and 30 seconds of rest for 5 minutes is helpful in the acute and sub-acute phase of a muscle tear. Lastly, the side lying position is probably the best position to deliver MRE for the hamstrings. The reason is that the hip position is more easily adjusted in side lying as compared to the prone position. Placing the hip in more or less flexion will change the tension on the hamstrings as manual concentric and eccentric resisted exercise is applied. For a significant tear, MRE begins to come into place somewhere in the neighborhood of three weeks post injury.

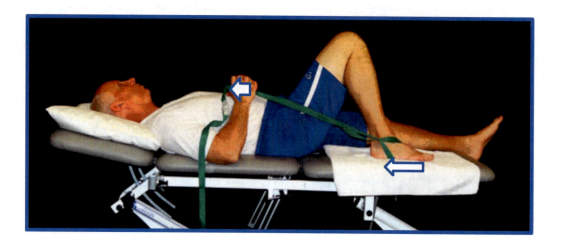

Figure 14-29: Assisted Heel Slide:

This is the old fashion heel slide exercise which is prescribed in many different venues of PT practice. The supine heel slide exercise is a good procedure for moving a knee into flexion. In this case we are going to use a looped strap in order to deliver either PROM or AAROM. Similar to the Swiss Ball Assisted Knee Flexion procedure, a therapist can prescribe short oscillatory passive knee flexion at the point of restrict knee flexion or a longer slower flexion and extension motion for swelling impairments.

Therapeutic Exercise

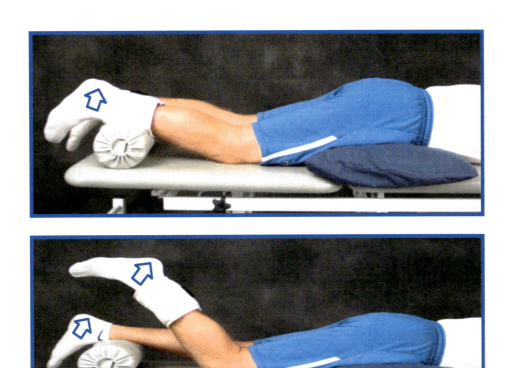

Figure 14-30: Resisted Hamstring Muscle Training-Prone - Open Kinetic Chain:

This is the classic short arc hamstring strength building exercise (SAH). For muscle strength building purposes I like to prescribe a rep max program for this short arc isotonic hamstring muscle training exercise as seen above. I believe this classic exercise should usually be prescribed in an alternating fashion. Also, manual resistive concentric and eccentric muscle training can be applied in the prone position. Manual resistive eccentric muscle training is quite important after a muscle tear especially in athletes involved in sprint activities This is one possible therapeutic progression after a hamstring muscle tear once the side lying gravity eliminated movement (exercise 14-28) has been successfully accomplished. (See Chapter 6, for tissue healing time frames). As the muscle heals, AROM against gravity is initiated. If AROM is pain free and as the hamstring muscle continues to heal, RROM should be applied (See Chapter 3 Therapeutic Motions and Movements).

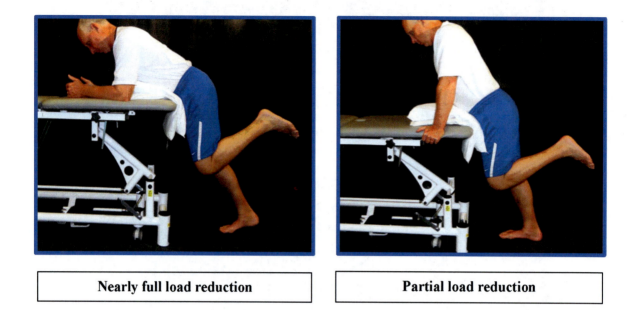

| Nearly full load reduction | Partial load reduction |

Figure 14-31 The Standing Bottom Kick Exercise:

The prone lying SAH exercise (14-30) is an excellent way to build strength in a load sensitive knee. One potential problem though is a patient's ability to transition into the prone lying position. The standing bottom kick exercise seen above helps to solve this potential problem. Note how the patient can be positioned with virtually no compressive loading through the knee(s) or just reduced load through the knee(s). If we reduce load through the knee we can often improve (increase) our patient's LE strength without provoking pain. For a patient with post-surgical or post-injury pain and swelling. When your patient performs bottom kicking as shown above he/she can also improve flexibility and reduce his/her sensation of knee stiffness.

Therapeutic Exercise

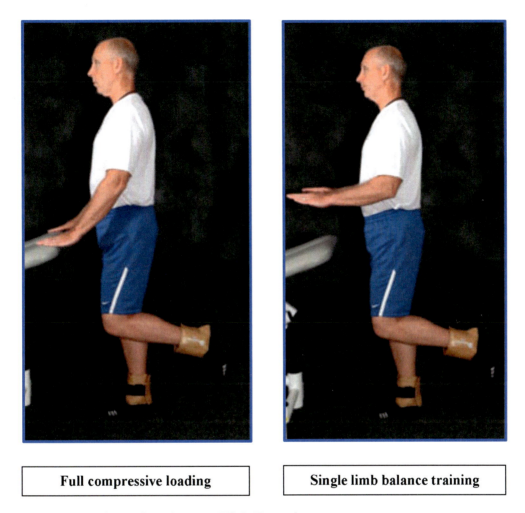

Full compressive loading **Single limb balance training**

Figure 14-32: The Standing Bottom Kick Exercise:

One final point of discussion regarding a very useful exercise. Hamstring strengthening, anterior knee soft tissue stretching, and balance training can all be achieved with the great therapeutic exercise. For strength building purposes, add cuff weights around the ankles and have your patient perform quick alternating isotonic movements with isometric knee flexion interspersed. Next, take the cuff weight off and teach your patients to attempt to kick their bottom with their heels any time his/her knees feel tight or stiff. Your older arthritic patient can perform this movement slowly and your athletic patients can perform this motion with speed before, during, and after a competition. Lastly, if balance impairment exists, have your patient perform alternating knee flexion very slowly with hands offs a table.

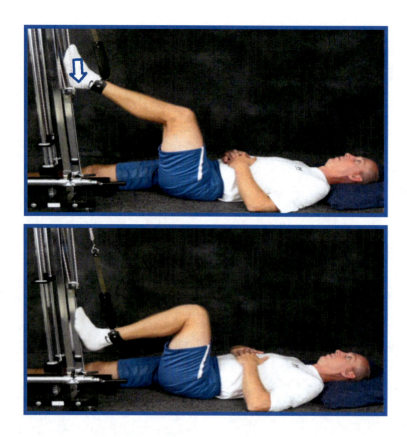

Figure 14-33: Resisted Knee Flexion- Supine- Open Kinetic Chain:

Back to open kinetic chain (OKC) for one last strength building exercise. This resisted motion incorporates a pulley system. While closed kinetic chain (CKC) therapeutic exercise motions align more closely with daily function, the fact is that many of our elderly patients with degenerated joints and many of our post-injury and post-surgical patients are in need for OKC training at least on a temporary basis. Orthopedic conditions such as total knee replacement, ACL reconstruction and various meniscal repair and excision procedures will have associated weakness, stiffness, and swelling impairments. That being said, we can isolate a precise amount of resistance and range (arc) of movement with OKC exercise. The exercised shown above does just that for the conditions listed above.

Therapeutic Exercise

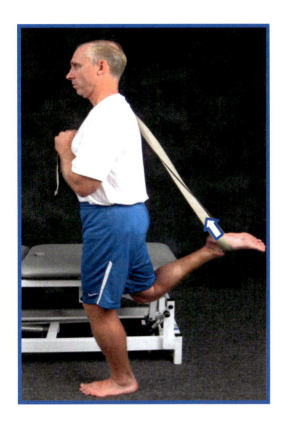

Figure 14-34: Rectus Femoris Self-Stretching – Standing:

Let's conclude the chapter with self-stretching related to knee flexion, and review correct body positioning and movement sequence. First, the patient is to elongate the posterior aspect of the neck and lift their chest bone (sternum) up and forward. Next, flex the knee joint on the side to be stretched and then extend the femur at the hip joint until the anterior aspects of both thighs are in line or, better yet, extended posteriorly beyond the stance leg. At this point the patient is to perform a posterior pelvic tilt with a firm abdominal drawing motion (the lower tummy is pulled upward and inward). The movement emphasis is hip extension and then a posterior tilting of the pelvis, not the forcing of additional knee flexion. Hold this muscular self-stretch for at least 30 seconds or up to a minute or more. The clinic based version of this self-stretch incorporates a mobilization belt as shown above and the home based version can incorporate a piece of rope.

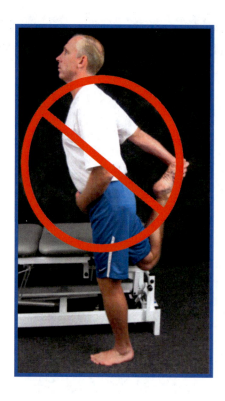

Figure 14-35: Rectus Femoris Self-Stretching – Incorrect Standing Position:

Well, the previous figure demonstrated the right way to stretch the Rectus Femoris muscle in a standing position, while this figure above shows the incorrect method. We need to look at the incorrect way to perform this exercise because it is a commonly prescribed stretch that is commonly performed the wrong way as shown in figure 14-35. Note the anterior pelvic tilting and lumbar hyperextension. This position is not only a poor one for the lumbar spine, but it will also slacken the Rectus Femoris muscle and is the main reason why most individuals must really flex their knee to end range in order to feel a stretching sensation. Also, be sure that the back of the cervical spine is elongated (lengthened) and thoracic spine is not in kyphosis during this stretch. Hold this muscular self-stretch for at least 30 seconds or up to a minute or more.

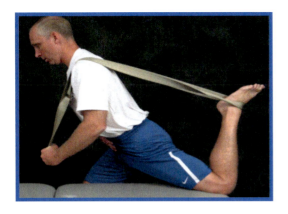 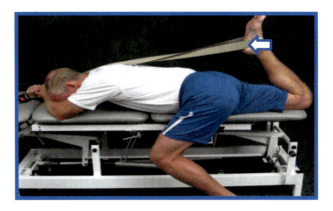

Figure 14-36: Rectus Femoris Self-Stretching – Prone:

The prone lying position is perhaps the best position to fully elongate the Rectus Femoris. First, have your patient pre-position the belt over the shoulder and passively flex their knee with a belt or rope. Next, the patient is to lay prone on a table or bed keeping the opposite LE off the table and drawing that LE as far forward as possible. Stabilize the foot placement on the ground with a thoracic wedge. This LE placement will stabilize the proximal attachment point of the Rectus Femoris muscle. Once positioned, the patient should draw the lower abdomen upward and inward to better separate attachments points of this muscle. Do not allow the cervical and lumbar spine to hyperextend. Hold this muscular self-stretch for at least 30 seconds or up to a minute or more. If your patient has a history of low back pain, and flexibility impairment affecting this muscle, this is the version to choose. Place a pillow in the abdominal region to further support the lumbar spine.

Chapter 15

Therapeutic Exercise for the Ankle-Foot

Chapter 15 will look at exercises for patients with various Ankle-foot impairments. Here is a bulleted list of some of the more important topic areas that will be covered in this chapter.

- Building strength to support the medial longitudinal arch while controlling weight bearing.
- Key self-stretches for common orthopedic foot pathology.
- After the sprain, ankle joint stabilization exercises.
- Reducing tensile load on key tendons while performing CKC exercise training.

Therapeutic Exercise

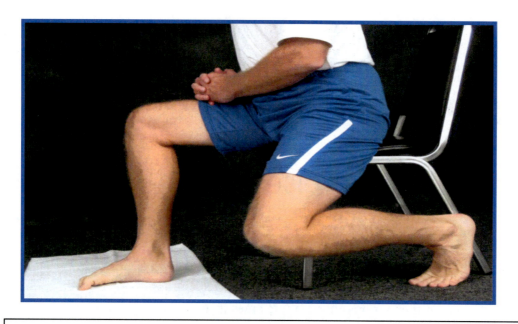

The exercise motion can be a combination of toe flexion and ankle inversion.

Figure 15-1: Isometric and Isotonic Foot Intrinsic Muscle Training- NWB:

This is a simple, well known, and important therapeutic motion often called the Arch Dome or Towel Scrunch exercise. We will start this chapter by presenting this exercise and two simple progressions which incrementally increase the load on the ankle-foot during the performance of this exercise motion. This procedure is important to prescribe in cases of generalized ankle-foot hypermobility, excessive pronatory motion, and weakness impairments affecting the toe flexor muscles. This exercise along with orthotic fabrication constitutes two of the principal interventions for the hypermobile over pronating ankle/foot. For isometric training the patient should hold the muscle contraction for a minimum of 6-10 seconds and perform a minimum of 6 to 10 repetitions. This would constitute one set and multiples sets should be performed in order to enhance muscular based stability. Regarding isotonic training, active toe flexion should occur at a fairly quick pace. A pace consistent with their normal walking cadence often works well.

Therapeutic Exercise

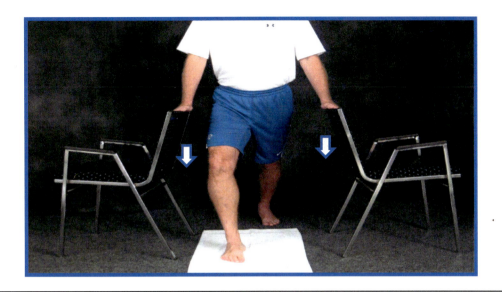

The exercise motion can be a combination of toe flexion and ankle inversion.

Figure 15-2: Isometric and Isotonic Foot Intrinsic Muscle Training- PWB:

The first progression of the arch dome exercise involves exercise prescription in a partial weight bearing position incorporating a split stance position and using the UE's to press down on the backs of two chairs. The amount of trunk weight that should be unloaded is dependent upon the patient's pain intensity and the stage of the patient's condition or injury. Patients should be instructed to press down on the backs of two chairs to a point where load produced symptoms are alleviated and then begin the isometric or isotonic training of the target muscles. For isometric training the patient should hold the muscle contraction (toe flexion) for a minimum of 6-10 seconds and perform a minimum of 6 to 10 repetitions. Regarding isotonic toe flexion, this toe curling exercise motion should be performed at a fairly quick pace. A pace consistent with their normal walking cadence often works well.

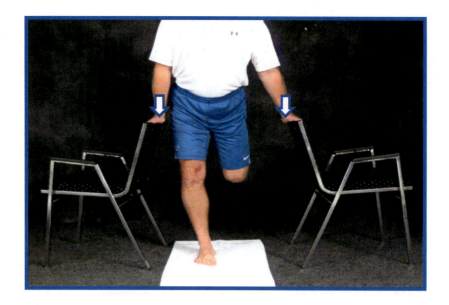

Figure 15-3: Isometric and Isotonic Foot Intrinsic Muscle Strength Training- FWB:

Figure 15-3 shows the next progression of the arch dome/towel scrunch exercise now performed in single leg stance and with full weight bearing. Note; now the chairs are used to assist with balance and unloading of the ankle-foot can still occur by pressing downward should pain be encountered during muscle training. Foot intrinsic muscle training may be helpful for the plantar and plantar-medial foot pain that is at times associated with cases of plantar fasciitis or posterior tibial tendonitis. For isometric training the patient should hold the muscle contraction for a minimum of 6-10 seconds and perform a minimum of 6 to 10 repetitions. This constitutes one set. One to three sets should be performed. Regarding isotonic training and this exercise technique, the patient should perform this motion at a fairly quick pace. A pace consistent with their normal walking cadence often works well. Sixty to 100 reps should be the goal.

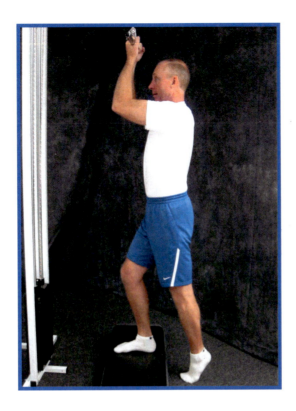

Figure 15-4: Assisted Plantar Flexor Muscle Training- Unilateral with Pulley System:

Weakness in the calf muscle group is not uncommon in cases of lumbar S1 nerve root compression, after immobilization of the ankle-foot, after Achilles tendon repair, and in association with Achilles tendinopathy. In the clinic, using a pulley system and a pull down bar, the patient is instructed to perform a simple step up with a focus on propelling themselves up onto the step with their calf muscle group (left in this figure). A 5 to 10-minute exercise program with with rest breaks as needed or a multi-set, multi-rep program can be prescribed if weakness impairment dominates the clinical presentation. In cases involving pain impairment affecting the Achilles tendon, have the patient use his/her upper extremities and "lead leg" (quad muscle) to a point where symptoms are not felt in the involved achilles tendon. Use rest breaks to monitor the pain level in the achilles tendon.

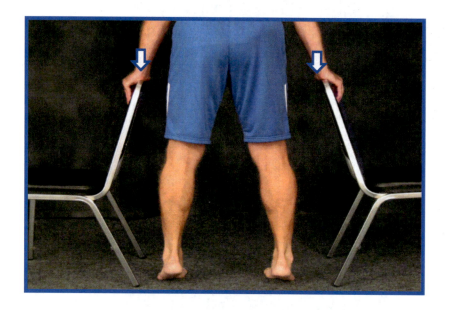

Figure 15-5: Assisted Plantar Flexor Muscle Training - Bilateral

Now we will have our patient build calf muscle and achilles tendon strength bilaterally and between two chairs. Weakness impairment affecting the plantar flexor muscles can occur in relation to any of the conditions mentioned in 15-4. In this exercise the patient is instructed to push downward with both hands in order to achieve assisted motion (AAROM) so that the muscle and achilles tendon(s) are stimulated but pain secondary to overloading is controlled. A 5-10-minute timed program with rest breaks or a multi-set, multi-rep program is a typical prescription. In order to facilitate eccentric stimulation of the tendon(s) the patient is instructed to slowly lower hi/her heel back to the ground. The speed of the concentric portion of the muscle contraction can vary based on the patient's strength and pain status.

Therapeutic Exercise

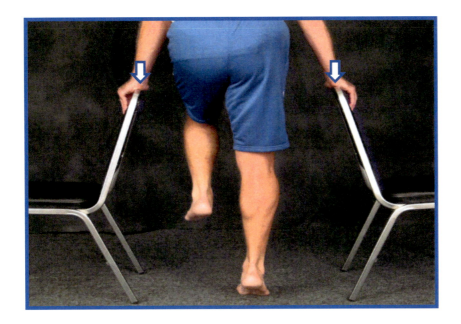

Figure 15-6: Assisted Plantar Flexor Muscle Training - Unilateral Emphasis

This exercise represents a progression from exercise 15-5. In our patients who hope to return to more vigorous occupational and recreational endeavors, sound single leg ankle plantar flexion strength is essential. Typically, exercise progression from bilateral to unilateral will initially require greater assistance from the UE's as shown above. Similar to exercise 15-5, as strength improves the contribution from the UE's should be reduced. As always, ensure good quality motion and little to no discomfort during the strength re-building process. A 5-10-minute timed program with rest breaks or a multi-set, multi-rep program is a typical prescription. In order to facilitate eccentric stimulation of the tendon(s) the patient is instructed to slowly lower hi/her heel back to the ground. The speed of the concentric portion of the muscle contraction can vary based on the patient's strength and pain status.

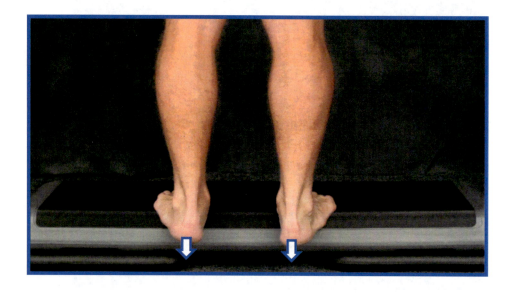

Figure 15-7: Concentric and Eccentric Plantar Flexor Muscle Training:

Slow eccentric heel lowering was mentioned in the previous two exercises and is an important part of tendinopathy management. The emphasis of this exercise procedure is a slow eccentric lowering of the patient's heels below the step. Full range concentric plantar flexion can also be prescribed as part of this exercise. This exercise can lead a patient toward more demanding pylometric jumping drills. This exercise can be performed with the 30-second work 30-second rest protocol or a more standard multi-set, multi-rep program can be prescribed. In cases involving pain impairment the therapist and patient should evaluate pain status and if necessary, modify the rate, amplitude, and amount of assistance/unloading required.

Therapeutic Exercise

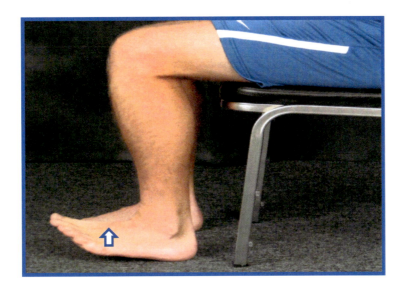

Figure 15-8: Active Ankle Dorsi-Flexor Muscle Training- Seated NWB:

Bilateral or alternating ankle-foot dorsiflexion, (the toe tapping) exercise performed in a non-weight bearing open kinetic chain position plays an important role in patients with pre-tibial muscle weakness secondary to less severe forms of L4 and L5 nerve root compression, post ankle-foot injury, and post cast immobilization due to fracture or other ankle-foot surgical procedures. A standard multi-set, multi-rep exercise dosage usually applies with non-weight bearing pre-tibial muscle training. This probably goes without saying, but a safe, stable gait pattern in part requires ankle dorsiflexion and a solid heel strike. This exercise and exercises 15-9 and 15-10 can be an important component of a safe walking/gait training program.

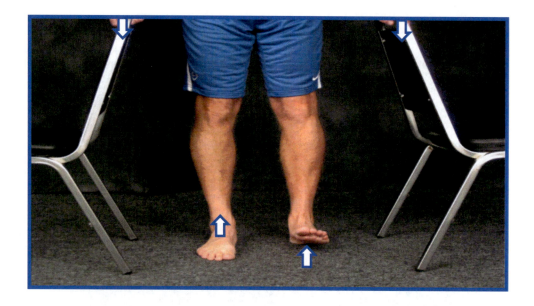

Figure 15-9: Active Ankle Dorsi-Flexor Muscle Training- Standing with Support PWB:

This exercise is a progression from 15-8 in that the ankle-foot joints are now partially weight bearing. If pre-tibial muscle weakness is present and there is ankle-foot pain due to an injury or surgical procedure, the patient is instructed to use their UE's to reduce weight bearing through the involved LE in order to provide for symptom free CKC concentric and controlled eccentric lowering movement. This exercise can be performed with a 5-10-minute timed program using rest breaks as needed or a multi-set, multi-rep program can be prescribed. In cases involving pain associated with weight bearing the patient is encouraged to minimize weight bearing through the involved LE during the rest break, and the therapist and patient evaluate pain status and if necessary, modify the rate, amplitude, and amount of assistance/unloading required.

Therapeutic Exercise

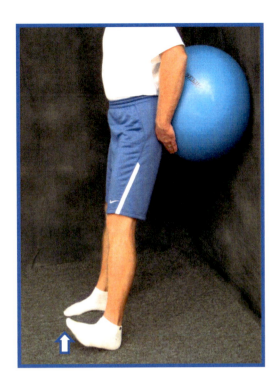

Figure 15-10: Active Ankle Dorsi-Flexion- Assisted with Wall and Swiss Ball, FWB

This version of pre-tibial muscles adds a balance requirement and full weight bearing status through the ankle-foot joints. In this exercise the patient is taught to shift weight back and forth while concentrically activating their pre-tibial muscles. In effect, the patient is taught to shift weight to the left and right while alternately lifting his/her forefoot off the ground. Again, this exercise adds an element of balance training which further increases the demand on the patient. This version of pre-tibial muscle training can be performed as a 5-minute timed exercise with rest breaks as needed or a standard multi-set, multi-rep program can be prescribed. One additional point of review, slow lowering of the plantar surface of the foot down to the ground in order to build eccentric muscular control is an important aspect of this exercise.

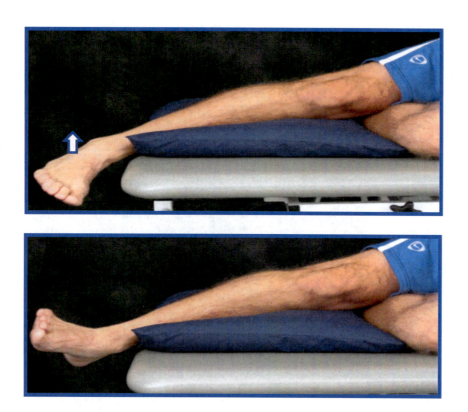

Figure 15-11: Active Ankle Eversion Muscle Training, NWB:

Open kinetic chain NWB muscle contractions are not consistent with the primary way muscles function in the LE. That being said there are still times when a basic therapeutic motion such as this needs to be prescribed. Immediate post-surgical and post injury management may be two such scenarios. I have shown this figure above to reinforce the importance of and the patient position where manual resistive exercise (MRE) can be performed. Clinicians can easily apply manual concentric and eccentric exercise training to the peroneal muscle group with their patient in this position. Regarding exercise dosage and MRE it is often good to provide manually resisted training until the quality of the desired motion begins to deteriorate and the patient feels a sense of fatigue in the target muscle group. Peroneal muscle strength building can be important post inversion ankle sprain.

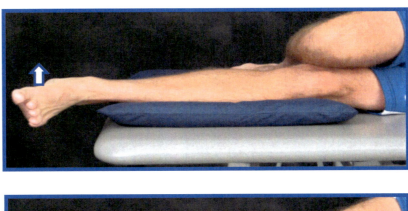
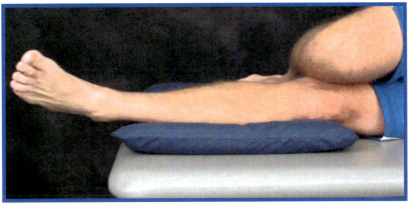

Figure 15-12: Active Ankle Inversion Muscle Training-NWB

Similar to the discussion associated with figure 15-11, OKC NWB concentric contraction is certainly not the most important function of the ankle-foot inverter muscle group. That being said there are still times when a basic therapeutic motion such as this needs to be prescribed. Immediate post-surgical and post injury management where weight bearing is not tolerated or allowed may be two such scenarios. Again, this figure above is shown here to demonstrate the patient position and the importance of manual resistive exercise (MRE). Clinicians can easily apply manual concentric and more importantly eccentric exercise training to the tibialis posterior and other synergistic muscle groups with their patient in this position. Regarding exercise dosage and MRE it is often good to provide resisted training until the quality of the desired motion begins to deteriorate and the patient feels a sense of fatigue in the target muscle group. Consider manual eccentric muscle training in cases of posterior tibial tendinopathy.

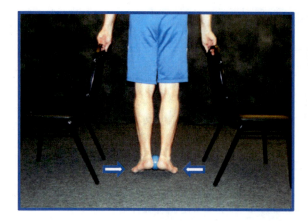 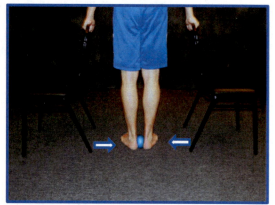

Figure 15-13: Concentric-Eccentric Muscle Strengthening for Tibialis Posterior:

Let's move into a closed chain exercise training position and discuss an important strength building exercise procedure for the tibialis posterior. The idea here is to have your patient perform a bilateral heel raise. As your patient performs the concentric heel raise and as he/she slowly (eccentrically) lowers his/her heels downward to the ground they are instructed to firmly squeeze (compress) a foam ball, rubber ball, hand-held medicine ball, or even a rolled towel. Compressing a ball with the medial aspect of heels with cause a strong contraction of the tibialis posterior muscle and build strength in this important medial longitudinal arch stabilizing muscle. The backs of two chairs or a walker can be used to assist with balance or two unload the medial aspect of the ankle if painful.

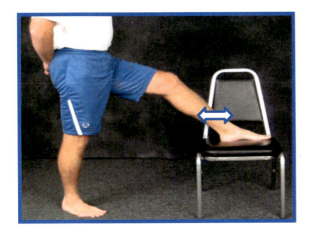 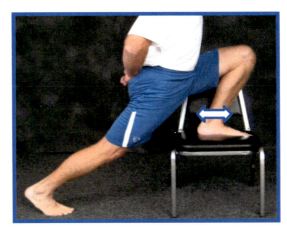

Figure 15-14: Talocural Self- Mobilization-PWB:

Exercise 15-14 will provide clinicians with an excellent way to initially re-mobilize the talocural joint after a period of ankle-foot immobilization. This therapeutic movement also provides a patient with a sound procedure to maintain restored mobility after manual stretching/mobilization. The patient is instructed to place the involved ankle onto a chair, preferably one without arms. The ankle joint is placed in mid-position and gently rocked back and forth into both plantar flexion and then dorsiflexion by advancing the mortise over the top of the talus. The concave member of the joint is moved back and forth until a mild stretching sensation is perceived. At that point the patient is to hold the stretch for a minimum of 30 seconds or up to a minute.

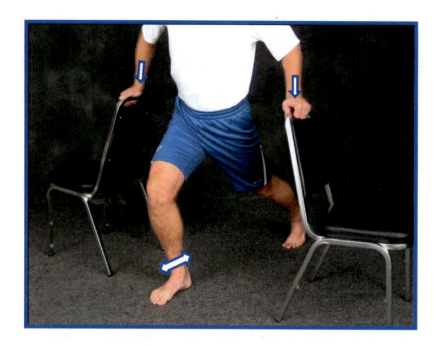

Figure 15-15: Talocural Self-Mobilization with UE Support-PWB:

This exercise is similar to 15-14 only now there is increased weight bearing through the LE. The upper extremities press down upon the backs of two chairs to reduce ankle-foot loading as the patient passes the mortise over the top of a fixed talus. The body movement here is not the same as a lunge. The body movement is forward as opposed to straight downward which is more consistent with a lunge/split stance squatting motion. The concave member of the joint (the tibia and fibula) is advanced forward and then backward until a mild stretching sensation is perceived. At that point the patient is to hold the stretch for a minimum of 30 seconds or up to a minute.

Therapeutic Exercise

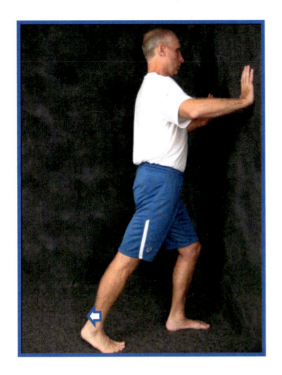 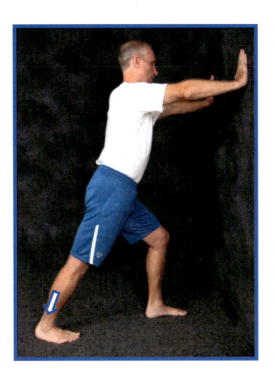

Figure 15-16: Gastrocnemius Self-Stretching- Unilateral:

This would not be a complete ankle-foot section without some discussion of the gastrocnemius muscle. This is a very common stretch often applied prior to athletic and recreational activities. Shortening of this muscle-tendon group is fairly common so here is a quick point. When performing this self-stretch on a unilateral basis, first instruct your patient to slide their foot backward until their heel just comes off the ground. At that point, the patient should extend (straighten) their elbows and attempt to "drive" the plantar surface of the calcaneus onto the ground. This muscular stretch should only be felt in the target area and should be held for a minimum of 30 seconds or up to a minute or more. If discomfort is felt over the anterior aspect of the talocural joint, the amount of dorsi-flexion should be reduced.

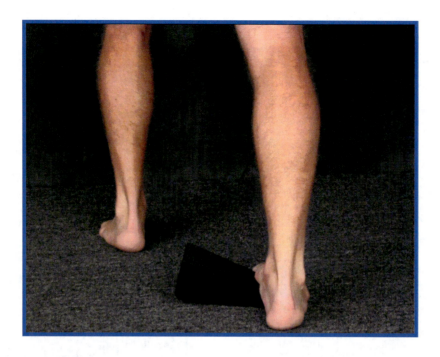

Figure 15-17: Gastrocnemius Self-Stretching-Lateral Head:

The movement pattern for this exercise is the same as figure 15-16. To better isolate the lateral head of this muscle, a spinal mobilization wedge is placed under the medial fore-foot to add a degree of ankle-foot inversion. This stretch should only be felt in the target area and should be held for a minimum of 30 seconds or up to a minute or more. If discomfort is felt over the anterior aspect of the talocural joint, the amount of dorsi-flexion should be reduced.

Therapeutic Exercise

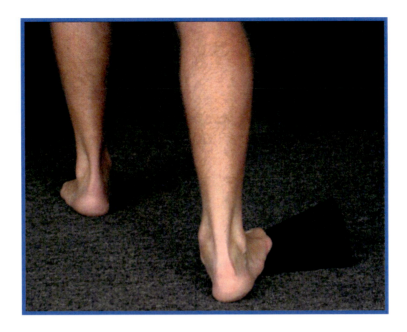

Figure 15-18: Gastrocnemius Self-Stretching-Medial Head:

To better isolate the medial head of this muscle, a spinal mobilization wedge is placed under the lateral fore-foot to add a degree of ankle-foot eversion. This muscular self-stretch should only be felt in the target area and should be held for a minimum of 30 seconds or up to a minute or more. If discomfort is felt over the anterior aspect of the talocural joint, the range of dorsi-flexion should be reduced. Note: this movement pattern and end position for this self-stretch is also useful when prescribing low load, long duration therapeutic stretching for a rigid, supinated foot.

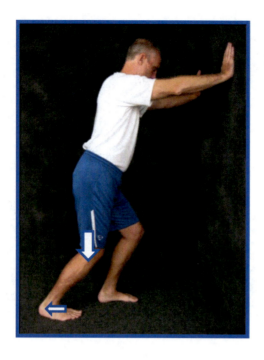

Figure 15-19: Soleus Self-Stretching:

The movement sequence for this stretch varies slightly as compared to the gastrocnemius muscle. The patient is instructed to slide their foot back to a point just before the plantar surface of the heel comes off the ground. At that point, the patient is to bend their knee which slackens the gastrocnemius muscle and further dorsiflexes the ankle joint. This muscular self-stretch should only be felt in the target area and should be held for a minimum of 30 seconds or up to a minute or more. If discomfort is felt over the anterior aspect of the talocural joint, the amount of dorsiflexion should be reduced.

Therapeutic Exercise

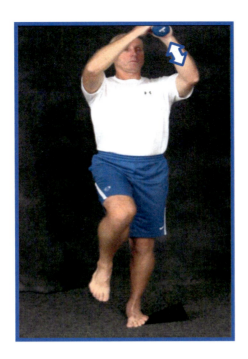

Figure 15-20: Ankle Stabilization Training, Protecting the Anterolateral Capsule:

Closed Kinetic Chain:

This is a single limb stance strength, balance, and proprioceptive stabilization exercise most often used after the very common inversion ankle sprain. The patient's B of S is reduced and C of G is elevated during this rapid UE diagonal elevation and depression movement pattern. Note, how the spinal mobilization wedge is placed in relation to the patient's foot. Placement of the wedge in this way will slightly dorsi-flex and evert the foot which slackens the ankle's anterolateral capsule. A single dumbbell weight is held with both hands during the rapid UE movement pattern. This exercise can be performed for up to 5-10 minutes with the 30 second work and 30 second rest protocol.

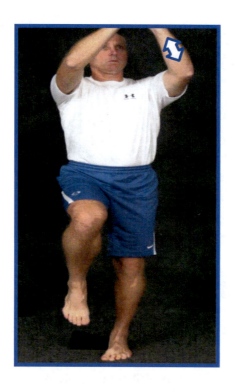

Figure 15-21: Ankle Stabilization Training, Protecting the Posterior Tibialis Tendon: Closed Kinetic Chain:

CKC ankle-foot strength, balance and proprioceptive training can be very challenging when there is irritation of the posterior tibialis tendon. This exercise set up allows for a single leg stance rapid UE movement patterns which will force the patient's LE muscles to constantly react to changes in the C of G. Note the placement of the spinal mobilization wedge. Insertion of the wedge as shown passively plantar flexes and inverts the foot and as a result, slackens the posterior tibialis tendon. In cases of strength or balance impairment and medial ankle pain due to inflammation or pathological degeneration of the posterior tibialis tendon this exercise can be helpful. A single dumbbell weight is held with both hands during the rapid UE movement pattern. This exercise can be performed for up to 5-10 minutes with the 30 second work and 30 second rest protocol.

Therapeutic Exercise

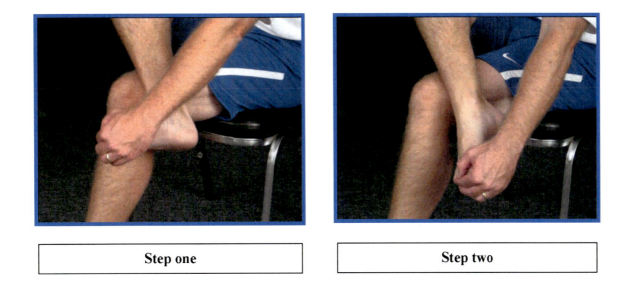

| Step one | Step two |

Figure 15-22: Pre-Tibial Self–Stretching- NWB:

These next two figures are self-stretching procedures for the pre-tibial muscles. Shortening of the pre-tibial muscles is not tremendously common, but irritation due to overuse is. The first version is performed in a seated position and the movement sequence is as follows. First, the patient is to passively flex their toes while the ankle is dorsi-flexed. Having done that, the patient should hold the toe flexion and then passively plantar flex the ankle. Stretching should be held for at least 30 seconds or up to a minute or more. This stretch may be helpful in cases of shin splints.

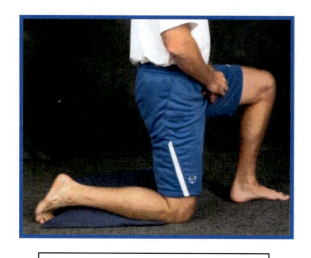 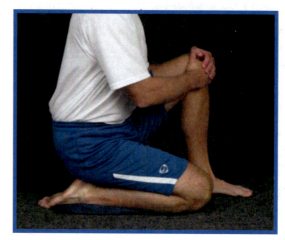

Start Position   **End Position**

Figure 15-22: Pre-Tibial Self – Stretching, PWB:

This stretch is more aggressive and should only be performed on stable and non-arthritic ankles. The patient is instructed to place themselves in a half kneeling position and then set themselves back onto their lower leg and ankle-foot area. This will force the ankle into a greater degree of plantar flexion and will elongate some of the pre-tibial muscles. Some patient or athletes may also passively flex their toes in order to elongate the remainder of the pre-tibials. A second pillow can be inserted into the popliteal region if end range knee flexion is painful. Muscular self-stretching should be held for at least 30 seconds or up to a minute or more and this stretch may prove useful in some cases of shin splints.

Therapeutic Exercise

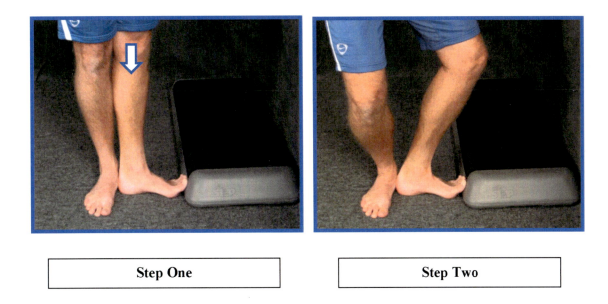

Figure 15-23: Flexor Digitorum and Flexor Hallucis Longus Self-Stretching:

These two muscle groups are best stretched in a standing position. The patient is instructed to place the toes in an extended position and up against a step, brief case or hard cover book. The toes are to be comfortably extended and not forced beyond their first stop for this particular motion. Once positioned, the patient is asked to bend their knees. Knee flexion will promote increased ankle dorsiflexion and fully elongate this muscle group. Muscular self-stretching should be held for at least 30 seconds or up to a minute. In cases of plantar foot pain with associated flexibility impairment of theses muscles, this stretch may be helpful.

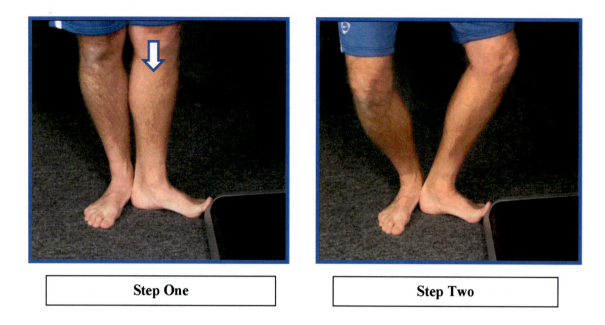

| Step One | Step Two |

Figure 15-24: Flexor Hallucis Longus Self-Stretching:

With a similar movement sequence, the Flexor Hallucis Longus muscle can be isolated by extending the great toe up against a step, brief case or hard cover book. The great toe is to be comfortably extended and not forced beyond the first stop of this particular motion. Once positioned, the patient is asked to bend their knees. Knee flexion will dorsi-flex the ankle joint and fully elongate this muscle. Muscular self-stretching should be held for at least 30 seconds or up to a minute. In cases of plantar foot pain with associated flexibility impairment this stretch may be helpful. Also in cases of Hallux Limitus, carefully applied self-stretching may improve ROM. Note in cases of Hallux Rigidus, this stretch should not be applied.

Therapeutic Exercise

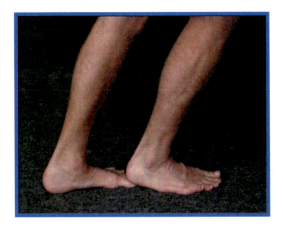 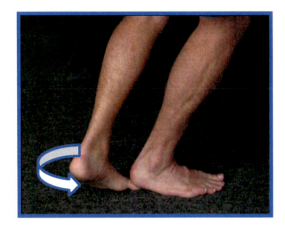

Figure 15-25: Adductor Hallucis Self-Stretching:

Self-stretching early in the management of Hallux Valgus may slow the progression of this condition and prevent some degree of capsular contracture, muscle shortening and painful symptoms. The patient is instructed to carefully and gently step onto the dorsal surface of their great toe with the plantar surface of the calcaneus. Next the patient is told to move their stabilized foot in a dorsal direction. This will promote a degree of traction-separation at the first MTP joint. The final step involves the patient turning their heel inward toward their other foot which will provide for a passive varus motion at the first MTP joint. This self-stretch should be held for at least 30 seconds or up to two minutes or more.

Chapter 16

Therapeutic Exercise for the Cervical Spine

Chapter 16 will look at exercises for patients with various cervical impairments. Here is a bulleted list of some of the more important topics covered in this chapter.

- Cervical Stabilization Exercises
    - Deep Cervical Extensor Muscle Training
    - Deep Cervical Flexor Muscle Training
- Cervical Self Mobilization Exercises
    - Active Self - Mobilization
    - Passive Self- Mobilization
- Cervicothoracic Postural Reinforcement Exercises
- Cervical Movement Patterns with Injury Potential

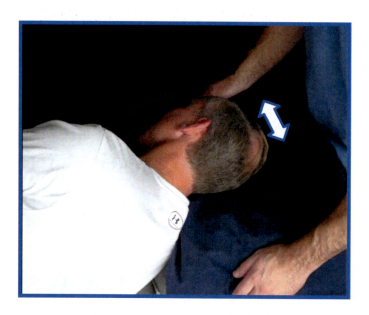

Figure 16-1: Side lying and Supported Cervical Flexion and Extension – PROM to AAROM to AROM Progression

The start position for this exercise is mid-line and mid-position with the patient's head and neck well supported and comfortable. This is especially important after an injury to the cervical spine. Slow short arc passive cervical flexion and extension is applied to the patient's segments as the clinician passively moves the pillow back and forth. The patient is asked to relax and rest their head and neck on the pillow. All therapeutic motion is kept in the pain free range. Progression of this exercise involves active assistance by the patient through use of their cervical flexor and extensor muscles. Post injury; apply a 15 second work (PROM) and 45 second rest period where the patient evaluates their cervical symptoms during the rest period. Adjust the arc and speed of motion based on feedback from the patient. Ensure that the patient's head and neck muscles are completely relaxed and that the full weight of the head is resting on the pillow. Take care that the arc of your therapeutic most is not repetitively placed through the C4-C6 segments post-injury or secondary to a painful flare up of discogenic instability.

Therapeutic Exercise

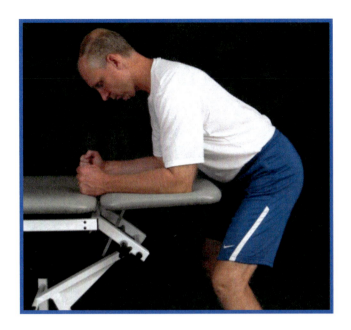

Figure 16-2: Cervical Stabilization- Isometric Cervical Extensor Muscle Training – Supported Hip Hinge Position:

Figure 16-2 shows our principal or beginning position for light isometric cervical extensor muscle training. The patient is instructed to widen their base of support by abducting their hip and then hip hinge over the edge of a treatment table. This will bring the head, neck, and trunk in front of the vertical plane facilitating isometric contraction of their cervical extensor muscles. Patients are instructed to move the chin down and in toward the anterior aspect of their neck (Adams Apple in this text), and elongate the posterior aspect of their neck (make the back of their neck long). This small movement of the chin will contract the cervical flexor muscles so that co-contraction is achieved during this exercise. This exercise can be the first step in strength building for the cervical extensor muscles. Isometric hold times should be a minimum of 6 -10 seconds and repeated a minimum 6 -10 times with two to three sets prescribed. To minimize patient position changes, the isometric muscle contractions could be held for longer periods of time; four times for 30 seconds works well. In terms of manual resisted exercise (MRE), manual isometric pressures can be applied by the therapist and held for 6-10 seconds. The manual isometric pressures should be applied from various angles against the various portions of the posterior aspect of the head.

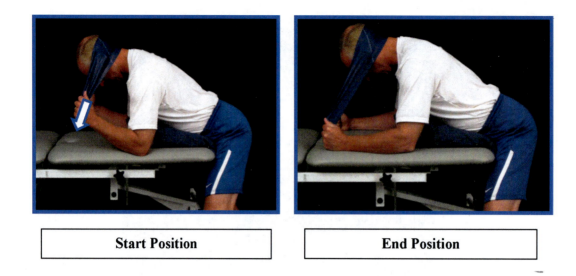

| Start Position | End Position |

Figure 16-3: Cervical Stabilization- Isometric Cervical Extensor Muscle Training- Supported Hip Hinge Position:

This figure shows the incorporation of elastic band in order to increase the level of isometric contraction. Note, how the elastic band is wrapped around the patient's head, and how the tension of the band is increased by extending the elbows. As the elbows are straightened, the increased elastic tension from the band will cause a greater degree of resultant isometric muscle contraction. Again, regarding pre-positioning of the cervical spine prior to the application of the isometric muscle training, the patient is asked to gently bring their chin down and in toward their Adams Apple in order to elongate the back of their neck. This small movement of the chin will contract the cervical flexor muscles so co-contraction is achieved during the exercise. I use exercises 16-2 and 16-3 as a starting point for stability training when mid- cervical segments demonstrate discogenic symptomatic hypermobility[34, 35]. Isometric hold times should be held a minimum of 6 -10 seconds and repeated a minimum 6 -10 times with two to three prescribed. To minimize patient position changes, the isometric muscle contractions could be held for longer periods of times; four times for 30 seconds works well. Regarding home-based exercise carry over; hip hinging can be performed over the edge of a table or counter top. Be sure to incorporate a pillow to reduce edge pressure in the abdominal area and to support the lumbar spine.

Therapeutic Exercise

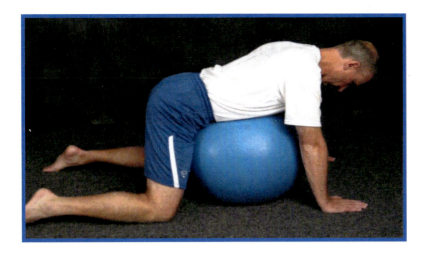

Figure 16-4: Cervical Stabilization- Isometric Cervical Extensor Muscle Training- Quadruped:

If the patient prefers, the four-point position can be used to achieve improved isometric cervical extensor muscle strength. Again, the patient is asked to elongate the back of their neck by moving their chin down and in toward their Adams Apple. Light isometric training of the cervical extensors is achieved as these muscles must hold up the weight of the head against gravity. This version of light isometric training is a good starting point for stability training when mid- cervical segments demonstrate symptomatic hypermobility[34, 35]. When treating in the four-point position my preference is to have the patient hold this head-neck position for 30 seconds and repeat the isometric training at least four times.

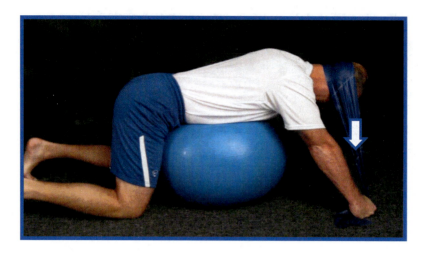

Figure 16-5: Cervical Stabilization- Isometric Cervical Extensor Muscle Training- quadruped:

Similar to figure 16-3 the level of isometric strength training can be increased when treating in the four-point position by incorporating elastic band. The patient is asked to elongate the back of their neck by moving their chin down and in toward their Adams Apple. Note, how the elastic band is wrapped around the patient's head, and how the tension of the band is increased by extending the elbows. As the elbows are straightened, the increased elastic tension from the band will cause a greater degree of resultant isometric muscle contraction. Isometric muscle contractions should be held for a minimum of 6-10 seconds and repeated at least 6-10 times. To minimize patient position changes, the isometric muscle contractions could be held for longer periods of times; four times for 30 seconds works well.

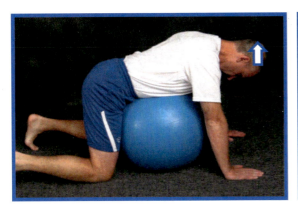 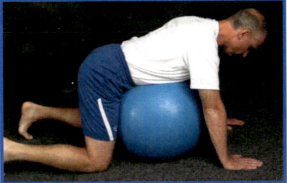

Figure 16-6: Cervical Stabilization- Short Arc Isotonic Cervical Extensor Muscle Training – Quadruped:

After a platform of isometric strength has been built, further cervical extensor muscle training can now be developed by incorporating short arc isotonic cervical extension. Often I begin this exercise by keeping the isotonic motion isolated to the upper cervical (UC) segments only while the remainder of the lower cervical spine is kept in a neutral or mid-position. This short arc movement pattern will build cervical extensor strength while at the same time protecting symptomatic lower cervical segments that may be degenerated, hypermobile, or painful[34, 35]. The arc of motion can be carefully increased to incorporate movement of lower cervical (LC) segments. Two quick notes, first placement of the Swiss ball as shown in these quadruped stabilization exercises will add support to the lumbar segments (Chapter 18). Second and this is a point of review, resistance training for the cervical extensor muscles is achieved as the patient lifts the weight of their head against gravity. Three sets of 6-10 short arc isotonic motions are typically prescribed and if well tolerated additional reps can be added.

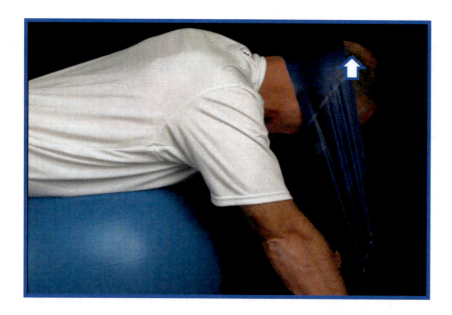

16-7: Cervical Stabilization-Short Arc Isotonic Cervical Extensor Muscle Training - Quadruped:

Now elastic band is added to increase resistance and as a result cervical extensor muscular strength. If cervical stabilization training has progressed to short arc isotonic motions, and if these motions are well tolerated, the patient is progressed to resisted short arc isotonic cervical extension. In cases of cervical pathology, it is important to keep the arc of movement small. Note, when the head and neck is in front of the vertical plane in this quadruped position the head never falls behind the neck and usually, we are able to prevent pathological posterior translation of cervical segment(s) during active or resisted short arc isotonic cervical extension. In cases of cervical injury or discogenic/degenerative hypermobility, cervical extension is typically less painful in these two exercise positions as compared to the upright position. One last note, if the "preciseness" of the short arc movement pattern becomes compromised when elastic band resistance is added the patient may need to revert back to the isometric training procedure and simply pull the elastic band down over their head by changing their elbow angle. Three sets of 6-10 short arc isotonic motions are typically prescribed.

Therapeutic Exercise

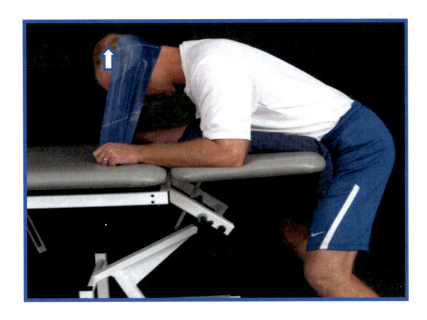

Figure 16-8: Cervical Stabilization- Short Arc Isotonic Cervical Extensor Muscle Training - Supported Hip Hinge Position:

Now we are back to the patient supporting himself over the edge of a table. Note how the pillow will reduce edge pressure from the table and will also support the lumbar segments. To expand on my comments in figure 16-7, if short arc isotonic movement against elastic band resistance is prescribed, monitor the quality of movement. The resisted cervical extension should look "angular" and be recruited from cranial to caudal. If the movement of the head and neck looks translatory in a posterior direction, then too much resistance has been added. To repeat, if the preciseness of the short arc movement pattern becomes compromised when elastic band resistance is added the patient may need to revert back to the isometric training procedure and simply pull the elastic band down over their head by changing their elbow angle. Three sets of 6-10 short arc isotonic motions or are typically prescribed.

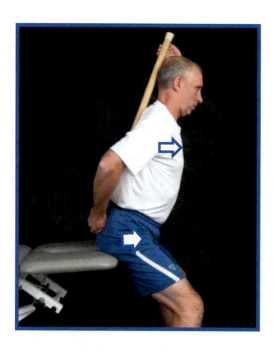

Figure 16-9: Cervical Stabilization, Isometric Co-contraction of Extensor and Flexor Muscles – Hip Hinge Movement Pattern:

There are a number of different ways to hip hinge. Most of which we will cover in the lumbar spine chapter. Seated in an elevated position and using a stick for tactile reinforcement, in other words keeping your chest up and the back of your neck long, is one way to hinge form the hips. I mentioned earlier in this chapter that when the head and neck are moved in front of the vertical plane, the extensor muscles will contract (dynamic stabilization). This is one of the main reasons for hip hinging. Hinging will build strength in all of the spinal extensor muscles including the cervical extensors. So have your patient lift their chest up and forward, lengthen the back of their neck by bringing their chin down and in toward their Adams Apple (cervical flexor contraction) and have them execute a hip hinge. Movement of the trunk in front of the vertical plane will cause isometric extensor muscle contraction. Hold this position for a minimum of 6-10 seconds and repeat a minimum of 6-10 times. To minimize position changes the prescription of four 30 second isometric co-contractions in the position just described will also improve dynamic (muscular based) stability.

Therapeutic Exercise

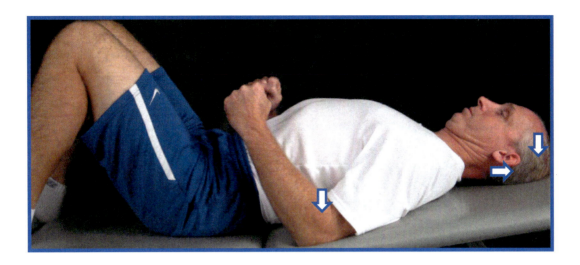

Figure 16-10: Cervical Stabilization- Isometric Tripod Exercise – Supine:

This is a slightly more aggressive cervical and thoracic extensor muscle strength training exercise. The patient is asked to isometrically contract their deep cervical flexors by sliding the back of their head up the table and bringing their chin down and in toward their Adams Apple. After this, have your patient press the back of their head and both elbows into the table. At this point there will be isometric contraction of the cervical flexors and extensors. This is the Tripod exercise and it is an excellent training procedure for athletes and even some of our patients. Note, be careful when prescribing this exercise if there is a greater degree of arthritic and degenerative change. Instruct your clients to hold this position for a minimum of 6-10 seconds and repeat a minimum of 6-10 times.

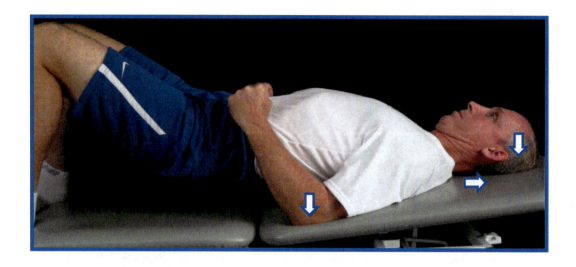

Figure 16-11: Cervical Stabilization Isometric Tripod Exercise – Advanced Position

This is the Tripod Advanced Position procedure. Similar to exercise 16-10, the patient is asked to isometrically contract their deep cervical flexors by sliding the back of their head up the table and bringing their chin down and in toward their Adams Apple. Next, the patient is to press the back of their head and both elbows into the table. After accomplishing these first two aspects of this exercise, the patient is then instructed to perform a bridge which will increase the level of isometric contraction of the lumbar extensor muscles. Again, the Tripod exercise and it is an excellent training procedure for athletes and even some of our less complicated patients. Note, be careful with this exercise if there is a greater degree of arthritic and degenerative change. Instruct your clients to hold this position for a minimum of 6-10 seconds and repeat a minimum of 6-10 times. Athletes with young healthy cervical spines can hold this position for 30 seconds or more.

Therapeutic Exercise

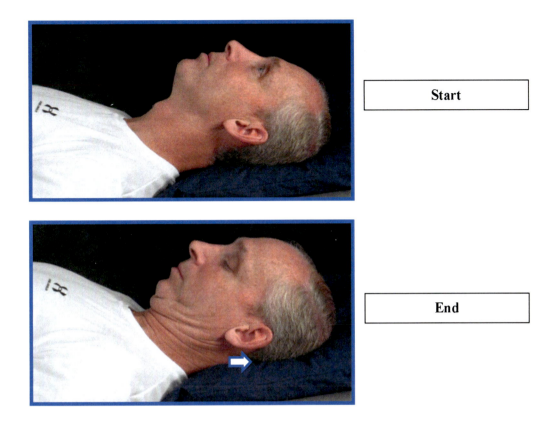

Figure 16-12: Cervical Stabilization- Isotonic Cervical Ventral Flexor Muscle Training - Supine Head Slide:

We have mentioned the deep cervical flexor muscles already; now let's look at a few more exercises directed toward building strength in that same muscle group. This is the isotonic head slide exercise where the patient is asked to slide the back of their head up the table (pillow) while bringing their chin down and in toward their Adams Apple. This exercise is performed at a comfortable rate of speed and with a short arc of movement. The head and neck should be well supported and the start position for the exercise should be slight cervical extension such that the patient's eyes are just above the horizontal. The end position of the exercise should find the eyes just below the horizontal with the back of head still resting on the pillow. Three sets of 6-10 short arc isotonic motions are typically prescribed hold the end position isometrically for 6-10 seconds.

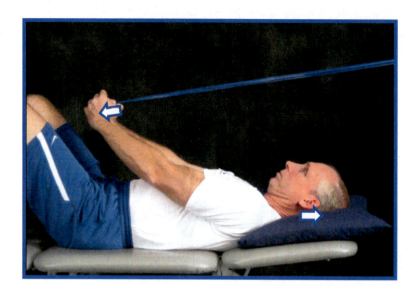

Figure 16-13: Cervical Stabilization, Isometric Deep Cervical Flexor Training with UE Depression, Cervical Supported Position:

This exercise brings UE movement into the equation. The UE pattern is resisted depression with assisted elevation. Now, there are a couple of points to make regarding the value of this exercise. UE elevation will at times provoke cervical pain particularly if it is accompanied by cervical extension. Given this, we assist the UE elevation with elastic band to minimize pain provocation during the UE movement. Next, patients will often unnecessarily extend their neck when elevating their UE's during common daily activities. This procedure trains the patient to keep the back of their neck long during UE elevation by using the cervical flexor muscles. The isometric head slide exercise is performed and held during multiple sets of UE elevation and depression. In cases of more acute, sub-acute flares of cervical discomfort, keep the head and neck well supported with pillows. Also, if a patient has a more rigid thoracic kyphosis, this position is preferred over figure 16-14.

Therapeutic Exercise

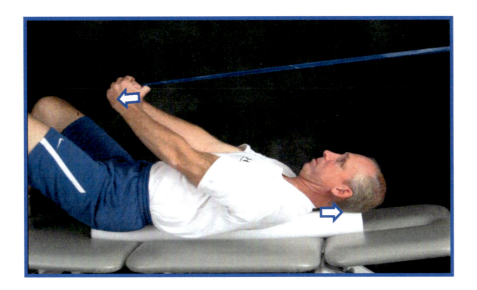

Figure 16-14: Cervical Stabilization, Isometric Co-contraction of Extensor and Ventral Flexor Muscles – Advanced Position

This exercise is similar to 16-13. In cases of less symptomatic cervical injury or degenerative hypermobility[34,35] and when the thoracic segments are able to flatten (extend) the firm foam roller can be used to reinforce good posture while isometrically training the cervical flexor muscles to contract and lengthen the posterior aspect of the neck during UE elevation. At the same time this exercise provides assisted motion training to the UE elevator muscles. Therapists should help their patients to understand that elongation of the posterior aspect of the neck through ventral flexor muscle contraction during UE elevation and lifting will enhance dynamic (muscular based) segmental stability.

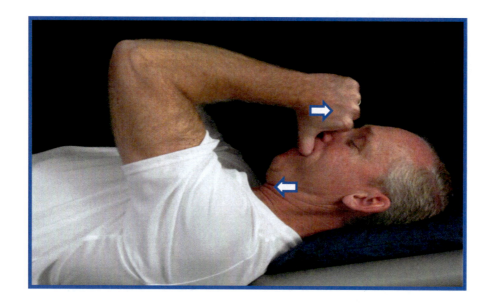

Figure 16-15: Cervical Stabilization, Isometric Cervical Ventral Flexor Muscle Training

I know this exercise looks a little weird, but I can explain it and we will go over it again in figure 16-18. The supine head slide stabilization exercise (figure 16-12) is an excellent way to build strength in the deep cervical flexor muscles. This procedure is an isometric version. The patient is instructed to look down at their belly button but the head slide motion is resisted by the palmar surfaces of both thumbs which are placed against the back upper molars. You might ask, why use this contact point? Over many years I have tried various contact points to isometrically exercise the cervical flexors, and with all things considered, I find this the best one. The point of fixation (the thumbs) is very close to the anterior aspect of the cervical vertebral bodies where the deep flexor muscles attach, the teeth are separated which is good for the TMJs and some of the smaller superficial cervical flexor muscles are placed in a relaxed and slackened position by opening the mouth. Hold this isometric strength building position for a minimum of 6-10 seconds and repeat a minimum of 6-10 times.

Therapeutic Exercise

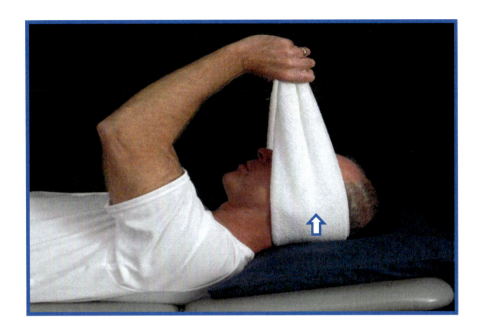

Figure 16-16: Cervical Stabilization - Assisted Isotonic Cervical Ventral Flexor Muscle Training

This procedure is an assisted short arc isotonic exercise that facilitates contraction of both the superficial and deep cervical flexors. The word short is to be taken literally here. We are not looking or asking for a large degree of cervical flexion. Large amplitude cervical flexion can irritate and injure the spinal cord in the presence of spondylotic changes and is generally not helpful for the posterior cervical ligaments. The patient who may need this exercise is the one who expresses that their head feels very heavy and may need their hands to assist bringing their head and neck along with their trunk during transitional movements such as supine to sitting or side-lying to sitting. The patient is instructed to lift the back of their head off the pillow. Both hands lightly pull forward to assist this motion. Standard multi-set, multi-rep strength training procedures apply to this exercise.

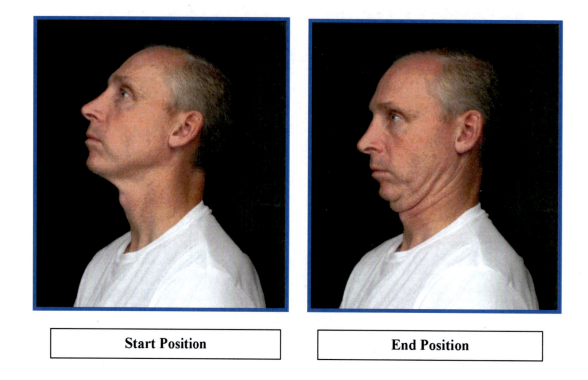

| Start Position | End Position |

Figure 16-17: Cervical Stabilization-Isotonic Ventral Flexor Muscle Training
Cervical Wall Slide Exercise:

This head slide exercise is really the same as the supine head slide. So, you might ask why we need it. First, I usually don't prescribe this procedure unless the patient's cervical spine is essentially pain free. The supine version is unloaded and is much better when symptomatic degenerative or injury based hypermobility is present. The positive point about the standing version of this exercise is that it may help a patient to better understand how to posture their neck when in an upright position and during ADLs. So, while this is a strength building exercise, I also look upon this procedure as neuromuscular re-education. One last note, bringing the chin down and in towards the Adams Apple, the upper right figure, will provide your patient with enhanced muscular based stability during all UE ADLs and transitional movement patterns. Posturing the neck in this way is an important aspect of teaching patients "dynamic" muscular based stability during daily movement patterns. Note, in patients with rigid and excessive thoracic kyphosis, the cervical spine will have to be significantly extended in order for the head to reach the wall and in that scenario prescription of this exercise is not a good idea.

Therapeutic Exercise

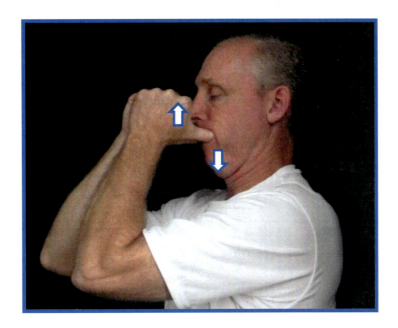

Figure 16-18: Cervical Stabilization, Isometric Cervical Ventral Flexor Muscle Training-Standing:

Here is that weird position again with the thumbs in the mouth. Instruct your patient to look down at their belly button. The head slide motion is resisted by the palmar surfaces of both thumbs which are placed against the back upper molars. Note the back of the neck should be in a lengthened position. Let me repeat the virtues of this manual resistance contact point. The point of fixation (the thumbs) is very close to the anterior aspect of the cervical vertebral bodies where the deep cervical flexor muscles attach, the teeth are separated which is good for the TMJs and some of the smaller superficial cervical flexor muscles are placed in a slackened position when the mouth is opened. Hold this position for a minimum of 6-10 seconds and repeat a minimum of 6-10 times. Remember, have the patient keep their chest (sternum) in an upward and forward position (thoracic extension) during this and all other cervical stabilization and self-mobilization exercises.

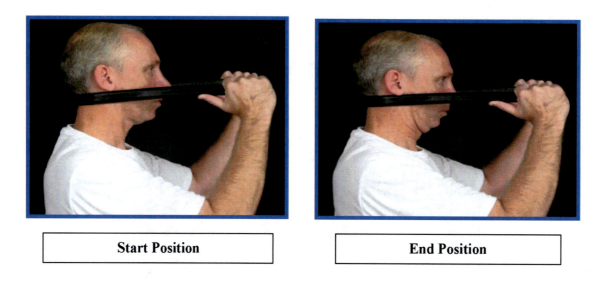

| Start Position | End Position |

Figure 16-19: Active Cervical Self-Mobilization, C0/C1 Flexion:

Now we are going to start a fairly long section on cervical self-mobilization. The first several exercises are termed active self-mobilizations because the patient is taught to use their own neuromuscular system to perform an isolated motion in a particular direction to select levels of the spine. You will also note that a belt is used to help isolate movement as well as possible. In general, for motions involving flexion the patient will be instructed to press their neck back into the belt. For movements involving extension, the patient is instructed to move their neck over the top edge of the belt. C0/C1 flexion self-mobilization is instructed by having the patient lift their chest up and forward, lengthen the back of their neck, and repetitively bring their chin down and in toward their Adams Apple. The start position is one where the eyes are just above the horizontal and during the motion the eyes move down even with the horizontal plane. The patient is to lightly press backward into the belt during the exercise. The axis of motion for this exercise is right through the ears (external auditory meatus). Six to ten reps are typically performed and repeated as needed when the patient perceives this motion to be limited and painful.

Therapeutic Exercise

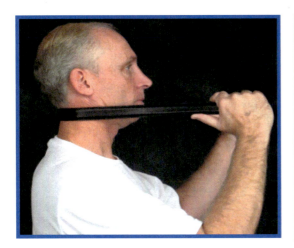 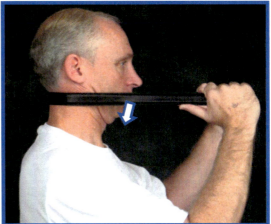

Figure 16-20: Active Cervical Self-Mobilization, C1/C2 Flexion:

C1/C2 flexion self- mobilization is instructed by having the patient lift their chest up and forward, lengthen the back of their neck, and repetitively bring their chin down and in toward their Adams Apple. The start position is one where the eyes are level with the horizontal plane and during the motion the eyes move down just below the horizontal plane. The patient is to lightly press backward into the belt during the exercise. The axis of motion for this exercise is right through the ears. Six to ten reps are typically performed and repeated as needed when the patient perceives this motion to be limited and painful. Note, for all of these active self-mobilizations the remainder of the neck that is below the belt is to remain vertical. Also, it is important for the patient to not shrug their shoulders during the exercise motion. Let's talk above moving the belt to different segments. For self-mobilization of the C0/C1 segment the top edge of the belt should be in contact with the base of the skull. For C1/C2 teach the patient to slide the belt down a half of an inch. For C2/C3 slide the belt down another half of an inch. Each half inch increment will approximate the posterior aspect of each cervical vertebra. Last note, exercise 16-9 and 16-10 may prove useful in cases of cervicogenic headache, particularly when UC extension is noted as a postural impairment.

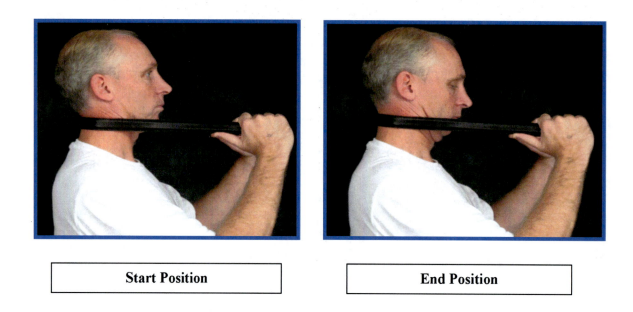

| Start Position | End Position |

Figure 16-21: Active Cervical Self-Mobilization, C2/C3 Flexion:

C2/C3 flexion self-mobilization is instructed by having the patient lift their chest up and forward, lengthen the back of their neck, and repetitively bring their chin down and in toward their Adams Apple. The start position is one where the eyes are level with the horizontal plane and during the motion the eyes move down just below the horizontal plane. The therapist should palpate the C2/C3 interspinous space and the patient is taught to stop the movement when motion is palpated at this level. The patient is to lightly press backward into the belt during the exercise. The axis of motion for this exercise is right through the ears. Six to ten reps are typically performed and repeated as needed when the patient perceives this motion to be limited and painful. Usually I do not have patients perform cervical self-mobilization below the C2/C3 segment. Often, patient's move less specifically than we would like and motion is carried into the C3/C4 segment when performing this exercise. Discogenic break down leading to segmental hypermobility is most commonly found at the C4/C5, C5/C6, and C6/C7 segments therefore in most cases, I do not recommend repetitive self-mobilization at these levels.

Therapeutic Exercise

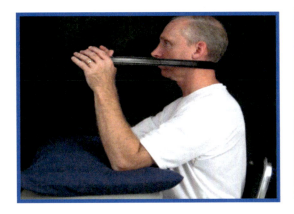
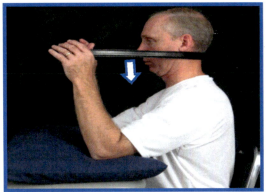

Figure 16-22: Active Cervical Self-Mobilization, C0/C1, C1/C2, and C2/3 Flexion UE Supported on a Pillow and Table:

Figure 16-22 demonstrates a different and very useful patient position. The therapeutic motion is the same as the previous three exercises and is isolated to the segment or segments where pain and motion impairment is found. Patients with more widespread cervical and shoulder girdle discomfort or a tension sensitive cervical radiculitis will find this position, where the shoulder girdles and upper arms are supported, to be much more comfortable when performing active self-mobilization. Now, to repeat an important point made with the last exercise, with the exception of the C7/T1 segment, I do not recommend repetitive self-mobilization below the C2 or the C3 segment in most cases. If on the other hand a patient has advanced cervical spondylotic changes with multi-segment hypomobility, then other mid-cervical segments may also require self-mobilization.

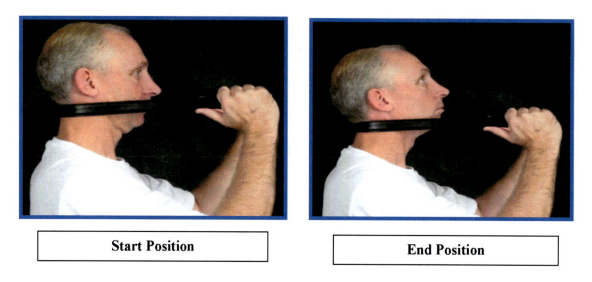

| Start Position | End Position |

Figure 16-23: Active Cervical Self-Mobilization, Upper Cervical C0/C1, C1/C2 and C2/C3

Extension

The extension self-mobilization series is very similar in terms of basic patient instruction. First, have the patient lift their chest up and forward and lengthen the back of their neck. Now the top edge of the belt is used as a fulcrum point and the patient is instructed to repetitively bring lift their chin up and away from their Adams Apple. The start position is one where the eyes are just below the horizontal and during the motion for C0/C1 the eyes move up even with the horizontal plane. For C1/C2 the eyes are to move just above the horizontal plane and for the C2/C3 segment, the motion is stopped as it is felt to arrive at the C2/C3 interspace. The axis of motion for this exercise is remains through the external auditory meatus (ears). Six-ten reps are typically performed and repeated as needed when the patient perceives this motion to be limited and painful.

Therapeutic Exercise

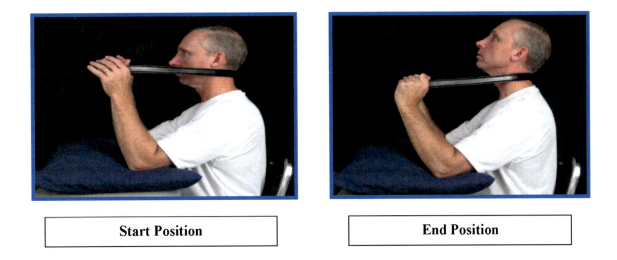

Start Position | End Position

Figure 16-24: Active Cervical Self-Mobilization, C0/C1, C1/C2, and C2/C3 Extension UE Supported on a Pillow and Table:

The therapeutic motion and patient instructions are the same as found in the previous exercise. Patients with more widespread cervical and shoulder girdle discomfort or a tension sensitive cervical radiculitis will find this position, where the shoulder girdles and upper arms are supported, to be much more comfortable when performing active self-mobilization. Remember, the top edge of the belt is used as a fulcrum point to backward bend (extend) each individual segment over the belt. Make sure that the patient's sternum (chest and rib cage) is in an upward and forward position. Instruct the patient to repetitively lift their chin up and away from their Adams Apple with a very small motion (short arc isotonic). The start and end position are the same as discussed in figure 16-23. The axis of motion should remain through the ears and six-ten reps are typically performed and repeated as needed when the patient perceives this motion to be limited and painful.

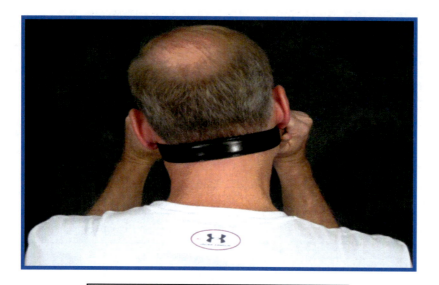

Left side bending and right rotation

Figure 16-25: Active Cervical Self-Mobilization, C0/C1 Coupled Rotation:

It is generally agreed that the direction of motion coupling at the Occiput-Atlas joints is opposite side bending and rotation. Coupled motion is motion that is mechanically forced to occur together during an active movement. This means that left side bending at C0/C1 will produce right rotation at that same segmental level and right side bending will produce a left rotation. Regarding this self-mobilization, note that the belt is placed just under the occiput wrapping around the posterior arch of C1. The belt will constrain the movement of the C1 vertebrae. This will allow greater soft tissue stretching between the occiput and atlas. The patient is to pull forward on both ends of the belt in order to stabilize the caudal vertebra of the segments being mobilized. Using both demonstration and passive motion applied by the therapist, the patient is taught to left side bend and right rotation occiput on atlas as seen above. Remember, both motions are to occur together and the arc of this movement is very small at C0/C1. Six to ten reps can be performed and then right side bending with left rotation is performed if coupled rotation is restricted in that direction. As a general rule, 6-10 reps per motion segment is usually about right in terms of these active belt stabilized self-mobilizations.

Therapeutic Exercise

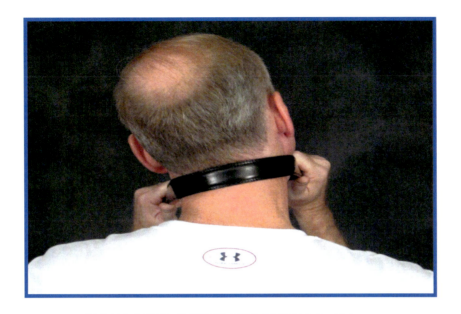

Left side bending and right rotation

Figure 16-26: Active Cervical Self-Mobilization, C0/C1 and C1/C2 Coupled Rotation:

Now the belt is moved downward a half of an inch and is wrapped around the posterior arch of C2. Through visual demonstration of the motion and passive movement applied by the therapist's hands on the patient's head, the patient is taught to couple side bending and rotation through both the C0/C1 and C1/C2 levels. Except in cases of severe cervical motion loss, usually due to severe spondylotic hypertrophy, there should be significantly more coupled rotation available when both of these upper cervical levels are actively mobilized. The belt is now wrapped around the posterior arch of C2 and the patient is to pull forward on the belt with both hands. Active upper cervical side bending and rotation will allow the occiput and atlas to rotate on a stabilized C2. Six to ten reps can be performed and then repeated on the opposite side if needed. Remember, the objective here is too gently self-mobilize (loosen) the upper cervical segments without placing excessive rotational movement through the UC region and without excessively loading the upper cervical ligamentous structures.

Therapeutic Exercise

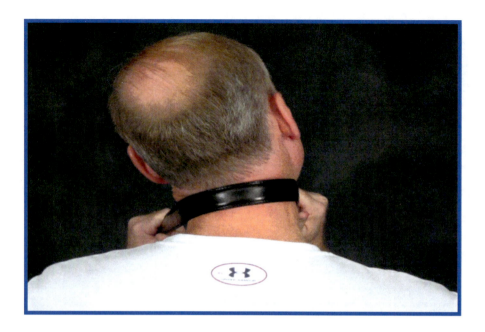

Left side bending and right rotation

Figure 16-27: Active Cervical Self-Mobilization, Upper Cervical Coupled Rotation, Non-Coupled Lower Cervical Rotation and Resultant Facet Distraction at C2/C3:

Look carefully at this figure and note that the belt has been dropped another half of an inch so that it is wrapped around the vertebral lamina of C3. This will allow for movement at three segments now. The patient will be able to perform coupled rotation at C0/C1, C1/C2, and non-coupled rotation at the C2/C3 segment which is part of the lower cervical spine. The leather belt wrapped around the vertebral lamina will prevent motion in the segments below the belt. This will protect sensitive, symptomatic hypermobile/degenerated mid-cervical segments. Through visual demonstration of the motion and passive movement or active assisted movement applied by the therapist, the patients is taught to side bend and rotate in the opposite direction through three motion segments. Verbal cues may also assist your patient to better understand this movement pattern. For example, instruct your patient to look backward, upward and to the right to facilitate this rotational movement. Six to ten reps can be performed and then repeated on the opposite side if needed. Non-coupled motion placed through a lower cervical segment will cause rotational motion through the disc joint and gapping (distraction) and resultant capsular stretching at the facet joint on the same side to which the head-neck is rotating.

Therapeutic Exercise

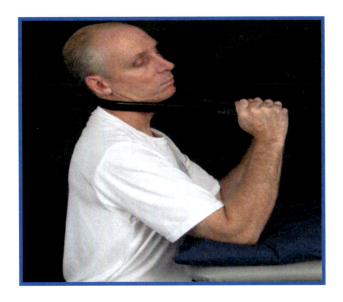

Right side bending and right rotation

Figure 16-28: Active Dorsal Caudal Glide Self Mobilization, C2/C3 UE Supported:

Note that the belt is wrapped around the vertebral lamina of C3. This will allow for movement at three segments again. Non-coupled rotation will occur at C0/C1, C1/C2, and coupled rotation at the C2/C3 segment which is part of the lower cervical spine. Verbal cues may also assist your patient to better understand this movement pattern. For example, instruct your patient to look backward and downward as they side bend and rotate over the top edge of the belt combining side bending and rotation in the same direction through the C2 segment. Six to ten reps can be performed and then repeated on the opposite side if needed. Given the anatomical construction of the C2 segment, segmental hypermobility secondary to disc degeneration is not commonly seen. Self-mobilization exercise applied through the C2/C3 segment can assist in improving cervical rotation. Remember, to assist your patient in the performance of the correct movement pattern, have them look backward, downward, and to the right or left as they actively rotate over the top edge of the belt. If your patient struggles with the performance of lower cervical coupled rotation in extension (dorsal/caudal gliding), have him or her perform transverse plane rotation instead.

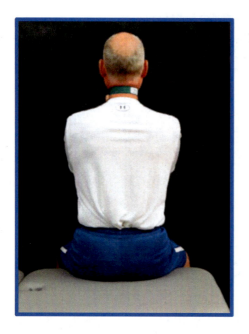 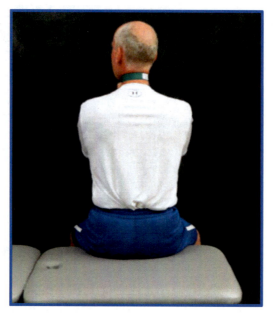

Figure 16-29: Lower Cervical Transverse Plane Rotation Self-Mobilization:

Exercises 16-27 and 16-28 ask our patients to perform non-coupled and coupled lower cervical rotation for the purposes of self-mobilizing restricted motion segments. While the biomechanical theory of facet joint distraction and facet gliding causing facet joint capsular stretching is sound, the actual motor performance of these two exercises can be quite challenging. Therefore, having your patient perform pure transverse plane rotation, seen above, with a belt stabilizing the caudal vertebrae of a given motion segment gives our patients with limited lower cervical rotation a very good stretching procedure that is much easier to perform correctly. Generally speaking, the main idea behind these lower cervical self-mobilizations is to protect the often degenerated and often hypermobile C4, C5, and C6 motion segments. Rotational self-mobilization of the C2 and C3 segments will usually improve our patient's cervical rotation without irritating the lower segments in the lower cervical region.

Therapeutic Exercise

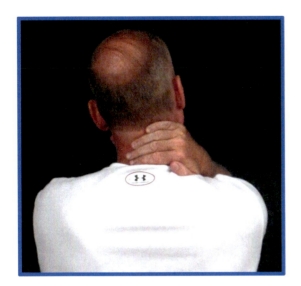 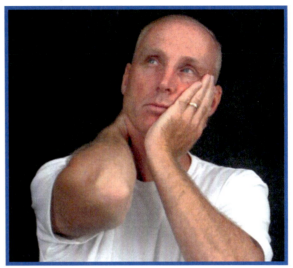

Figure 16-30: Passive Coupled Rotation Self Mobilization C0/C1, C1/C2, and C2/C3

Note the word passive and note that there is no belt any longer. In general, when it comes to the smaller and more delicate cervical segments, my preference is to start with active self-mobilization techniques. Active self-mobilization techniques train the neuromuscular system to better control cervical segmental motion and this is more easily translated into improved cervical movement patterns where we can train the patient to stop extra and unnecessary mid-cervical motion. Through visual demonstration of the motion and passive movement applied by the therapist to the patient's head and neck, the patients are taught to side bend and rotate in the opposite direction through each of the upper three motion segments. Note the position of the hand on the lower portion of the chin. After the patient has performed a side bending motion with an axis through the tip of the nose, the chin is passively moved upward to create passive rotation in the opposite direction. The patient's other hand acts similar to the belt in terms of constraining and minimizing motion in the mid-cervical segments. Six to ten reps of passive rotation can be performed and then repeated on the opposite side if needed.

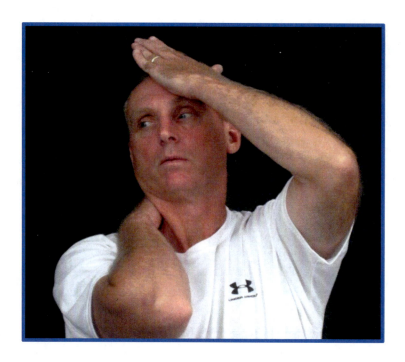

Figure 16 -31: Passive C2/C3 Dorsal Caudal Glide Self- Mobilization

This is another passive self-mobilization which incorporates the patient's hand to push and other hand to stabilize segments below C2. To repeat one additional time, in general, when it comes to the smaller and more delicate cervical segments, my preference is to start with active self-mobilization techniques (Figures 16-19 -16-28). Active self-mobilization techniques train the neuromuscular system to better control cervical segmental motion and this is more easily translated into improved cervical movement patterns where we can train the patient to stop extra and unnecessary motion through mid-cervical segments which often show degenerative break down and associated hypermobility. For this passive self-mobilization exercise, the patient is instructed to place one hand on their forehead (temple region) while the ulnar aspect of the other hand wraps around the vertebral lamia of C3 on the opposite side. The patient is instructed to look backward and downward and to gently push their head and neck in that same direction over a stable C3 segment. Six to ten reps can be performed and then repeated on the opposite side if needed. No significant amount of rotation or extension should be seen below C3.

Therapeutic Exercise

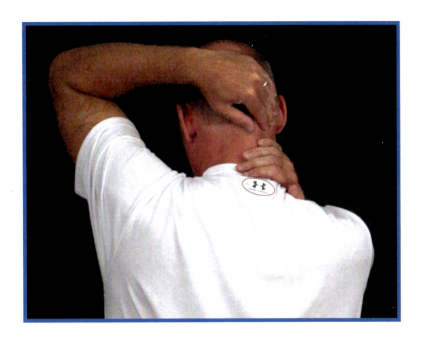

Figure 16-32: Passive C2/C3 Ventral Cranial Glide Self-Mobilization

The last passive self-mobilization for the C2 segment is a ventral-cranial gliding motion of the C2 inferior facet. Again, have your patient lift their chest up and forward and make the back of their neck long. The ulnar aspect of the stabilizing hand is wrapped around the bilateral vertebral lamina of C3. The self-mobilizing hand is placed on the lamina and inferior facet of C2 and passively pulls one side of this segment in and upward and forward (ventral/cranial) direction. As with all of these self-mobilizations, the remainder of the cervical spine must remain vertical. Very little motion should be seen to occur below the C2/C3 segment. In order to keep the axis of movement close to the C2 disc, the patient must be shown how to "pull" the opposite side of their chin inward and downward as the self-mobilizing hand pulls the C2 lamina and facet upward and forward. Six to ten reps can be performed and then repeated on the opposite side if needed.

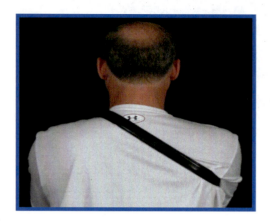
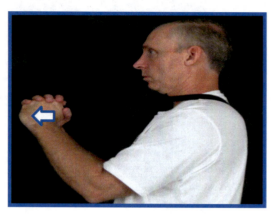

Figure 16-33: Passive Cervical Self-Mobilization, C7/T1 Ventral/Cranial Self-Mobilization, Cervical Segments in Mid-Position:

The C7/T1 segment is prone to the development of motion loss (stiffness impairment) as people age. Therefore, we will devote several self-mobilization exercises to this particular segment. This first procedure will keep the upper and mid cervical segments in a mid-position. The patient is shown to place a standard 1-inch belt with the buckle just in front of the axilla. Next the patient adducts their arm down onto the belt to stabilize it in the axilla. The remainder of the belt is placed over the nape of the neck on the opposite side so that it crosses over the lamina of the C7 vertebrae. Using both hands the patient is taught to pull the end of the belt forward. This motion will drag the lamina of C7 forward producing a passive rotation of C7 on T1. The patient should pull forward on the belt until the belt compresses the over lying soft tissues which will press against the lamina and move the vertebrae. This exercise should be performed in an oscillating manner six to ten times and repeated on the opposite side if necessary. Remember, rotational motion loss at the C7 segment will prevent rotational motion recruitment into the upper thoracic segments. T1-T3 need to contribute to our patient's total cervical rotation.

Therapeutic Exercise

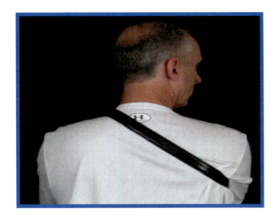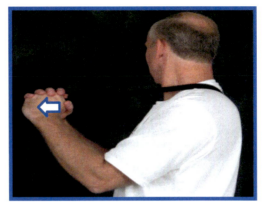

Figure 16-34: Passive Cervical Self-Mobilization, C7/T1 Ventral/Cranial Self-Mobilization,

End range rotation:

To repeat, as compared to the C4, C5, and C6 segments, the C7/T1 segment is prone to a greater degree of motion loss (stiffness impairment) as people age. This second procedure seeks to take up segmental soft tissue slack in the direction of cervical rotation restriction prior to loosening the C7/T1 segment. The patient is shown to place a standard 1-inch belt with the buckle just in front of the axilla. Next, the patient adducts their arm down onto the belt to stabilize it. The remainder of the belt is placed over the nape of the neck so that it crosses over the lamina on the opposite side. Using both hands the patient is taught to pull the end of the belt forward. This motion will drag the lamina of C7 forward producing a passive rotation of C7 on T1. The patient should pull forward on the belt until the belt compresses the over lying soft tissues which will press against the lamina and move the vertebrae. This exercise should be performed in an oscillating manner six to ten times and repeated on the opposite side if necessary.

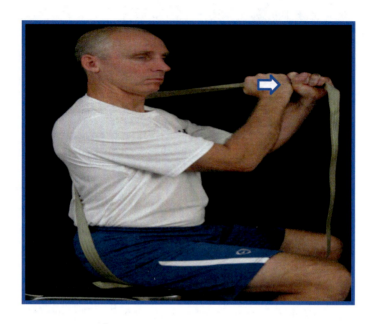

Figure 16-35: Passive Cervical Self-Mobilization, C7/T1 Ventral/Cranial Self-Mobilization, Clinic Based Version:

This version of C7/T1 self-mobilization works well in the clinic prior to the application of manual mobilization applied to the C7 segment. The procedure is essentially the same as versions 16-32 and 16-33, but now the patient places the buckle of a mobilization belt medial to their thigh, sits on the belt to stabilize it, and then pulls forward to mobilize the C7 inferior facet in an upward and forward or ventral/cranial direction. This exercise should be performed in an oscillating manner six to ten times and repeated on the opposite side if necessary. Note, the T1 segment is stabilized to some extent by that vertebra's connection to the rib cage.

Therapeutic Exercise

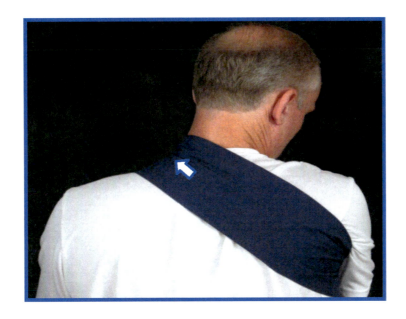

Figure 16-36: Cervical Self-Massage, Ventral/Cranial Motion

Use a repeating (oscillating) motion and a towel or pillow case with a broad, diffuse surface. Stabilize one end of the towel in the axilla. Use a light repetitive pulling motion to massage shoulder girdle elevator tissues. This will give the patient a nice self-massage when the shoulder girdle elevator muscles are sore perhaps due to overuse or pain referral from the cervical spine. Repeat the massaging motion until the soft tissue in this area becomes less painful.

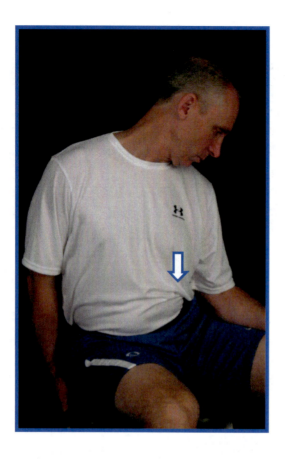

Figure 16-37 Cervical Axioscapular Muscle Self-Stretching- Levator Scapula

There are a couple of points to discuss with regard to this first axioscapular muscle self-stretch. First, I do not care for versions which have the patient pull forcibly on their head with their hand. There is a great potential for segmental irritation in the presence of spondylotic hypertrophy, radicular irritation, or segmental laxity due to disc degeneration. My preference is to position the cervical segments in flexion, side bending and rotation to the same side and then position the thoracic and lumbar spine in a side bent position as well. The additional side bending of the trunk, left in this case, will shift the position of the head and neck further from a vertical/ upright position and this will allow the weight of the head to more effectively elongate this axioscapular muscle. Instruct the patient to move their head to the first stop of all three movements, side bend their trunk and hold this position for at least 30 seconds.

Therapeutic Exercise

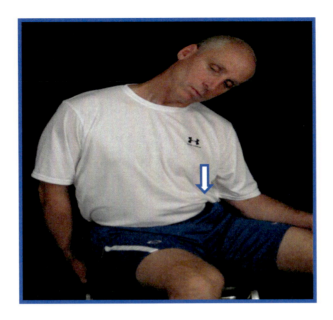

Figure 16-38: Cervical Axioscapular Muscle Self-Stretching-Upper Trapezius

To repeat the same comment from the last figure, I do not care for axioscapular self-stretching which have the patient pull forcibly on their head with their hand. Therefore, you don't see my hand on top of my head. There is a great potential for segmental irritation in the presence of spondylotic hypertrophy, radicular irritation, or segmental laxity due to disc degeneration. My preference is to position the cervical segments in flexion, side bending and rotation to the opposite side and then position the thoracic and lumbar spine in a side bent position as well. The additional side bending of the trunk, left in this case, will shift the position of the head/neck further from a vertical/ upright position and this will allow the weight of the head to more effectively elongate this axioscapular muscle. Instruct the patient to move their head to the first stop of all three movements, side bend their trunk and hold this position for at least 30 seconds.

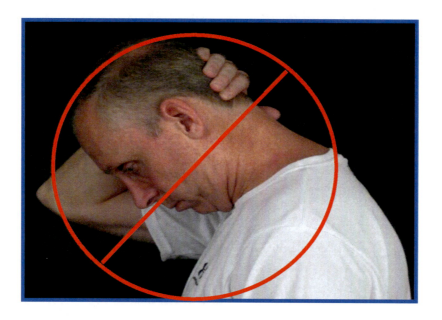

16-39: Cervical Motions with Injury Potential, Repetitive or End Range Passive Flexion

The last section of this chapter offers a word of caution regarding the over performance of generalized range of motion (ROM) exercises applied to on a repetitive basis through the mid and lower-cervical segments. Studies demonstrate that early grade disc degeneration is associated with increased angular and translational motion in certain spinal motion segments. Disc degeneration and increased segmental motion appears to occur on a more consistent basis in the C4-C6 segments[34,35]. This being the case, the question arises as to whether we should support the use of generalized ROM exercises in the presence of mild neck ache when the root cause may be early grade disc degeneration and associated increased segmental motion? As demonstrated earlier in this chapter, I believe that self-mobilization of the neck should minimize motion through the mid-cervical region and focus on active and some passive movements applied to only certain key segments that don't tend to be subject to degenerative hypermobility. So, figure 16-38 is not a movement I would support individuals applying on a repetitive basis to the cervical segments particularly if there is spondylotic hypertrophy of the posterior aspect of the vertebral body. Just think of how the spinal cord moves within the vertebral canal during flexion and you may agree with me.

Therapeutic Exercise

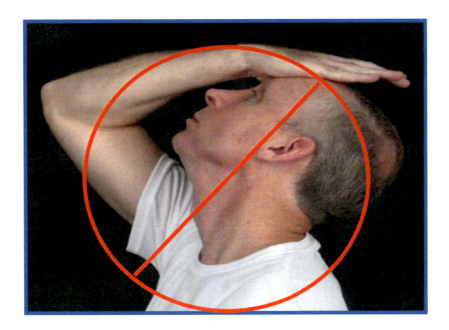

Figure 16-40: Cervical Motions with Injury Potential, Repetitive or End Range Passive Extension

I cringe when I see this movement prescribed for the neck. Pain sensitive structures are being compressed and excessive angular and translational motion in a posterior direction is likely to occur through the mid and lower cervical segments particularly after injury or in the presence of early grade disc degeneration. Excessive vertebral posterior translation can cause cervical nerve root compression and with enhance the telescoping of a superior facet up into the IVF which is not a good thing. I see no therapeutic value to the repeated application of a cervical motion I often find this motion to be quite painful when examining patients after a neck injury, with known instability, or with a painful flare up of a chronic neck condition.

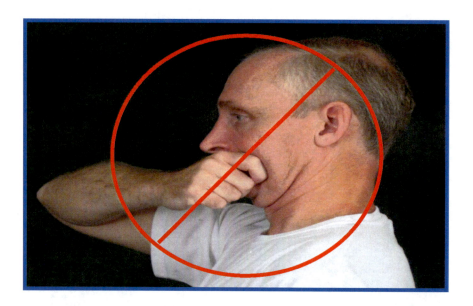

Figure 16-41: Cervical Motions with Injury Potential, Repetitive Dorsal Gliding

This therapeutic exercise motion came into being many years ago and was associated with several fairly prominent therapists. I suppose one positive attribute to this motion is that the neck is not hyper extended. Unfortunately, the lengthening of the posterior portion of the neck is achieved incorrectly. In essence, this exercise reduces the cervical lordosis (flexes) the neck, but does so in a biomechanically incorrect fashion. In other words, a forced posterior translational movement is applied to flatten the cervical lordosis. Posterior translation is a component of cervical extension. Flexion of the neck (lordotic reduction) should occur through activation of the cervical flexor muscles. These muscles will produce both angular and translational movement in an anterior direction. If this motion is applied repetitively, a forced posterior sheering of the lower cervical segments could eventually could structural damage to the intervertebral disc and other passive restraining structures. This may result in too much segmental motion in a posterior direction and irritation of structures mentioned in figure 16-40.

Therapeutic Exercise

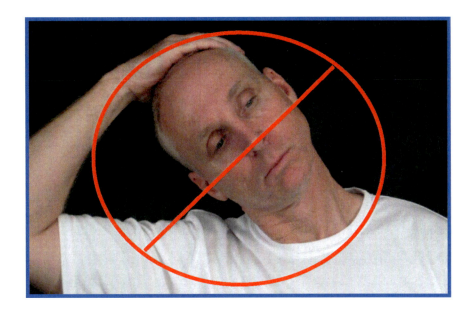

Figure 16-42: Cervical Motions with Injury Potential, Repetitive or End Range Passive Side Bending

Well I don't dislike this motion quite as much as the previous two but why would we want to repetitively compress potentially pain sensitive structures on a unilateral basis in order to affect a temporary soft tissue stretch on the opposite side. I don't believe that most therapists typically prescribe this particular motion on any kind of consistent basis but I do observe many people applying this motion to their neck. This movement and this movement applied with cervical rotation is a typical "self-cracking" motion that many folks find themselves addicted to. It does not help! Don't do it and stop your patients from doing it! Self-popping of a spinal segment will only give temporary relief of cervical discomfort and it will have no lasting beneficial effect. This is why many people must continually repeat this movement pattern.

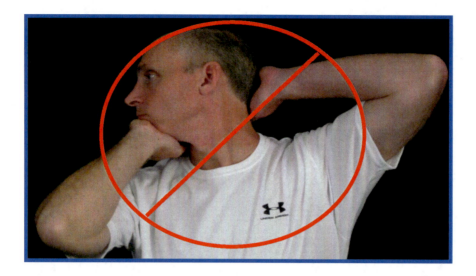

Figure 16-43: Cervical Motions with Injury Potential, Repetitive or End Range Passive Rotation

There are many different versions of this self-ROM/popping/cracking movement pattern with slight differences in hand position and amount of side bending. I offer the same perspective and comments as written in figure 16-42. It does not help! Don't do it and stop your patients from doing it! The self-popping of a spinal segment will only give temporary relieve of cervical discomfort and it will have no lasting beneficial effect in terms of pain relief. This is why many people continually repeat this movement pattern. It is my strong opinion that this type of motion will only aid in the process of structural breakdown of the cervical intervertebral disc[34, 35]. Remember, the disc is the principal stabilizing structure of the spinal motion segment, and initially when it degenerates and in some cases even latter grades of degeneration are associated with increased segmental motion.

Chapter 17

Therapeutic Exercise for the Thoracic Spine

Chapter 17 will look at exercises for patients with various thoracic impairments. Here is a bulleted list of some of the more important topics covered in this chapter.

- Thoracic Self Mobilization Exercises
    - Clinical decision making regarding using of self-mobilization equipment.
- Thoracic Extensor Muscle Strength Training
    - Clinical decision making regarding use of the Swiss Ball.
- Thoracic Intra-Scapular Muscle Strength Training

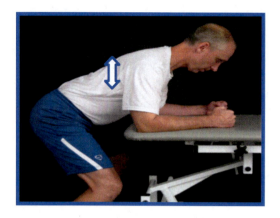 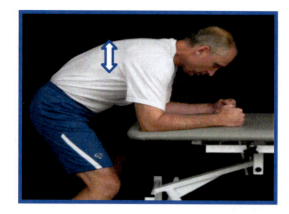

Figure 17-1: Thoracic Self-Mobilization, Flexion and Extension:

I wanted to briefly discuss an exercise which is more commonly performed in the quadruped position. We don't typically have to self-mobilize the thoracic spine into a more flexed position. An increase in the thoracic kyphosis is the last thing that most of our orthopedic spinal patients need. That said, I still think this exercise has merit as a general multi-segment range of motion procedure that can be applied to move the spinal segments back and forth in the sagittal plane provided the segmental motion restriction is not too significant. If on the other hand a thoracic segment or segments have become stiffened due to advanced degenerative change, this exercise will not likely restore motion. Now just a couple of more points regarding this exercise, have the patient focus on their sternum and use light tactile cueing on their chest and mid-thoracic segments (AAROM) to assist the patient in understanding this movement pattern. One thought would be to have the patient move their sternum away from and towards the table. Make sure that the patient's head and neck stay as still as possible. Again, I do not believe that repetitive full range flexion and extension through the cervical segments is wise when degenerative change or injury has occurred. This thoracic motion can be performed repetitively or held in one position or the other for several seconds for light stretching purposes.

Therapeutic Exercise

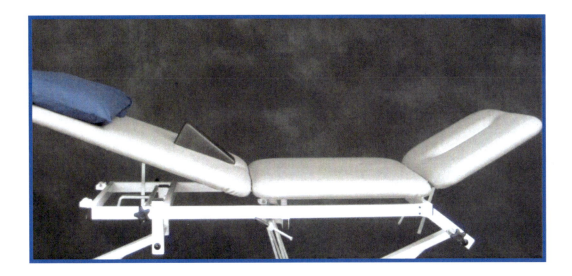

Figure 17-2: Typical Clinical Set Up for Thoracic Self-Mobilization

Now let's discuss more significant stiffness impairment in thoracic motion segments. Similar to other regions of the spine, a thoracic segment with grade V (end stage) disc degeneration is not likely to improve (increase mobility) regardless of the movement intervention applied. Unlike the cervical or lumbar region, given the morphological structure of the thoracic segment and vertebral attachments to the rib cage, early stage disc degeneration does not appear to be consistently associated with increased segmental motion (hypermobility) and because of this, prescription of self-mobilization can be a bit more aggressive. Figure 17-2 shows a thoracic mobilization wedge placed on a manual therapy table. This wedge serves to stabilize the caudal vertebrae of a thoracic segment where self –mobilization intervention is to be applied. Further, if the patient's thoracic segment(s) are painful the table is initially angled upward to reduced body weight loading on the sensitive segment during the therapeutic exercise motion. A pillow is placed on the foot section of the table to support the cervical spine and the patient's feet are often placed on the head section of the table which is also angled upward. Other variations of this exercise set up are certainly acceptable but if you have tables that move in this fashion, this represents a good clinic-based exercise set up.

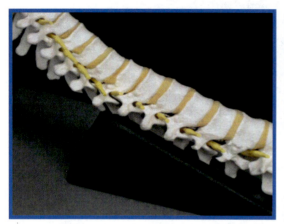 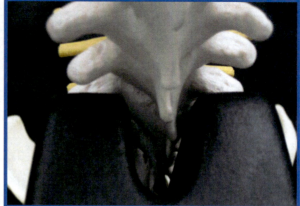

Figure 17-3: Vertebral Positioning on the Thoracic Wedge

On the left, figure 17-3 demonstrates how the peaks of a thoracic wedge support the transverse processes of the caudal vertebrae in a thoracic segment. This will allow the cranial vertebrae of the thoracic segment to move in a more isolated and specific fashion. The picture on the right demonstrates how the spinous processes are relieved of any pressure as they fit into the open section of the wedge. This will allow for dorsal translation and backward bending (extension) of the thoracic segment. These are the principal translational and angular movements we hope to achieve (restore) in most all cases when assisting a thoracic patient with postural and stiffness impairments.

Therapeutic Exercise

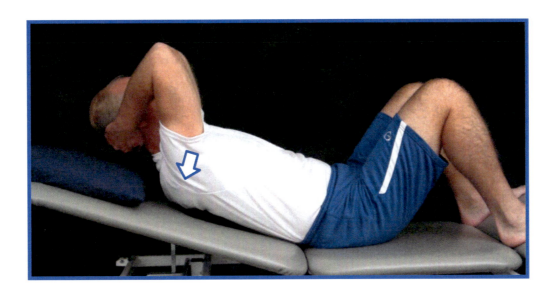

Figure 17-4: Thoracic Self-Mobilization, Posterior Translation and Facet Separation

The transverse processes of the caudal vertebrae of a stiff thoracic segment are placed on the peaks of a thoracic wedge and the patient is taught to "sink or melt" straight backward (posterior translation) over the top of the wedge. This is a fairly small motion and should not be initially accompanied by segmental thoracic extension. If more than one segment is going to be self-mobilized the caudal most segment is typically stretched first. In order to move from segment to segment, the patient can use their UE's and LE's to assist in scooting down the wedge in approximate one inch increments. The stretching position at each segment can be held for as little as 7-10 seconds or up to 30 seconds. Note how the cervical spine in essentially in line with the trunk. The patient is instructed to keep their neck muscle relaxed and to let the weight of his head rest in one or both hands as they self-mobilize their thoracic segments.

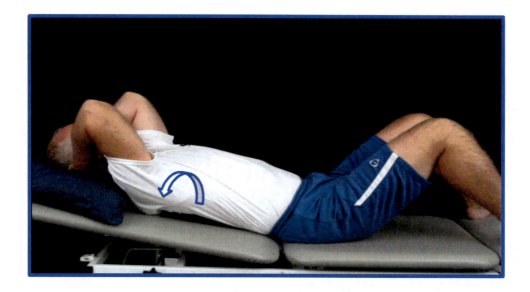

Figure 17-5: Thoracic Self-Mobilization, Segmental Extension

Again, the transverse processes of the caudal vertebrae of a stiff thoracic segment are placed on the peaks of a thoracic wedge and the patient is now taught to perform a short arc gravity assisted segmental backward bending (extension) motion over the top of the wedge. The wedge act as a fulcrum and as such promotes a larger and more specific form of this segmental motion. The patient's head and neck should be supported by their hand(s) and not allowed to extend backward. If more than one segment is going to be self-mobilized the caudal most segment is typically stretched first. In order to move from segment to segment, the patient can use their UE's and LE's to assist in scooting down the wedge in approximate one inch increments. The stretching position at each segment can be held for as little as 7-10 seconds or up to 30 seconds.

Therapeutic Exercise

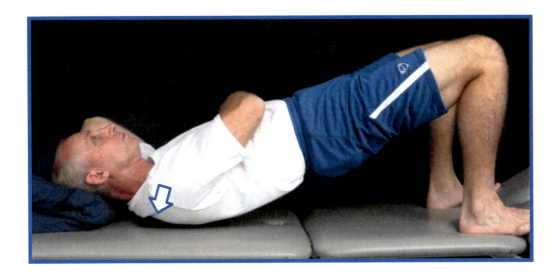

Figure 17-6: Thoracic Self-Mobilization, Posterior Translation and Facet Separation- Upper Thoracic Segments

Let's go back to a translational motion again for the purposes of self-mobilization with facet separation/distraction. The set up and patient instruction is very similar to the lower and mid thoracic self-mobilization shown in figure 17-4. Over many years of prescribing this exercise, I have found that in the upper thoracic region having the patient add a simple bridging procedure will improve contact with the peaks of the wedge. Therapists will find this helpful at the T1 and T2 segments if there is an increase in the upper thoracic kyphosis. Remember, there is only a small degree of thoracic posterior translation and segmental extension, your patient should not expect to feel a great deal of movement. If more than one segment is going to be self-mobilized, start with the most caudal segment and move segment by segment in a cranial direction. The patient should use their UE's and LE's to assist in scooting down the wedge in approximate one-inch increments. The stretching position at each segment can be held for as little as 7-10 seconds or up to 30 seconds.

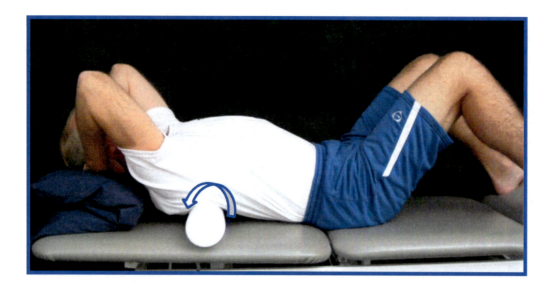

Figure 17-7: Thoracic Self-Mobilization, Short Arc Segmental Extension

- Firm Foam Roller

Now we can discuss a less specific (semi-specific) form of thoracic self-mobilization or segmental extension. This exercise incorporates a firm foam roller which is placed in the neighborhood of the caudal vertebrae of a thoracic segment that demonstrates restricted extension. The patient is now taught to perform a short arc gravity assisted backward bending motion over the top of the foam roller. I do not recommend that the segment be forcibly moved beyond the first stop in the direction of extension. The patient's head and neck should be supported by their hand(s) and not allowed to extend backward. If multiple segments are going to be self-mobilized the caudal most segments are stretched first. In order to move the roller from a more caudal position in the thoracic region to a more cranial position the patient can use their UE's and or LE's to roll on the foam roller. This stretching (extended) position can be held for up to 30 seconds.

Therapeutic Exercise

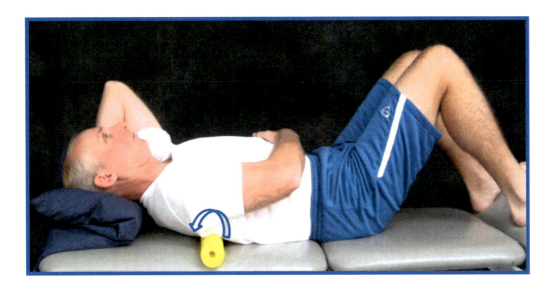

Figure 17-8: Thoracic Self-Mobilization, Short Arc Segmental Extension- Swimming Noodle:

This is a second form of semi-specific thoracic self-mobilization performed in the direction of thoracic extension. This version incorporates a swimming noodle which is placed on the caudal vertebrae of a segment that is restricted in the direction of extension. The patient is now taught to perform a short arc gravity assisted backward bending motion over the top of the noodle. I do not recommend that the segment be forcibly moved beyond the first stop in the direction of extension. The patient's head and neck should be supported by their hand(s) and not allowed to extend backward. Remember, if multiple segments are going to be self-mobilized the caudal most segments are stretched first. In order to move from segment to segment, the patient can use their UE's and or LE's to roll on the swimming noodle in approximate one inch increments. The extended position can be held for 7-10 seconds and up to 30 seconds. Note if the patient is more stiffness dominant a wooden dowel is inserted into the swimming noodle which stiffens this object. If the patient's thoracic segments are more painful and less stiff only the noodle is used. No dowel is inserted. This will allow the noodle to compress during the therapeutic motion and this will be more comfortable for a patient with thoracic pain impairment.

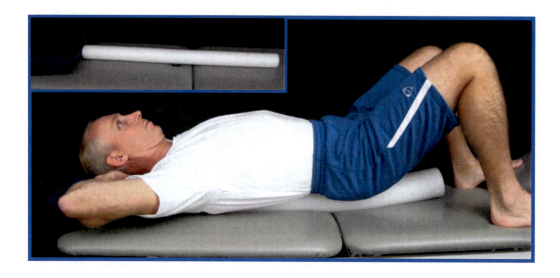

Figure 17-9: Thoracic Postural Reinforcement Exercise:

If the thoracic kyphosis is "loosened" and now better able to flatten as a result of the previous self-mobilization exercises, good posture can be reinforced with this procedure. Typically, the patient is instructed to lie in this position for 2-5 minutes. Patients with more advanced cervical degenerative disease or tissue trauma secondary to an injury will need cervical support with additional pillows. In other words, in these cases, the head and neck are not to lie directly on the firm foam roller. The idea here is to have the patient relax and let their shoulders and shoulder girdles sink backward toward the table. This figure shows a three-inch firm foam roller which is commonly found in many outpatient clinics. Additional stretching of the abdominal portion of the pectoral muscles can be achieved by placing the UE's in the position shown in figure 17-11.

Therapeutic Exercise

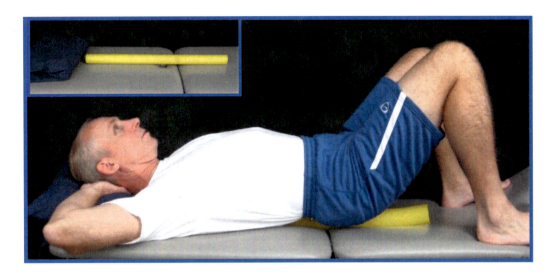

Figure 17-10: Thoracic Postural Reinforcement Exercise:

If the thoracic kyphosis is "loosened" and now better able to flatten as a result of the previous self-mobilization exercises, good posture can be reinforced with this procedure. Typically, the patient is instructed to lie in this position for 2-5 minutes. Patients with more advanced cervical degenerative disease or tissue trauma secondary to injury will need further cervical support with additional pillows. In other words, in these cases, the head and neck are not to lie directly on the swimming noodle. The idea here is to have the patient relax and let their shoulders and shoulder girdles sink backward towards the table. This figure shows a swimming noodle with a wooden dowel inserted into the noodle. This is an inexpensive way to make this exercise part of a home based exercise program. Additional support for the cervical region can be achieved by placing the hands behind the head-neck region.

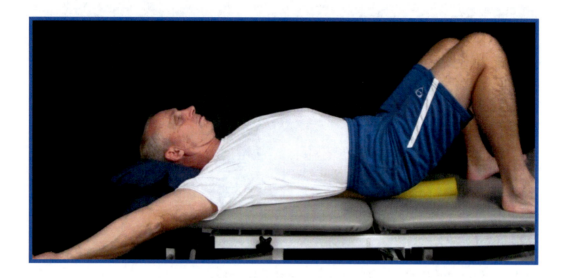

Figure 17-11: Thoracic Postural Reinforcement Exercise with Muscle Stretching:

For additional stretching of the various portions of the Pectoralis Major, the patient is placed in a similar position and instructed to position their UE's out to their side at approximately 90, 120, and 170 degrees of elevation in order to stretch the clavicular, sternocostal, and abdominal portions of the Pectoralis Major muscle. Stretching for each portion of the muscle should be held at least 30 seconds. To repeat, a firm foam roller or swimming noodle with dowel rod inserted is best tolerated if the thoracic kyphosis has a degree of flexibility and is able to flatten to some extent. Again, patients with more advanced cervical degenerative disease or tissue trauma secondary to injury will need further cervical support with a pillow or perhaps a folded pillow as shown above.

Therapeutic Exercise

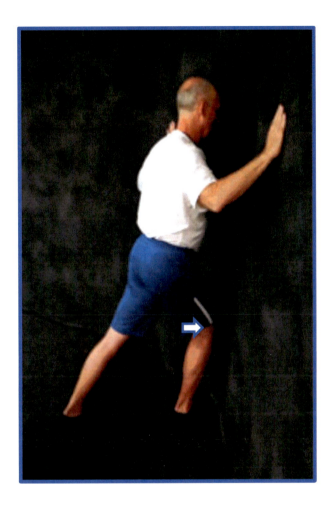

Figure 17-12: Pectoral Muscle Self-Stretching, The Corner Stretch:

After having improved your patient's passive thoracic extension mobility with exercises 17-4 - 17-9, and reinforced good posture with exercises 17-10 or 17-11, you might choose to prescribe the Corner Stretch. This exercise procedure will elongate the pectoral muscle and this can indirectly assist and improve our patient's spinal posture. Have your patient place his/her hands at shoulder height, place one foot in front of the other, and flex the front knee. Knee flexion will allow the trunk to lean in toward the corner.

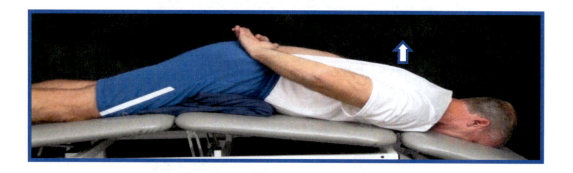

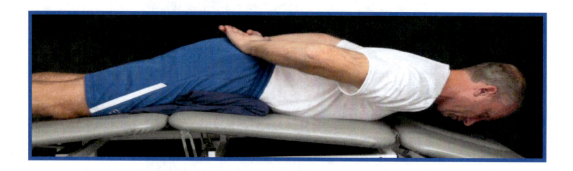

Figure 17-13: Thoracic Extensor Muscle Strength Training

There are many good ways to isometrically train the spinal extensor muscles. This is a clinic based version where the lumbar segments are pre-positioned in slight flexion with a pillow and over the moveable hinge section of a treatment table. The patient is instructed to lift their head, neck and chest upward and just off the table. The active motion is stopped prior to recruitment of movement into the lumbar region and the cervical segments are not allowed to extend. The therapist may manually stabilize the patient's lower extremities and also call for a concurrent bilateral gluteal muscle isometric squeeze. Isometric thoracic extensor strength training should be held for a minimum of 6-10 seconds and repeated a minimum of 6-10 times. For the more athletic client isometric training time can be increased.

Therapeutic Exercise

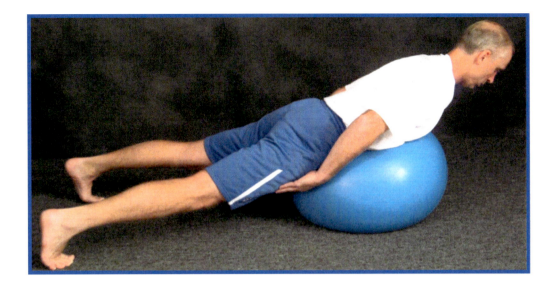

Figure 17-14: Thoracic Extensor Muscle Strength Training – Isometric Thoracic Extension

This is a second clinic-based version incorporating a Swiss Ball. You will see a similar figure again in our lumbar stabilization section. (Level 2 Swiss Ball Supported Lumbar Stabilization) The patient is instructed to separate their feet in order to achieve a wide base of support, extend their knees, perform a gluteal muscle squeeze, and lift their head, neck and chest upward without hyper extending their lumbar spine. Therapists should palpate and monitor for firm isometric contraction of the thoracic extensors. Remember to have your patient move his/her chin toward the anterior aspect of the neck (keep the back of the neck long).

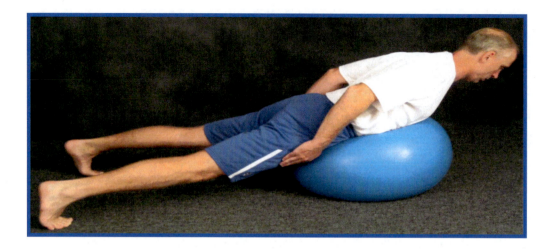

Figure 17-15: Thoracic Extensor Muscle Strength Training – Isometric and Isotonic Scapular Retraction

Isometric scapular retraction, note the UE and shoulder girdle position above, can also be added as the patient holds the training position for the thoracic extensors. Isometric strength training for the scapular retractors should be held for a minimum of 6-10 seconds and repeated a minimum of 6-10 times. Encourage your patient to maintain a wide base of support with their LE's, perform a bilateral gluteal muscle squeeze, and keep the back of their neck long by not looking upward.

Therapeutic Exercise

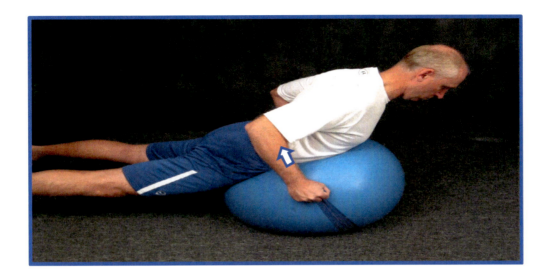

Figure 17-15: Thoracic Extensor and Resisted Scapular Retraction Muscle Strength Training:

Now a piece of elastic band is placed under the Swiss Ball to provide resisted scapular retraction. A standard multi-rep and multi-set exercise program can be prescribed by the therapist. Encourage your patient to maintain a wide base of support with their LE's, perform a bilateral gluteal muscle squeeze, and keep the back of their neck long by not looking upward.

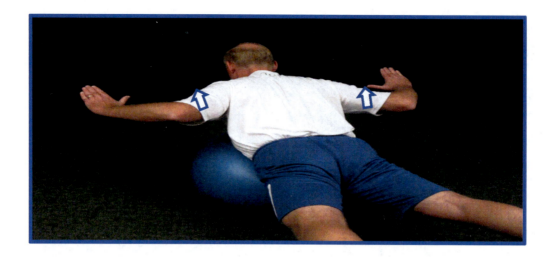

Figure 17-16: Thoracic Extensor and Superficial Spinal Muscle Layer Strength Training:

The following three therapeutic exercises (17-16 – 17-18) can be referred as the Alphabet exercises. The UE position that is adopted facilitates contraction of the Rhomboid (17-16), Lower Trapezius (17-17) and Middle Trapezius muscles (17-18). The first letter, and you have to use your imagination a little bit is a "W." When the UE's are held in this position isometrically or when repetitive isotonic contraction is performed, strength impairment in the Rhomboid muscle group can be affectively strengthened. Regarding isotonic training, the patient is to maintain their shoulder position just below 90 degree of abduction and their elbow position at 90 degrees of flexion. The medial aspect of one or both arms is dropped down to the Swiss Ball and then lifted away from the Swiss Ball. A standard multi-rep and multi-set exercise program can be prescribed by the therapist. Encourage your patient to maintain a wide base of support with their LE's, perform a bilateral gluteal muscle squeeze, and keep the back of their neck long by not looking upward.

Therapeutic Exercise

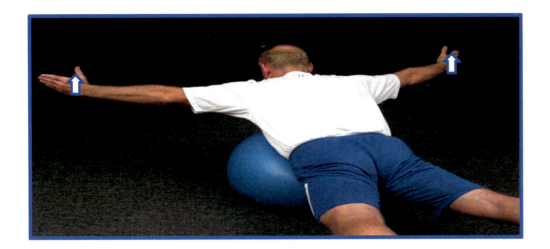

Figure 17-17: Thoracic Extensor and Superficial Spinal Muscle Layer Strength Training:

The next exercise in this short series for the superficial layer group is called the "Y" exercise. The second letter is a "Y" and this position/motion can be used to facilitate contraction of the Lower Trapezius. The patient is instructed to elevate their upper extremities in the frontal plane to approximately 120 degrees, externally rotate their arms, and perform a unilateral or bilateral lifting motion such that the ulnar aspect of their hand(s) touches the ground and then is lifted off the ground. A standard multi-rep and multi-set exercise program can be prescribed by the therapist. Encourage your patient to maintain a wide base of support with their LE's, perform a bilateral gluteal muscle squeeze, and keep the back of their neck long by not looking upward.

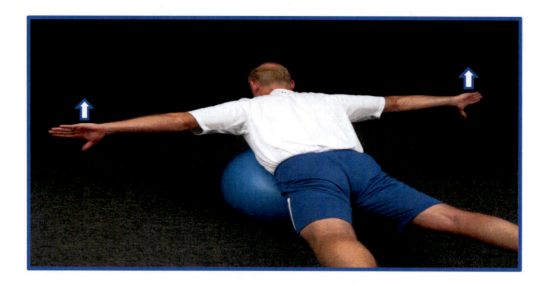

Figure 17-18: Thoracic Extensor and Superficial Spinal Muscle Layer Strength Training:

The third and last letter is a "T" and this position/motion can be used to facilitate contraction of the middle trapezius. The patient is instructed to elevate their arms to 90 degrees in the frontal plane, internally rotate their arms, and perform a unilateral or bilateral UE lifting motion. The patient's thumb can touch the ground and then be lifted away from the ground. A standard multi-rep and multi-set exercise program can be prescribed by the therapist. Encourage your patient to maintain a wide base of support with their LE's, perform a bilateral gluteal muscle squeeze, and keep the back of their neck long by not looking upward.

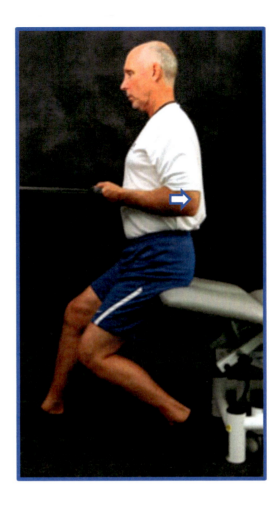

Figure 17-19: Isotonic Scapular Retractor Strengthening:

As you can see, there are a number of very nice Swiss Ball thoracic extensor and scapular muscle strength building exercises. Don't forget this simple one which works very well for our older patients who might not be able to transition onto and off of a Swiss Ball. Start by having the patient seated with hips higher than knees, and then have the patient lift his/her chest up and forward and move his/her chin down and in toward the anterior aspect of his/her neck. Prescribe isotonic scapular retraction using a multi- rep and multi-set program.

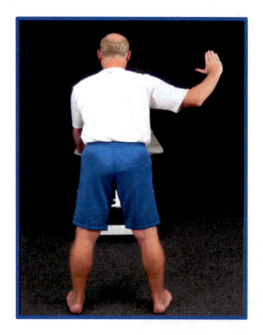 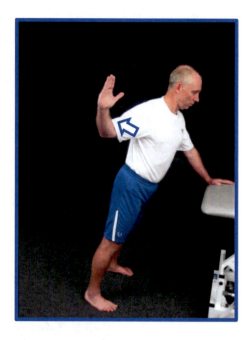

Figure 17-20: Thoracic Superficial Spinal Muscle Layer Strength Training:

We need to consider patients who cannot or do not wish to lie prone on a Swiss Ball. The modified plantigrade position can be used for unilateral isometric or unilateral isotonic superficial layer muscle training. This is the "W" exercise and this version offers some patients a way to perform light muscle training for strength impairments affecting this muscle group. This isotonic exercise is performed unilaterally, on the right side as seen above. Instruct the patient to lean forward and contact a table or counter top with one hand. On the training side have him/her move their shoulder to just below 90 degrees of abduction and position the elbow at 90 degrees of flexion. The patient is instructed to move the medial aspect of their UE downward toward the table and then lift the UE upward back to the start position. A standard multi-rep and multi-set exercise program can be prescribed by the therapist.

Therapeutic Exercise

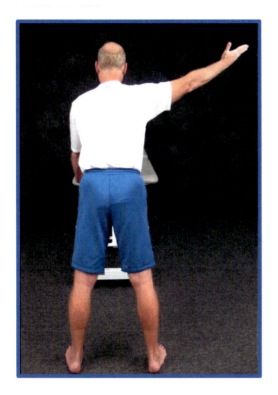 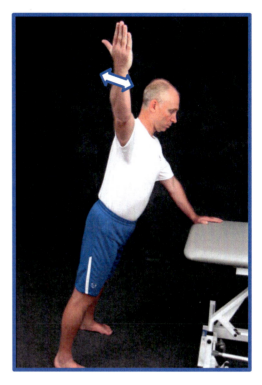

Figure 17-21: Thoracic Superficial Spinal Muscle Layer Strength Training:

Again, in consideration of those patients who are not able to perform superficial layer muscle training on the Swiss Ball the "Y" exercise can be performed in the modified plantigrade position. This UE motion will target the lower portion of the trapezius muscle. The patient is instructed to elevate his/her UE in the frontal plane to approximately 120 degrees, externally rotate their arm, and perform a unilateral motion which moves the UE in front of and behind the frontal plane. A standard multi-rep and multi-set exercise program can be prescribed by the therapist.

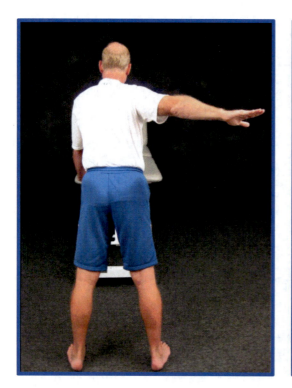 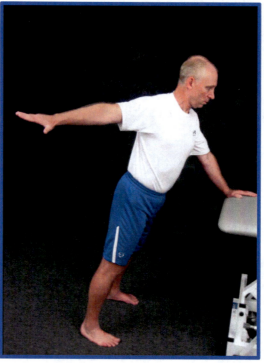

Figure 17-22: Thoracic Superficial Spinal Muscle Layer Strength Training:

Lastly and with regard to the third and last letter, the "T" position/motion can be used to facilitate contraction of the middle trapezius. The patient is instructed to lean forward and contact a table or counter top and then elevate their arm to 90 degrees in the frontal plane. The arm is then internally rotated and unilateral UE motion in front of and behind the frontal plane is performed. A standard multi-rep and multi-set exercise program can be prescribed by the therapist.

Chapter 18

Therapeutic Exercise for the Lumbar Spine

Chapter 18 will look at exercises for patients with various lumbar impairments. Here is a bulleted list of some of the more important topic areas that will be covered in this chapter.

- Lumbar Stabilization Exercise Training
    - Controlling excessive lumbopelvic motion during gait
    - Swiss Ball Supported Stabilization Exercises
    - Swiss Ball Supported Abdominal Muscle Exercises
    - Hip Hinge Stabilization Exercises
    - Muscular (Dynamic) Stabilization During Lifting
    - Lateral Trunk Muscle Stabilization Exercises
- Correcting and Controlling Lumbopelvic Movement Patterns
- Reducing Lumbar Compression During Aerobic Training
- Therapeutic Exercises for Lumbar Stenosis
- Therapeutic Exercises for Lumbar Radiculitis
- Therapeutic Lumbar Self Mobilization Exercises

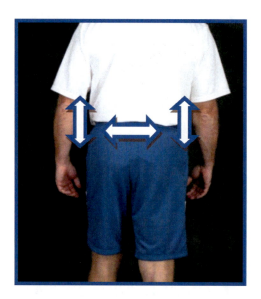

Figure 18-1: Lumbar Stabilization, Controlling Excessive Lumbopelvic Side Bending and Rotation during Gait:

Figure 18-1 and 18-2 relate to what I feel is a somewhat common finding in some lumbar pain patients who also demonstrate symptomatic segmental hypermobility. There is a subset of these patients who also demonstrate excessive pelvic motion in either the transverse plane, the frontal plane, or both while walking. This excessive motion maybe a perpetuating factor associated with their low back ache. The first step toward correction of this extra and unnecessary lumbopelvic movement is simple movement re-education advice. In other words, just make the patient aware of the extra motion and give them a simple cue such as not allowing their belly button or belt buckle if you like, to move left and right while walking. Next, increased pelvic motion during gait can relate to lack of hip extension, lack of gluteal muscle strength or lack both in some cases. If hip extension is passively limited due to capsular or muscular shortening the pelvis will demonstrate increased rotation in the transverse plane and self-stretching should be prescribed (Figure 18-2). Next, gluteal muscle weakness is an accepted cause of increased lumbopelvic motion in the frontal plane during gait. Neuromuscular re-education regarding the performance of a quick unilateral isometric gluteal muscle contraction during the contact phase of gait will assist in reducing this excessive pelvic motion in this plane.

Therapeutic Exercise

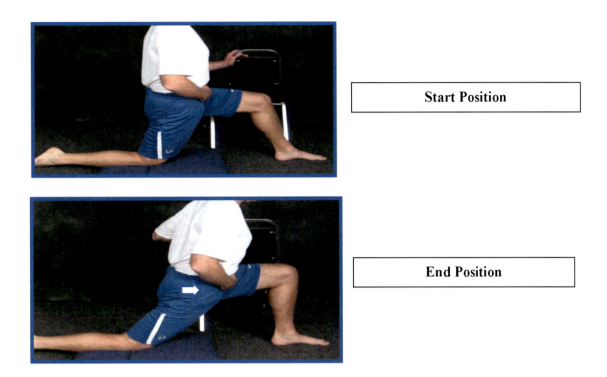

Figure 18-2: Hip Flexor Self-Stretching, Half Kneeling Position:

This self-stretch can be performed in half kneeling as shown or in a standing position. Regarding the discussion in associated with figure 18-1; this stretch will assist in reducing excessive pelvic motion in the transverse plane during gait by addressing passive hip extension restriction. In terms of movement sequence, the patient is instructed to perform a strong posterior pelvic tilt (PPT) incorporating a bilateral gluteal squeeze and firmly pulling their lower tummy upward and inward (up and in toward the "upper tummy" or up and in toward the belly button). Once the PPT is firmly established, instruct the patient to flex their front knee and "drag" their back hip into extension. Do not let the lumbar spine hyperextend as their body translates forward. This important self-stretch should be held for 30 seconds or up to a minute or more. We should make one other important point about this self-stretch and lumbopelvic position. Abnormal spinal structure (posture) is at times seen and may or may not be associated with low back pain. Excessive anterior pelvic tilt may be associated with hip flexor shortening. If a patient presents with low back pain and excessive anterior tilting of the pelvis, this stretch may be helpful.

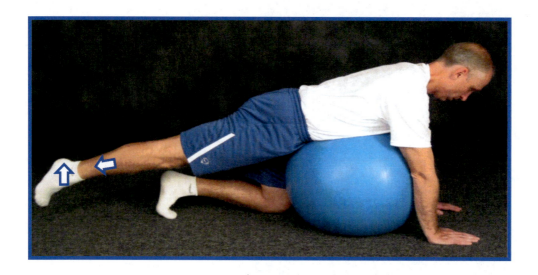

Figure 18-3: Lumbar Stabilization, Swiss Ball Supported Four Point Alternating Leg Extension - Quadruped:

This four-point spinal stabilization training exercise is an excellent way to build muscular strength and endurance in the proximal hip extensors and lumbar extensor muscles. Unfortunately, this exercise training movement has little practical carryover in terms of promoting dynamic stabilization during common upright movement patterns. That idea will be covered latter in this chapter. When prescribing this exercise, have the patient slide their LE's backward and keep the angle of the LE's low to minimize movement through the lumbar segments. The lumbar segments will be well supported through the abdomen by virtue of the Swiss Ball pressing up into this region. This exercise is a nice "starter" exercise in patients with chronic low back pain and associated muscular atrophy. Typically, I have the patient perform 30 reps with each LE. The exercise can be performed with a rhythmical alternating motion or the LE position can be held isometrically for 6-10 seconds and repeated as indicated by the therapist. Lastly, when the patient brings his/her thigh back toward the ball, make sure his/her femur gets back to a "vertical" position and fully presses up into the ball.

Therapeutic Exercise

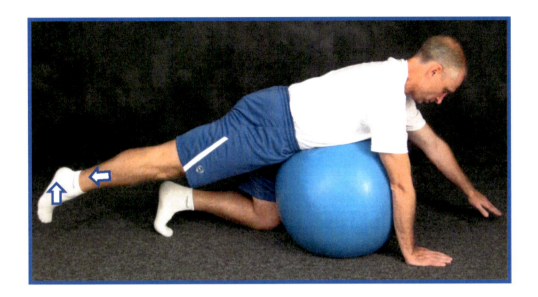

Figure 18-4: Lumbar Stabilization, Swiss Ball Supported Four Point Alternating Opposite Arm and Leg Extension - Quadruped:

This is a second and slightly more challenging four-point spinal stabilization exercise that is also an excellent way to build muscular strength and endurance in the proximal hip and lumbar extensor muscles. The patient is now asked to move from four points of reference on the ground to just two points of reference. When prescribing this exercise, have the patient slide their UE's and LE's forward and backward respectively and keep the angle of the UE's and LE's low in order to minimize movement through the lumbar segments. The lumbar segments will be well supported through the abdomen by virtue of the Swiss Ball pressing up into this region. Be sure that the patient's chin is moved down and in toward the Adams Apple in order to keep the back of the neck "long". Generally, have the patient perform 30 reps of this procedure with a rhythmical alternating motion or the extremity position can be held isometrically for 6-10 seconds and repeated as indicated by the therapist. Same as exercise 18-3, when the patient brings his/her thigh back toward the ball, make sure his/her femur gets back to a "vertical" position and fully presses up into the ball.

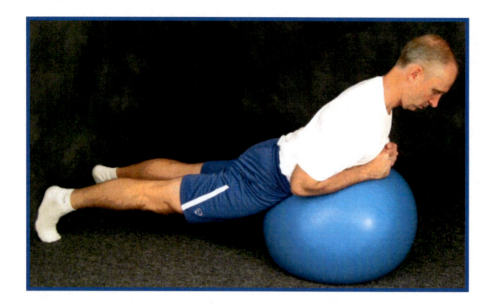

Figure: 18-5: Lumbar Stabilization, Swiss Ball Supported Stabilization Series;

Level 1 Training:

This is the first exercise in a comprehensive series of progressively more challenging lumbar stabilization exercises. Have the patient establish a wide base of support, extend their knees, perform a bilateral gluteal squeeze, lengthen the back of their neck and lift their chest upward without hyper extending their lumbar spine. Note how the patient's hands and distal UE's contact both the ball and their chest. This allows the UE's to assist the spinal extensors in preventing trunk flexion due to the effect of gravity. Assistance from the UE's is important in this first level stabilization exercise if the patient's condition is more acutely symptomatic or if their trunk extensor muscles are weak. Placing the UE's on the ball as seen above facilitates a light contraction of the spinal extensors. This next point is very important, keep the ball somewhat deflated so it will flatten and spread throughout the patient's entire abdominal region. This is not only more comfortable but it will also lend a greater degree of support to the lumbar segments. Have the patient hold this isometric training position for 6-10 seconds and repeat 6-10 times. While resting after their 6-10 second isometric repetition, the patient should move into one of two rest positions shown in the next figure.

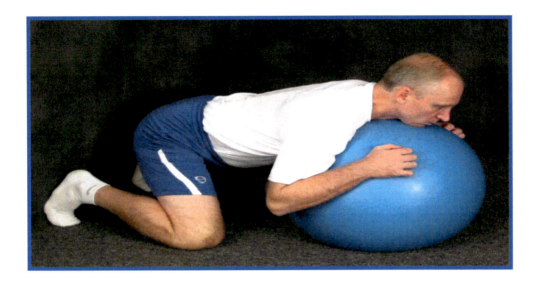

Figure 18-6: Lumbar Stabilization, Swiss Ball Supported Stabilization Series Starting/Rest Position 1:

This is one of two rest positions that are recommended when patients are performing the Swiss Ball Supported lumbar stabilization exercises. After the patient performs a repetition, they essentially roll backward by flexing their hips and knees. The ball comes to rest under the chin, neck and upper chest region. In younger back pain patients with less degenerative change, the recommendation is to have the patient gently push their tail bone upward toward the ceiling as their LE's flex. In effect the patient is performing a gentle anterior pelvic tilt which will keep the spinal extensors lightly activated and also keeps the lumbar segments in a mid-position as the hip progressively flex into this rest position. When in the rest position the therapist can chose to have the patient rate their intensity of low back pain using the 0-10 NPRS. This scale could also be used during the performance of any of the Swiss ball supported muscular training exercises. (See my comments on the next page, figure 18-7).

Therapeutic Exercise

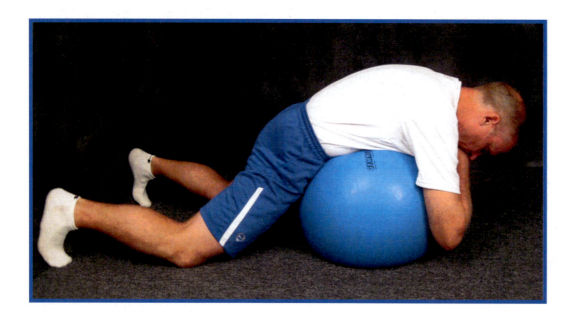

Figure 18-7: Lumbar Stabilization, Swiss Ball Supported Stabilization Series Starting/Rest Position 2:

This is the second rest position that can be used in between repetitions of Swiss Ball Supported lumbar stabilization exercise training. In essence, after a repetition the patient is instructed to flex their knees, hips and spine and "melt down" and drape themselves over the ball. All of the spinal extensor muscles will relax as the motion segments are supported over the ball in slight flexion. For patients with acquired lumbar stenosis and other more advanced forms of degenerative disc disease, this is the rest position to use. Rest time should be approximately equal to the isometric training time. Now, let's make an important point about the Swiss Ball. When placed in the abdomen, the Swiss Ball makes the lumbar stabilization exercises easier and safer. The Swiss Ball helps patients with back problems to build strength in their spinal muscles and when performed correctly and with the right exercise dosage without provocation of symptoms. Yes, the Swiss Ball can be used to make exercises more challenging which we will also see later in this chapter, but our goal for the Swiss Ball Supported exercises is to train without provocation of spinal or radicular pain.

Therapeutic Exercise

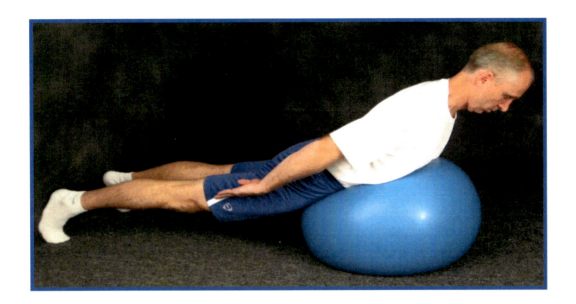

**Figure 18-8: Lumbar Stabilization, Swiss Ball Supported Stabilization Series
Level 2 Training:**

Have the patient establish a wide base of support, extend their knees, perform a bilateral gluteal squeeze, lengthen the back of their neck and lift their chest upward without hyper extending their lumbar spine. The patient is to first place their UE's in the level 1 position giving assistance to their spinal extensors. Once set in the level 1 position the patient is instructed to bring their arms down to their sides. At this point the patient will be relying on their spinal extensor muscles exclusively to keep their head, neck and trunk from breaking down into flexion over the top edge of the ball. If the patient experiences any discomfort or unpleasant sensation across their back in the level 2 position, they are instructed to move the ball upward toward their chin by an inch or two. Now less of their body will be over the top edge of the ball. Usually this will alleviate the spinal discomfort. Remember, keep the Swiss Ball partially deflated so it will flatten and spread throughout the patient's entire abdominal region. This will lend a greater degree of support to the lumbar segments. Have the patient hold this isometric training position for 6-10 seconds and repeat 6-10 times. While resting after the 6-10 second isometric repetition, the patient should move into one of two rest positions shown previously.

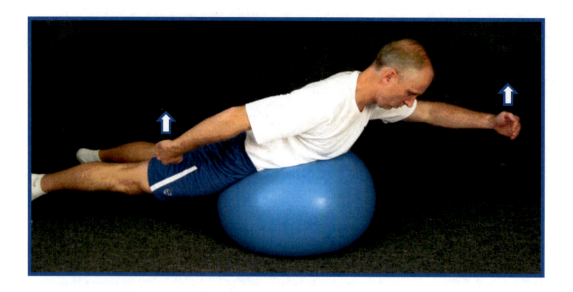

Figure 18-9: Lumbar Stabilization, Swiss Ball Supported Stabilization Series
Level 3 Training:

Have the patient establish a wide base of support, extend their knees, perform a bilateral gluteal squeeze, lengthen the back of their neck and lift their chest upward without hyper extending their lumbar spine. The patient is to first place their UE's in the level 1 position giving assistance to their spinal extensors. Once set in the level 1 position the patient is instructed to make an alternating UE swinging pattern. Swinging of the UE backward and behind the trunk will activate some of the more superficial spinal muscles and swinging the other UE out in front of the trunk will force the spinal extensor muscles to increase their level of contraction adding to the isometric strength building benefit of this exercise. This is also the first step in demonstrating to the patient how to hold the lumbar spine stable while making isolated UE movement. To repeat, if the patient experiences any discomfort or unpleasant sensation across their back in the level 2 through level 6 position, they are instructed to move the ball upward toward their chin by an inch or two. Usually this will alleviate the spinal discomfort. Remember, keep the Swiss Ball partially deflated so it will flatten and spread throughout the patient's entire abdominal region. Have the patient perform 6-10 reps with each arm and repeat this at least 3 times. The patient should rest in between sets in one of two rest positions shown previously.

Therapeutic Exercise

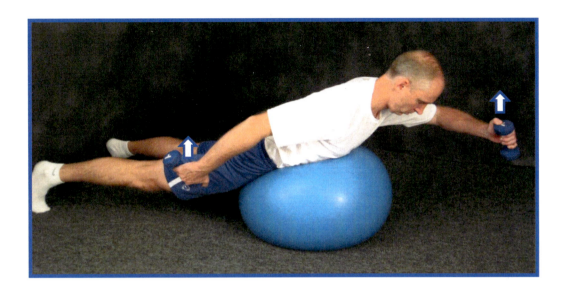

Figure 18-10: Lumbar Stabilization, Swiss Ball Supported Stabilization Series
Level 4 Training:

Have the patient establish a wide base of support, extend their knees, perform a bilateral gluteal squeeze, lengthen the back of their neck and lift their chest upward without hyper extending their lumbar spine. The patient is to first place their UE's in the level 1 position. Once set in the level 1 position the patient is instructed to make an alternating UE swinging pattern while holding onto 1-3 pounds of free weight. Swinging of the UE backward and behind the trunk will activate some of the more superficial spinal muscles and swinging the other UE out in front of the trunk will force the spinal extensor muscles to increase their level of contraction adding to the isometric strength building benefit of this exercise. It is important that patients eventually understand that their UE's can be moved without their lumbar spine having to move. To repeat, if the patient experiences any discomfort or unpleasant sensation across their back in the levels 2-6 position, they are instructed to move the ball upward toward their chin by an inch or two. Usually this will alleviate their lumbar discomfort. Remember, keep the Swiss Ball partially deflated so it will flatten and spread throughout the patient's entire abdominal region. Have the patient perform 6-10 reps with each arm and repeat this at least 3 times. The patient should rest in between sets in one of two rest positions shown previously.

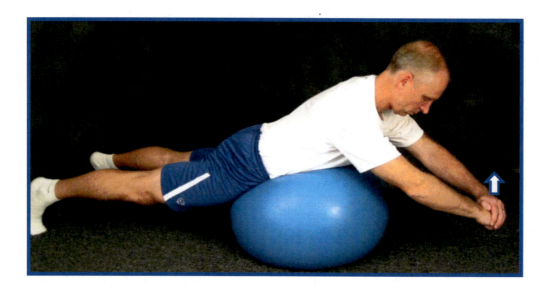

Figure 18-11: Lumbar Stabilization, Swiss Ball Supported Stabilization Series
Level 5 Training:

Have the patient establish a wide base of support, extend their knees, perform a bilateral gluteal squeeze, lengthen the back of their neck and lift their chest upward without hyper extending their lumbar spine. The patient is to first place their UE's in the level 1 position. Once set in the level 1 position the patient is instructed to place one hand over the top of the other and make a repetitive UE lifting motion. This bilateral UE position and movement will facilitate increased spinal extensor muscle contraction adding to the isometric strength building benefit of this exercise. This UE movement pattern also demonstrates to the patient a common UE lifting motion while the spine is held stable. If the patient experiences any discomfort or unpleasant sensation across their lumbar region while performing the levels 2-6 stabilization procedures, they are instructed to move the ball upward toward their chin by an inch or two. Usually this will alleviate their lumbar discomfort. Remember, keep the Swiss Ball partially deflated so it will flatten and spread throughout the patient's entire abdominal region. Have the patient perform 6-10 reps with each arm and repeat this UE movement pattern at least 3 times. The patient should rest in between sets in one of two rest positions shown previously. The bilateral "stacked" hand lift shown in this figure is a bit more challenging and ball placement in relation to the trunk must be exact.

Therapeutic Exercise

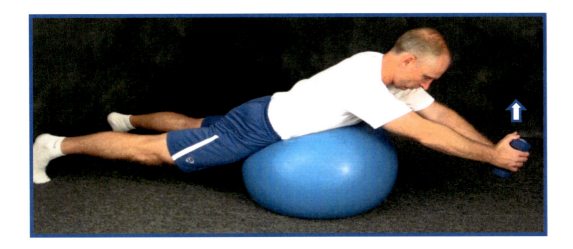

Figure 18-12: Lumbar Stabilization, Swiss Ball Supported Stabilization Series - Level 6 Training:

Have the patient establish a wide base of support, extend their knees, perform a bilateral gluteal squeeze, lengthen the back of their neck and lift their chest upward without hyper extending their lumbar spine. Once set in the level 1 position the patient is instructed to make a repetitive UE lifting motion while holding onto 1-3 pounds of free weight. This bilateral UE elevation will significantly facilitate increased spinal extensor muscle contraction adding to the isometric strength building benefit of these exercises. This UE movement pattern also demonstrates a common UE lifting motion while the spine is held stable. If the patient experiences any discomfort or unpleasant sensation across their back in the level 6 position, they are instructed to move the ball upward toward their chin by an inch or two. Have the patient perform 6-10 reps with a 1-3-pound weight and repeat this at least 3 times. The patient should rest in between sets in one of two rest positions shown previously. This completes the first phase of lumbar stabilization training. The prone lying Swiss Ball Supported Phase. Many patients with low back pain with various grades of disc degeneration and resultant segmental hypermobility[36, 37] will stop at this point in the stabilization series. Many patients should not have the support of the ball taken from them (out of contact with the abdomen) while training. Some patients and athletic clients can be advanced to the next level of stabilization training where the ball no longer contacts the abdomen.

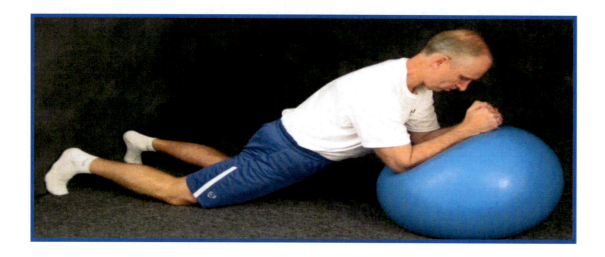

Figure 18-13: Lumbar Stabilization, Swiss Ball Stabilization Series - Level 7 (Advanced) Stabilization Training:

Now things get a bit more challenging. The next few stabilization exercises are termed advanced because the Swiss Ball has officially left the abdomen. One final point here about stabilization exercises 1-6. It is my opinion that when the Swiss ball is in the abdomen patients should not focus on any type of abdominal contraction. The ball will push the patient's abdomen in a posterior direction and support the lumbar segments. The focus for levels 1-6 should be on the spinal and hip extensors. There are many good stabilization exercises with an abdominal emphasis. This exercise for example (level 7) must be performed with a strong abdominal drawing or bracing now that the ball is no longer in the abdomen. This exercise begins with the patient positioned with his/her bottom (buttock) back toward their heels and hips and knees in flexion. The patient's hands are positioned close to the equator of the Swiss Ball. Instruct the patient to straighten their hips and knees and to roll their hands from the equator of the ball up the top of the ball. The end position for the UE's is one where the elbows rest on the ball. As the patient's hips are extending instruct the patient to perform a strong PPT with a strong bilateral gluteal squeeze and a very firm abdominal drawing. In the level 7 exercise, the patient is to keep their knees on the ground and just extend through the hips. Have the patient hold this isometric training position for 6-10 seconds and repeat 6-10 times. While resting after the 6-10 second isometric, the patient should move into one of two rest positions shown previously.

Therapeutic Exercise

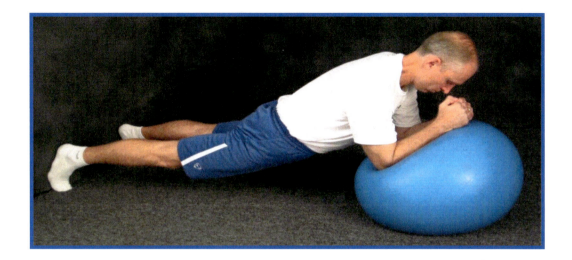

Figure 18-14: Lumbar Stabilization, Swiss Ball Supported Stabilization Series Level 8 (Advanced) Stabilization Training:

The level 8 exercise also begins by having the patient positioned with their bottom back toward their heels in hip and knee flexion. The patient's hands are positioned close to the equator of the Swiss Ball. Instruct the patient to straighten their hips and knees and to roll their hands from the equator of the ball up toward the top of the ball coming to rest on their elbows. As the patient's hips are extending instruct the patient to perform a strong PPT with a strong bilateral gluteal squeeze and a very firm abdominal drawing. To repeat, abdominal drawing can be easily understood by telling the patient to pull or draw their lower tummy (abdomen) up and in towards their upper tummy or to pull their lower tummy up and in toward their belly button. Don't just tell a patient to "tighten his/her stomach muscles," that verbal cue means very little. Now with the level 8 exercise, the patient is to extend their knees as their hips are extending. Have the patient hold this isometric training position for 6-10 seconds and repeat this stabilization movement pattern 6-10 times. As always, keep the cervical segments stable as well by having the patient bring the chin down and in toward the anterior aspect of the neck (Adam's Apple) as this will facilitate contraction of their cervical ventral flexors and assist in keeping posterior cervical structures safe and partially unloaded.

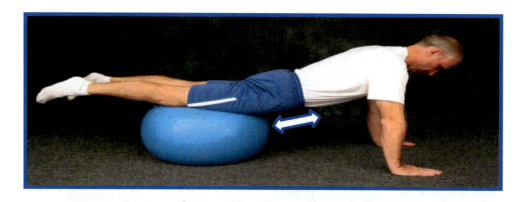

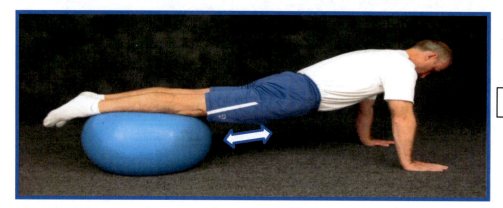

Advanced

Figure 18-15: Lumbar Stabilization, Swiss Ball Rolling Plank Stabilization Training, Abdominal Emphasis:

Now the patient's feet are up and off the ground. This exercise begins with the Swiss Ball in the patient's lower abdomen (not shown) and the patient is instructed to perform a strong bilateral gluteal and quadriceps isometric muscle contraction in order to keep their LE's parallel to the ground. Using both UE's the patient moves in a way that rolls the ball to a point where it is in contact with the anterior aspect of the thighs as shown above. At this point the ball is no longer supporting the lumbar spine and a strong posterior pelvic tilt with a firm abdominal draw must be performed and held. Isometric co-contraction of the principal trunk flexors and extensors will occur here and should be held for a minimum of 6-10 seconds or the patient can just have some fun continually rolling the ball back and forth from his/her abdomen to anterior thighs. For a greater degree of challenge and a more advanced training position, the patient is instructed to crawl forward to a point where the ball rolls down to and contacts the anterior aspect of the lower legs (lower picture).

Therapeutic Exercise

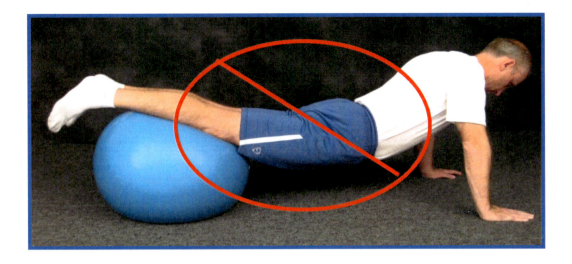

Figure 18-16: Lumbar Stabilization, Swiss Ball Rolling Plank Stabilization Training Abdominal Emphasis – Incorrect Position:

In this example the patient does not appear to have the trunk muscle strength to be progressed beyond the level 6 position where the ball can supports the lumbar segments. Note how the lumbar spine has "broken down" into a hyperextended position. Most all significant orthopedic problems affecting the lumbar spine eventually relate back to disc degeneration and disc herniation. This point must be understood by orthopedic clinicians. Loss of disc height, particularly posterior disc height is commonly seen and we don't need to aid and albeit the process by having our patients repetitively hyperextend their lumbar segments. Let's review another important point about disc degeneration. As the disc begin to degenerate, both angular and translatory segmental motion will increase. That comment is not theory, it is fact and is the main reason why I don't support repetitively applied large amplitude range of motion exercises for the lumbar spine. You will note, every stabilization exercise you have seen so far in this chapter minimizes excessive movement through the lumbar segments. As a patient's lumbar disc(s) degenerate, that is what we need to do[36, 37].

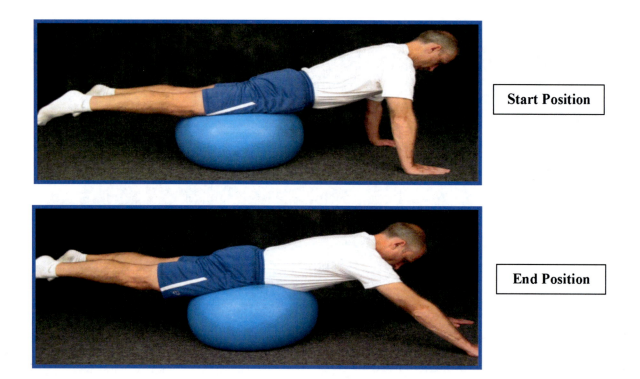

Figure 18-17: Lumbar Stabilization, Swiss Ball Rolling Plank Stabilization Training, Hip and Spinal and Hip Extensor Emphasis:

The lower extremities are up in the air again and held parallel to the ground with strong bilateral gluteal and quadriceps muscle contraction. The start position for the Swiss Ball is in contact with the upper anterior thighs (top photo). Both hands are in contact with the ground and the patient is instructed to push their UE's toward a more elevated position. As a result of this UE motion, the ball will roll up into the abdomen. In response, the patient will have to significantly increase the extent of their bilateral gluteal isometric contraction in order to maintain hip extension. The spinal extensor muscles will increase their level of isometric contraction as well. Have the patient hold this isometric training position for at least 6-10 seconds and repeat 6-10 times. Quick point about professional expertise. We (physical therapists) have to practice these exercises, all of the exercises we prescribe to our patients, not just the Swiss Ball exercises. In my opinion, clinicians prescribing therapeutic exercise should be experts at how a therapeutic movement is to be performed, how the exercise should "feel" and what the common movement and positioning mistakes are for each therapeutic motion.

Therapeutic Exercise

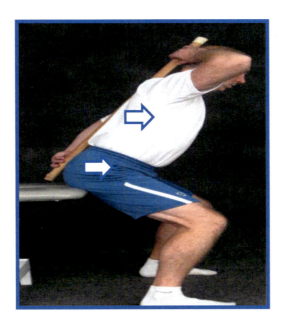

Figure 18-18: Lumbar Stabilization - Seated Hip Hinging Isometric Spinal Extensor Muscle Training Cane Reinforcement of Spine Position:

Hip hinging is a multi-purpose movement pattern that can be used to train the spinal extensors, enhance dynamic (muscular based) segmental stability during common daily movement patterns, and reduce spinal injury potential during lifting. As soon as an individual's trunk moves in front of the vertical plane all of the posterior spinal muscles including all of the spinal extensors will contract isometrically. Clinicians should palpate the patient's spinal extensor for muscular tone and bulk when their client is in this position. Patients can palpate the therapist's spinal extensors to develop an appreciation of how the extensors will contract and strengthen in this position. In this figure, note the position of the patient's hips in relation to his knees. Sitting with the hips higher than the knees will keep the pelvis in a more vertical alignment and the lumbar segments closer to a mid-position. The patient is instructed to lift their chest (sternum) up and forward and then place the cane in a vertical position behind their spinous processes. If the patient's thoracic or lumbar region begins to flex during this motion, the spine will press into the cane alerting the patient. With tactile cueing and passive or active assisted motion provided by the therapist, the patient is taught to move from their hip only bringing their trunk in front of the vertical plane. This motion can be performed in a more rhythmical manner or held isometrically for a minimum of 6-10 seconds and repeated 6-10 times.

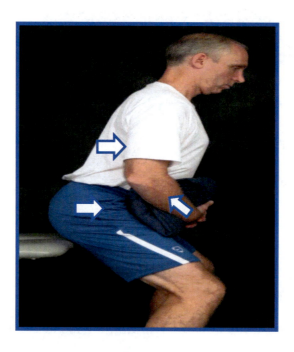

Figure 18-19: Lumbar Stabilization - Seated Hip Hinging Isometric Spinal Extensor Muscle Training with Passive Abdominal Drawing (Bracing):

Again note the position of the patient's hips in relation to his knees. Sitting with the hips higher than the knees will keep the pelvis in a more vertical alignment and the lumbar segments closer to a mid-position. In order to increase intra-abdominal pressure and provide support to the lumbar segments a pillow can be placed in the abdomen. The patient is instructed to either actively draw their abdomen inward, pull their abdomen inward with their hands, or both. Similar to the previous exercise, have the patient lift their chest (sternum) up and forward and maintain an awareness of where their chest is during the performance of the hip hinging motion. With tactile cueing and passive or active assisted motion provided by the therapist, the patient is taught to move from their hip only bringing their trunk in front of the vertical plane. This motion can be performed in a more rhythmical manner or held isometrically for a minimum of 6-10 seconds and repeated 6-10 times. If your patient reports an increase in discomfort, incorporate the seated self-traction between exercise shown latter in this chapter.

Therapeutic Exercise

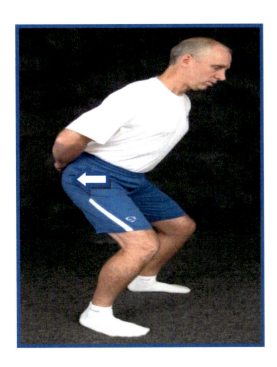

Figure 18-20: Lumbar Stabilization, Hip Hinge Isometric Spinal Extensor Muscle Training –Trunk Forward of the Upright Standing Position:

Now the patient is moved to the standing position, and in some ways the hip hinge movement pattern is more easily understood and often times better performed in this position as compared to the seated position. The instructional sequence is as follows: First, has the patient abduct at their hips to achieve a wide base of support. Second, instruct the patient to flex their knees. Third, and this is where the movement pattern changes, have the patient "push" their bottom straight backward (arrow) while keeping their chest up and forward. This last motion is repeated rhythmically and or held isometrically. Remember, the patient's bottom is not in contact with the table and can be pushed backward causing flexion at the hip joints without lumbopelvic flexion. Lastly, once in the hinge position, the patient is instructed to either actively draw their abdomen inward which enhances support to the lumbar segments and trains the abdominal muscles. Abdominal drawing likely reduces intra-discal pressure and likely assists with minimizing unwanted vertebral translation. This will often reduce or eliminate lumbar discomfort when training. After hip hinge spinal extensor muscle strength building has been performed, have your patient unload the lumbar segments with seated or hook lying self-traction seen later in this chapter.

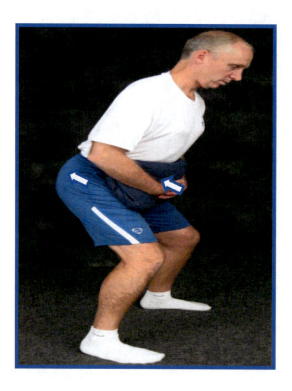

Figure 18-21: Lumbar Stabilization, Hip Hinge Series Isometric Spinal Extensor Muscle Training – with Active and Passive Abdominal Drawing:

Still in the standing position, first have the patient abduct at their hips to achieve a wide base of support. Second, instruct the patient to flex their knees. Third, have the patient "push" their bottom straight backward while keeping their chest up and forward. Remember, the patient's bottom is not in contact with the table and can be pushed backward causing flexion at the hip joints without spinal motion. Lastly, once in the hinge position, the patient is instructed to either actively draw their abdomen inward; pull their abdomen inward with their hands, or both. Pulling a pillow into the lower abdomen will support the lumbar segments and often reduce or eliminate discomfort when training the spinal extensors. This position should be held for a minimum of 6-10 seconds or to build additional isometric muscular endurance having the patient hold this position several times for 30 seconds each time. There is a tremendous amount of research that verifies lumbar multifidus muscle atrophy with first time back ache and fibro fatty replacement of this muscle in cases of chronic back pain. The various Swiss ball hip hinge exercise shown in this chapter can assist in building back an element of multifidus size and strength.

Therapeutic Exercise

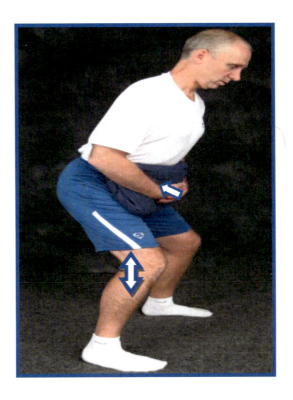

Figure 18-22 Lumbar Stabilization, Hip Hinge Standing Series – Mini Squats with Active and Passive Abdominal Drawing:

Again, have the patient abduct at their hips to achieve a wide base of support, flex their knees, and "push" their bottom straight backward while keeping their chest up and forward. Once in the hinge position, the patient is instructed to actively draw their abdomen inward and then support this position with their hands and a pillow. Once in the hinge position the patient is asked to perform short arc isotonic mini squats in order to add a component of LE strength training in addition to this isometric trunk stabilization exercise. It is not uncommon for our chronic lumbar pain patients and for patients with and disc degeneration and intermittent radiculitis to also demonstrate LE strength impairment. This exercise will enhance lumbar and LE muscle strength.

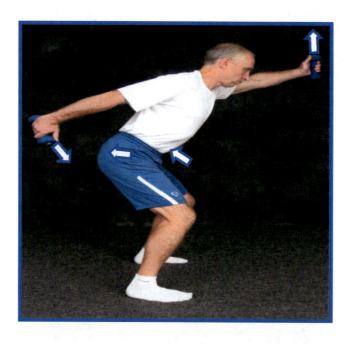

Figure 18-23: Lumbar Stabilization, Hip Hinge Series - Alternating Arm Swings

Similar to the Swiss Ball Supported exercise series, this hip hinge lumbar stabilization exercise can be progressed by incorporating UE movement. As before, have the patient abduct at their hips to achieve a wide base of support, flex their knees, and then push their bottom straight backward while keeping their chest up and forward. Once their trunk is in front of the vertical and their spinal extensors are contracting, have the patient actively pull their abdomen inward (abdominal drawing). At this point the patient is to initiate an alternating UE swinging motion without moving their spine. Holding and moving free weights will force the spinal extensor muscles to contract more aggressively as they attempt to hold the spinal segments stable. Six to ten arm swings constitute one set and one to three sets are typically performed. In terms of exercise carryover to other daily activities, teach your patient that isolated UE movements (reaching, lifting, carrying) can be performed during daily activities with their spine in a stable position hip hinge position, and without "mass movement" involving the lumbopelvic region. Again, we want to minimize lumbar angular and translatory motion in cases of early grade disc degeneration and resultant instability-hypermobility.

Therapeutic Exercise

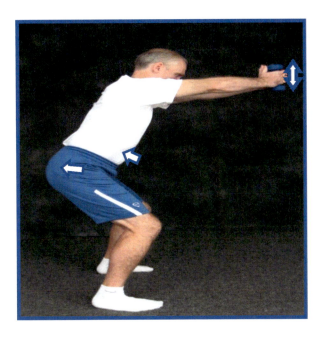

Figure 18-24: Lumbar Stabilization, Hip Hinge Series - Bilateral Arm Lifts:

Have the patient abduct at their hips to achieve a wide base of support, flex their knees, and have the patient "push" their bottom straight backward while keeping their chest up and forward. Once their trunk is in front of the vertical and their spinal extensors are contracting, have the patient actively pull their abdomen straight backward (inward). At this point the patient is to initiate a bilateral UE lifting motion while keeping their lumbopelvic region fixed in the hip hinge position. To repeat a comment made on the previous page, and in terms of exercise carryover to other daily activities, teach your patient that isolated UE movements (reaching, lifting, carrying) can be performed during daily activities with their spine in a stable position hip hinge position and the abdomen drawn inward. Remember, the IVD is the spine's principal ligament-stabilizing structure and our patients with discogenic instability-hypermobility should be preforming many daily movement patterns and activities in the hip hinge position.

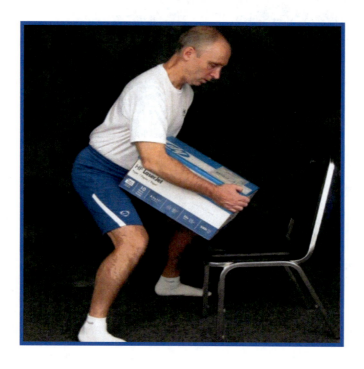

Figure 18-25: Lumbar Stabilization during Lifting, Hip Hinge Lift:

Here is a look at one of the practical applications of hip hinging. Note how the position of the body for this lift is almost identical as the hip hinge isometric spinal extensor strength building exercises. Your instruction to the patient should be the same. First, have the patient abduct at their hips to achieve a wide base of support. Second, instruct the patient to flex their knees. Third, have the patient push their bottom straight backward while keeping their chest up and forward. With the patient's trunk in front of the vertical plane, all of the posterior spinal muscles will be contracting isometrically and holding the spinal segments more stable during this lift. This position and movement pattern can be performed by rhythmically picking up various objects as part of a work hardening or a clinic based safe lifting program.

Therapeutic Exercise

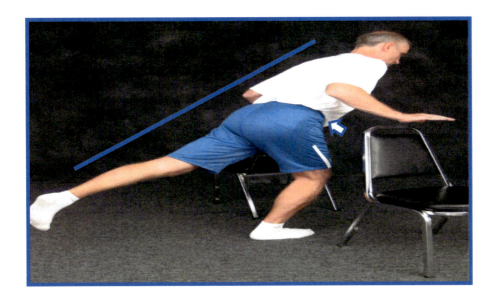

Figure 18-26: Lumbar Stabilization, Hip Hinge Series – Single Leg Hip Hinges with Balance Support:

You are looking at the single leg hip hinge stabilization exercise. The base of support is smaller and the balance requirement is more demanding. Position the patient close to the backs of two chairs so they can touch the chairs if they lose balance. The patient is instructed to flex their stance knee and hinge (flex) at the same hip. As the hip flexes the opposite LE extends backward at the hip while maintaining full knee extension. Again, once the patient's trunk is in front of the vertical plane their spinal extensors will contract isometrically. Also, once in this position, have the patient pull their abdomen inward (abdominal drawing). Note, the entire LE must remain in line with the trunk. This movement pattern and position can be held for 6-10 seconds and repeated a minimum of 6-10 times or performed more rhythmically by picking up various objects as part of a work hardening or clinic based safe lifting program. (See figure 18-27). The single leg hip hinge movement-lifting pattern allow an individual to pick up and move lighter objects in a safe and quick manner.

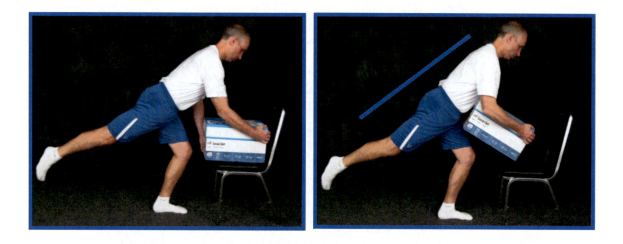

Figure 18-27: Lumbar Stabilization during Lifting, Single Leg Hip Hinge Lifting with Active Abdominal Bracing:

Using a similar single leg hip flexion movement pattern with full hip and knee extension for the LE in OKC, have the patient pick up various objects with this hip hinge movement pattern. Active and passive abdominal drawing can be performed as the object lifted is lifted and then pulled into the abdomen. Keep in mind that the rules for good overall spinal posture must be followed with single leg hip hinging. In other words, the patient is to keep the back of their neck long and their chest up and forward during all single leg hip hinge motions. Performance of exercises 18-26 - 18-28 will minimize lumbar segmental motion, and build LE strength and balance during the performance of this safe lifting movement pattern.

Therapeutic Exercise

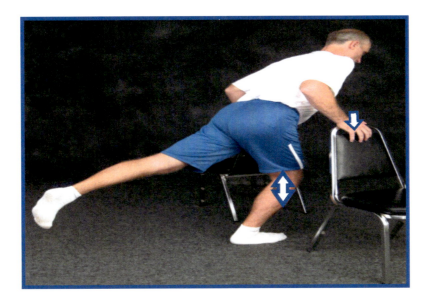

Figure 18-28: Lumbar Stabilization, Hip Hinge Series – Single Leg Hinges with Balance Support and Assisted Mini - Squat LE Strengthening

While building isometric spinal extensor strength and improved LE balance in the position shown above, this patient can also be taught to build additional LE strength and endurance with assisted single leg mini-squats. Short arc knee flexion and extension is performed with the LE in CKC and assisted if need be by the UE's which are in contact with the back of two chairs. This exercise technique is an excellent way to build LE strength and while building spinal extensor strength and practicing this important and useful lifting pattern. As a general point of review, remember that assisted motions, arms assisting the legs in this case, should be incorporated when strength impairment or pain impairment adversely affects a patient's ability to perform an active or resisted motion.

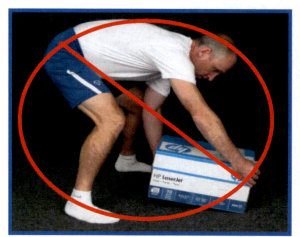 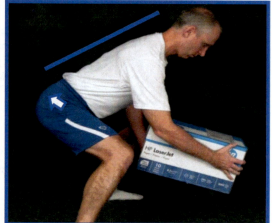

Figure 18-29: Lifting Position from Floor, Trunk Flexion Verses the Hip Hinge Position:

Patient involved with material handling or individuals that just have to lift objects occasionally should learn to feel the difference between the right and wrong spinal position during a lift. Regarding the figure on the left, note how the chest position has dropped causing excessive thoracolumbar flexion and how the chin has escaped forward causing a shortening of the posterior aspect of the cervical spine. The hip hinge position will promote isometric contraction all of the posterior spinal extensor muscles and this will hold the spinal segments stable during a lift. Having the patient draw their chin down and in toward the anterior aspect of the neck, (Adam's Apple) if your patient prefers, will activate the cervical flexor muscles and this will provide increased muscular based stability for the cervical segments as well.

Therapeutic Exercise

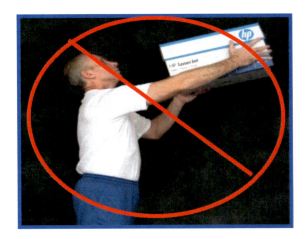 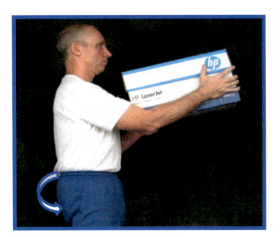

Figure 18-30: Spinal Positioning During an Overhead Lift and UE Reach Movement:

Let's finish this segment of the text, incorporating hip hinging into a safe lifting movement pattern by discussing a related and relevant point. When an object is lifted and held over head or when working with the upper extremities overhead, the lumbar and cervical spine should not be allowed to hyperextend if degenerative changes in the facets or loss of disc space are present (Figure on the left). To prevent lumbar hyperextension during overhead lifting, the patient should be instructed to perform a posterior pelvic tilt. Next, the patient's neck should not hyperextend. Regarding this, the patient is taught to lift their chest bone (sternum) up and forward and to elongate the back of their neck by moving their chin down and in toward their Adam's apple (Figure on the right).

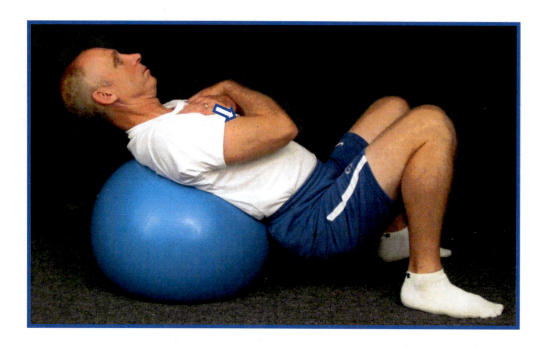

Figure 18-31: Swiss Ball Abdominal Muscle Training – Level 1:

The Swiss Ball offers many patients with significantly impaired abdominal muscle strength a means to begin the process of improving abdominal muscle control. Note the start position including the degree of hip flexion, UE position, and the angle of the trunk with respect to the horizontal plane. This type of positioning will allow a patient with reduced muscle strength the opportunity to begin upper abdominal strength building. The patient's breast bone or sternum should be a point of focus and the following bit of instruction is given. Tell the patient to move their sternum 1 to 2 inches downward toward their belly button and then move back to the start position with a nice rhythm. Isotonic gravity resisted movement with the trunk starting well in front of the horizontal plane should occur with multiple sets and reps dictated primarily by the quality of the patient's motion. As abdominal muscle strength improves, therapists should further challenge the patient's abdominal muscles by moving their UE's behind their head (Level 2).

Therapeutic Exercise

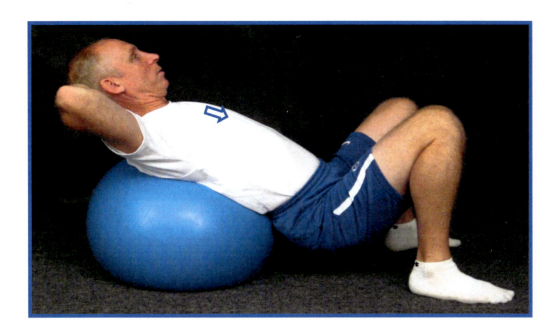

Figure 18-32: Swiss Ball Abdominal Muscle Training – Level 2:

The level 2 position begins to increase the demand on the abdominal muscles by placing a small amount of weight (the UE's) further from the axis of movement. The patient's breast bone or sternum should still be the point of focus and the instruction should be the same. Tell the patient to move their sternum 1 to 2 inches downward toward their belly button and then move back to the start position with a nice rhythm (Arrow above). Short arc isotonic gravity resisted movement with the trunk in front of the horizontal plane is performed. The therapist will determine the number of sets and reps based on strength and resultant movement quality. Progression toward the level 3 position will occur incrementally by teaching the patient to straighten (extend) their hips and knees and move their trunk progressively toward the horizontal plane.

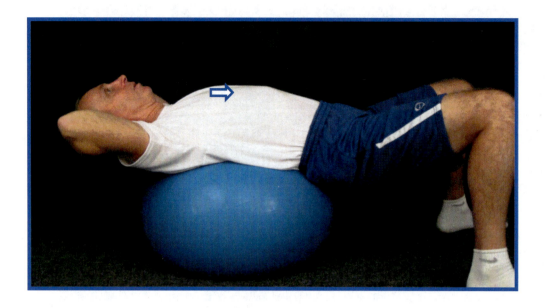

Figure 18-33: Swiss Ball Abdominal Muscle Training – Level 3:

Continue to instruct the patient to move their sternum 1 to 2 inches downward toward their belly button and then move back to the start position with a nice rhythm. Now their trunk is in the horizontal plane and this short arc isotonic gravity resisted movement will be much more challenging. Inform your patient and be sure that they understand that this training position is similar to lying flat on their back in bed. In other words, all of the vertical compressive loads have been taken off the lumbar segments making this training position very safe. Next, while the emphasis of movement can still remain on the upper abdomen, the lumbopelvic angle (tilt) should be held isometrically using the lower abdominal muscles and the gluteal muscles. The therapist should ask for constant isometric contraction of the lower abdomen (pulling the lower tummy up toward the belly button and inward) while also "squeezing" their gluteal muscles together. Note, the lumbopelvic angle (tilt) is held in the most symptom free position. Use this level 3 version where isometric lumbopelvic tilting (position) is held in cases of symptomatic lumbar instability.

Therapeutic Exercise

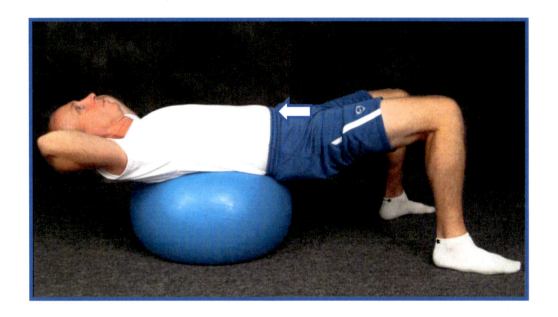

Figure 18-34: Swiss Ball Abdominal Muscle Training, Posterior Tilting – Level 4:

Now the emphasis of the movement pattern switches to the lower abdomen and our focus is the performance of isotonic pelvic tilting. In the same way, instruct your patient to perform rhythmical isotonic contractions of their lower abdomen (pulling the lower tummy upward toward the belly button and inward) while also "squeezing" their gluteal muscle together. The amount of lumbopelvic flexion and extension (tilting) should be determined based on symptoms. The movement pattern should be as pain free as possible. Make sure that your patient realizes that they control the movement pattern. If pain is encountered while dropping the pelvis downward over the lower edge of the ball (lumbar extension with anterior pelvic tilting) then this portion of the movement should be shortened! Also, the rate of isotonic lumbopelvic tilting should be set where pain is controlled or even reduced. Some patients find a slower motion more comforting whereas some patients find a quicker movement more helpful. To repeat, be sure that your patient understands that this training position is similar to lying flat on their back in bed. In other words, all of the vertical compressive loads have been taken off the lumbar segments making this training position very safe. In cases of discogenic lumbar segmental instability, hold the pelvic tilt isometrically (Level 3).

Therapeutic Exercise

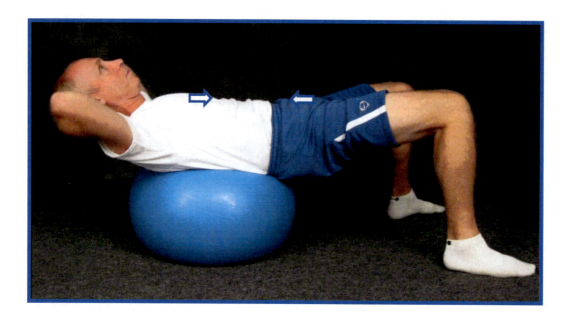

Figure 18-35: Swiss Ball Abdominal Muscle Training, Tilt-Mini Crunch Combo – Level 5:

To further improve abdominal muscle strength and lumbopelvic positional control in patients with symptomatic lumbar conditions, have the patient perform both upper and lower abdominal muscle training at the same time. Instruct the patient to move their sternum 1 to 2 inches downward toward their belly button and simultaneously pull their lower abdomen (pulling the lower tummy upward toward the belly button and inward) while also "squeezing" their gluteal muscles together. The end position for the lumbar segments should be close to neutral or slight lumbopelvic flexion. Once this position is reached, the patient is instructed to release their tilt, let their pelvis drop, and release their upper abdominal contraction as well so that the sternum moves back to its original position. Make sure that your patient realizes that they control the movement pattern. If pain is encountered while dropping the pelvis downward over the lower edge of the ball (lumbar extension with anterior pelvic tilting) then this portion of the movement should be shortened. Some patients find a slower motion more comforting whereas some patients find a quicker movement more helpful. Remind your patients that their lumbar spine is unloaded in this supine position as compared to the seated or standing position.

Therapeutic Exercise

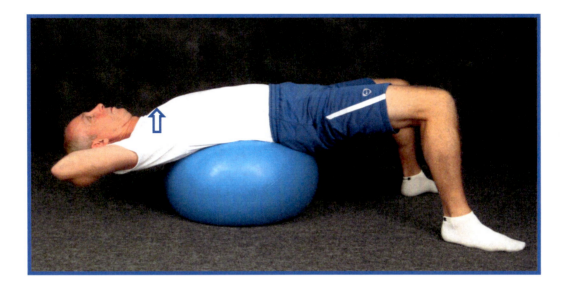

Figure 18-36: Swiss Ball Abdominal Muscle Training – Level 6

For our more well-conditioned lumbar pain patients or perhaps when training an athlete, challenge the abdominal muscle more so by having the patient drop their upper body further over the top edge of the Swiss Ball. From this more advanced starting position, instruct the patient to move their trunk upward and sternum downward in a rhythmical manner. At the same time the patient is to perform isotonic contractions of their lower abdomen (pulling the lower tummy upward toward the belly button and inward) while also "squeezing" their gluteal muscles together. The end position for the lumbar segments should be close to neutral or slight lumbopelvic flexion. Make sure that your patient realizes that they are in control of the arc and speed of movement. For the athletic client, perform a rep max program where repetitions are performed until muscle fatigue is reached.

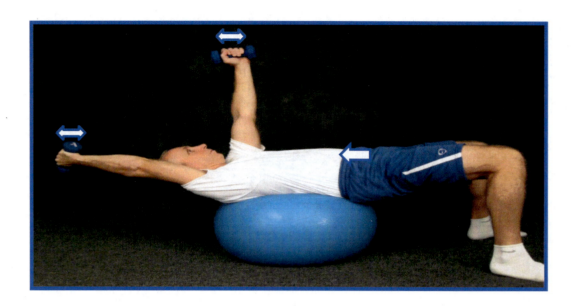

Figure 18-37: Swiss Ball Advanced Abdominal Muscle Training Activities:

This is a more advanced training exercise which can be prescribed in order to develop a higher level of abdominal strength. Isometric posterior pelvic tilting is held while various U/E movement patterns are performed. Free weight, elastic band resistance, or pulley system resistance can be incorporated. Note, for this and other Swiss Ball abdominal strength training exercises, the patient should maintain their cervical segments in a neutral or mid position. The patient should be instructed to bring the chin down and in toward their Adam's apple to facilitate contraction of the ventral flexor muscles. Multiple sets of alternating UE elevation can be performed while isometric lower abdominal and gluteal strength is improved by constantly holding a firm posterior pelvic tilt.

Therapeutic Exercise

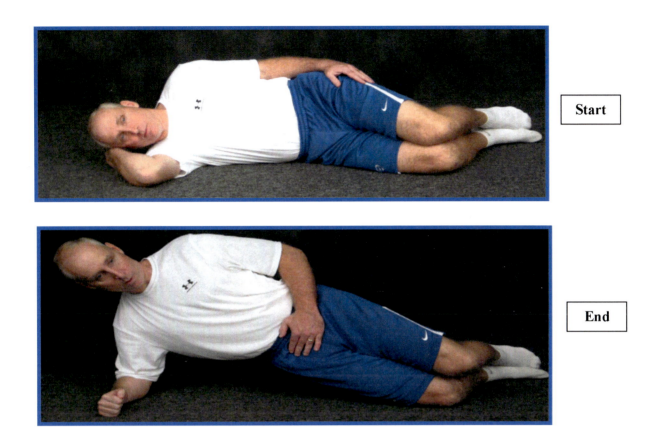

Figure 18-38: Lumbar Stabilization, Lateral Trunk Muscle Training – Level 1:

Now we move into the topic of developing isometric muscle strength in order to improve dynamic trunk stability using the Quadratus Lumborum, abdominal muscles, and the spinal extensors and proximal hip muscles. Note, during rest breaks, (top figure) side bending of the lumbar spine is not permitted and the patient should keep their lumbar spine in a mid-position with regard to the frontal plane. Through lumbopelvic tilting, and with regard to the sagittal plane, the lumbar segments may be placed in mid-position, slight lumbopelvic flexion, or slight lumbopelvic extension. Lumbopelvic positioning is based on which position is least symptomatic. Regarding this first level lateral trunk muscle training exercise, instruct your patient to move from the side lying rest position to this first level isometric training position. A 6-10 second isometric contraction should be held with longer isometric positioning determined by the therapist's evaluation of the patient's strength and clinical condition.

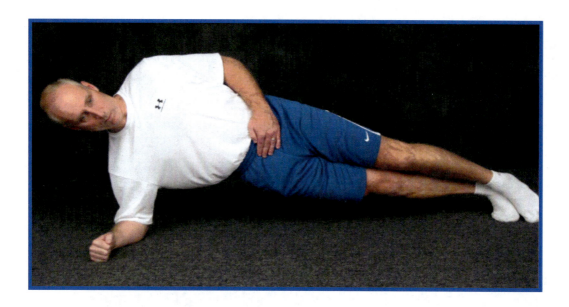

Figure 18-39: Lumbar Stabilization, Lateral Trunk Muscle Training – Level 2:

The level 2 position reduces the patient's base of support by extending their hips and knees. This will increase the balance requirement for this version of lateral trunk muscle training. Hold the training position for a minimum of 6-10 seconds moving into and out of the rest position (Top photo, Figure 18-38) or teach the patient to roll from one side to the other multiple times without coming out of the lateral trunk muscle training position and without relaxation of the abdominal drawing and or gluteal squeeze.

Therapeutic Exercise

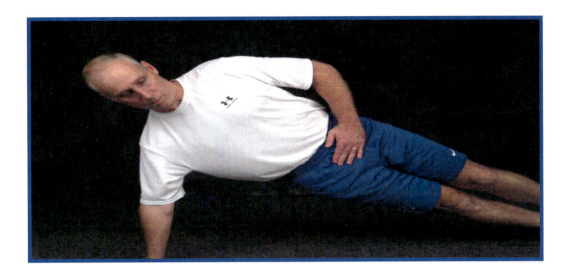

Figure 18-40: Lumbar Stabilization, Lateral Trunk Muscle Training – Level 3:

The level 3 position continues to reduce the patient's base of support by extending the elbow and placing the palm of the hand in contact with the floor. This position will require increased distal UE strength and proximal shoulder muscle control. Do not forget to have your patient position their lumbopelvic angle (tilt) so that their lumbar segments are placed in the least symptomatic position. Encourage active abdominal drawing to further support the lumbar segments. Abdominal drawing can be reinforced with the uppermost hand as shown above. Hold the training position for a minimum of 6-10 seconds moving into and out of the rest position (Top photo Figure 18-38).

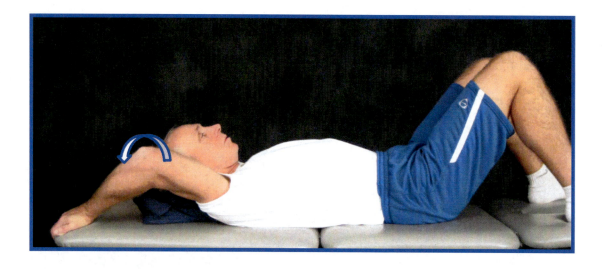

Figure 18-41: Lumbar Self-Traction, Hook lying

This self-traction exercise can be easily applied in your clinic and as part of a patient's home exercise program. It is an important exercise for pain impairments associated with central low back pain and sciatic nerve irritation. First, the patient lies in a hook lying position which will reduce compressive load on the lumbar discs. Next, the patient is instructed to take a deep breath in, and then gently tense his elbow flexors. Isometric elbow flexion is held during exhalation only. With the patient's pelvis acting as an "anchor" the isometric elbow flexion will impart a gentle therapeutic motion to the spinal segments which approximates a traction or elongation of the lumbar segments. This motion often reduces low back ache and in some cases LE sciatic pain referral. Remember, most cases of significant lower back ache involve, at some level, disc degeneration with or without radiculitis and instability. This procedure can also be used in conjunction with lumbar stabilization exercise training as a "rest break position" to unload the IVD. Again, the self-traction should only be applied during exhalation and multiple reps can be performed until there is symptomatic relief.

Therapeutic Exercise

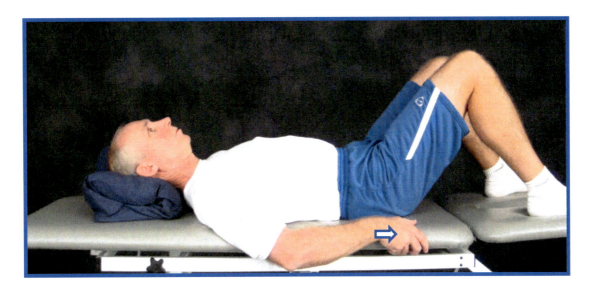

Figure 18-42: Lumbar Self -Traction, Hook Lying-Version 2:

This version of self-traction can be prescribed when an elevated shoulder position is painful or not possible. This procedure can be performed at home and in your clinic for pain management purposes and it is a key exercise when low back ache and nerve irritation is present. Similar to exercise 18-41, this procedure can be used for segmental unloading during a rest break in between sets of lumbar stabilization exercises. After having taken a deep breath, instruct the patient to isometrically contract their elbow extensor muscles during exhalation. The combination of the hook lying position and resultant movement due to UE muscle contraction will assist in reducing compressive loading on the lumbar discs. Remember, self-traction is applied during exhalation only and reps are performed until a treatment effect (reduced low back pain or sciatic irritation) is achieved.

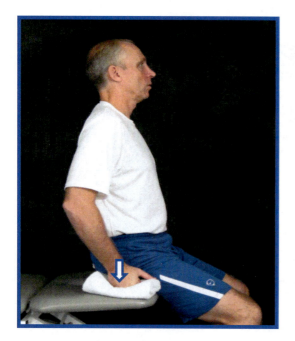 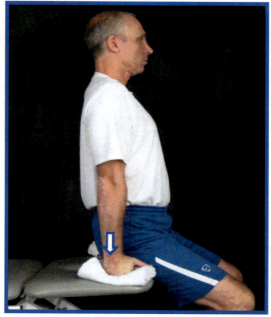

Figure 18-43: Lumbar Self-Traction – Seated:

The figure above demonstrates the seated version of lumbar self-traction. Note how the patient is seated with their hips higher than their knees. This is the ideal seating posture in that a more vertical pelvic position is promoted. Typically, the patient presses downward for 5-6 seconds and repeats the UE push down 5-6 times. The ideal amount of force unloads the patient's buttock from the surface they are sitting on. This lumbar unloading exercise can be performed many times daily particularly if the seated position appears to predispose your patient to lumbar or sciatic pain discomfort. A caudally directed pressure is applied into the seat of a chair or bench. Towel rolls may be used to "lengthen" a patient's arms and provide a soft surface for their knuckles to press into. The UE's should be tucked into the patient's side and right in line with the lumbar spine. For my money, this is our most "pure" form of self-traction in that the entire pelvis pulls down on the lumbar segments.

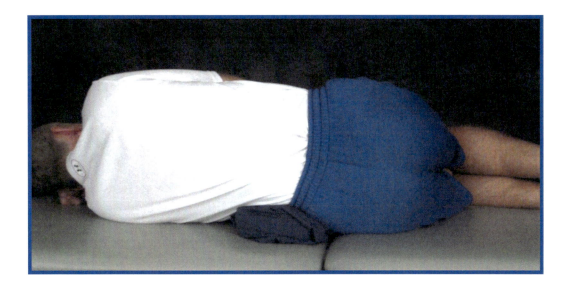

Figure 18-44: Lumbar Positional Distraction - Version 1

This exercise can be applied in the presence of lumbar nerve irritation causing referral of pain into a patient's LE. The objective of this therapeutic positioning exercise is to incorporate both lumbar flexion and side bending over a pillow roll in order to open the intervertebral foramen (IVF) and decompress an irritated, swollen nerve root.[38] Increased side bending can be achieved by moving the undermost shoulder forward and in effect have the patient lay on their scapula. Do not allow the uppermost shoulder to roll backward causing spinal rotation. Bilateral hip flexion of at least 60 degrees is used in order to reduce the lumbar lordosis which may also assist in opening the lumbar IVF. As the patient lies over the towel or pillow roll, they should determine if their LE pain improves. Note, the painful LE is uppermost. This positioning technique is used for unilateral LE radicular pain. This position may be held for 2-5 minutes and if effective can be repeated as needed throughout the day.

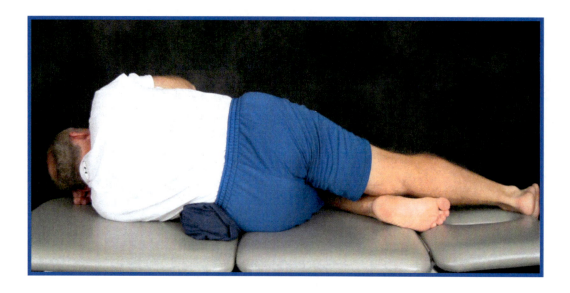

Figure 18-45: Lumbar Positional Distraction – Version 2

This version also seeks to incorporate therapeutic positioning in order to open lumbar intervertebral foramina and decompress an irritated, swollen nerve root.[38] The patient is to lie over a towel roll and determine if their LE pain improves. Similar to exercise 18-44, the painful LE is uppermost and this exercise position may be held for 2-5 minutes and if effective, repeated as needed throughout the day. Remember, exercise technique is used for unilateral LE radicular pain only, not bilateral neurogenic claudication often seen with lumbar stenosis. Note that in version 2, the uppermost LE is extended at the hip and knee. This will increase side bending over the towel or pillow roll and in so doing will increase the size of the exit zone which is medial to, under, and just lateral to the pedicle for each lumbar nerve root. Choice of version 1 or version 2 is based on which position provides the most symptomatic relief of LE pain. In both version 1 and 2, the patient should not lay directly on their "undermost" shoulder. The patient should in effect lie on their scapula which will increase the lumbar side bending over the pillow roll.

Therapeutic Exercise

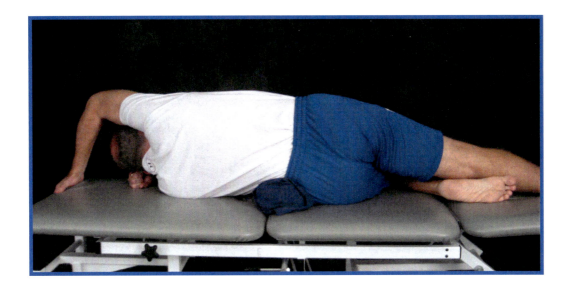

Figure 18-46: Lumbar Positional Distraction with Self-Traction

This variation of positional distraction incorporates self-traction as an additional means to provide a treatment effect. Similar to exercises 18-44 and 18-45 the patient is to lie over a towel roll and determine if their LE pain improves. If pain relief is noted, the patient is then instructed to tense their elbow flexor muscles. In doing this, increased side bending over the pillow roll is achieved and in some cases, additional LE pain relief is reported. To repeat, the painful LE is uppermost and the patient should not lie directly on their undermost shoulder. This position may be held for 2-5 minutes while self-traction is intermittently applied during exhalation only. Choice of LE positioning (version 1 or 2) is based on which position best relieves LE pain. In addition to separating the roof and floor of the lumbar IVF, lumbar side bending and flexion can temporarily move a hypertrophic superior facet downward and away from an existing lumbar nerve root.

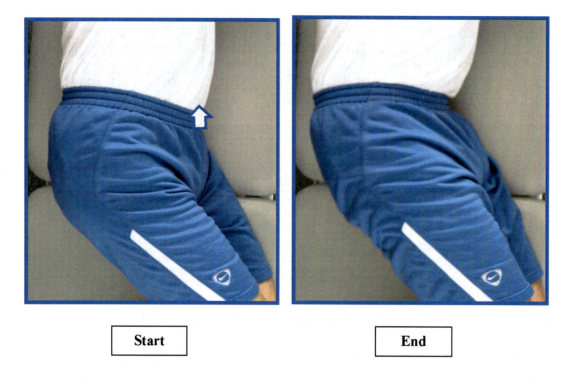

| Start | End |

Figure 18-47: Posterior Lumbopelvic Tilting – Side lying:

The next three figures discuss posterior pelvic tilting. We will frame our discussion of this basic exercise around a very common orthopedic condition, lumbar spinal stenosis. Acquired or degenerative stenosis is a commonly seen condition in orthopedic physical therapy practice. Perhaps the most common disability associated with this condition is reduced tolerance for the upright position and upright ambulation. In order to better tolerate the upright position patients must be able to flatten their lumbar lordosis (posteriorly tilt their pelvis) when in an upright position. Exercises 18-47 and 18-48 often need to be mastered in order for patients to become proficient at lordotic reduction in the upright position (Figure 18-49). The side lying and hook lying posterior tilt exercise can be instructed in either order. Some patients find it easier to learn lumbopelvic tilting in a side lying position, while some will find the movement pattern more easily performed in hook lying. Therapists will find that palpatory reinforcement (AAROM) of the movement pattern in side lying is much easier in terms of manual contact on the sacrum and lower abdominal region. Lastly, in terms of preparation for standing posterior tilting, this exercise in side lying can be performed with the patient's hips in various degrees of extension.

Therapeutic Exercise

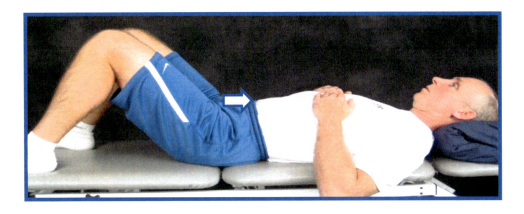

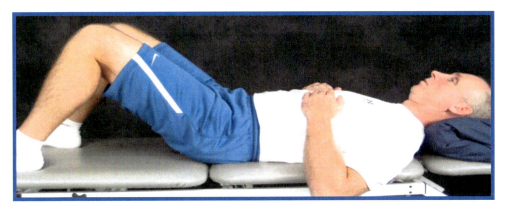

Figure 18-48: Posterior Lumbopelvic Tilting – Hook lying:

This is the more conventional exercise intervention position for isometric gluteal and lower abdominal muscle strength and endurance building. The patient with weakness impairments in these key muscle groups should be encouraged to perform side lying and hook lying posterior lumbopelvic tilting often throughout the day using various isometric hold times and or rhythmical short arc isotonic motions. As a patient's muscle strength and neuromuscular control improves, their ability to control their lumbopelvic position when upright (standing) will also improve. The ability to control and typically reduce the lumbar lordosis when performing common daily activities in the upright position is a key to symptom control when a patient presents with posterior disc space narrowing and other degenerative stenotic changes.

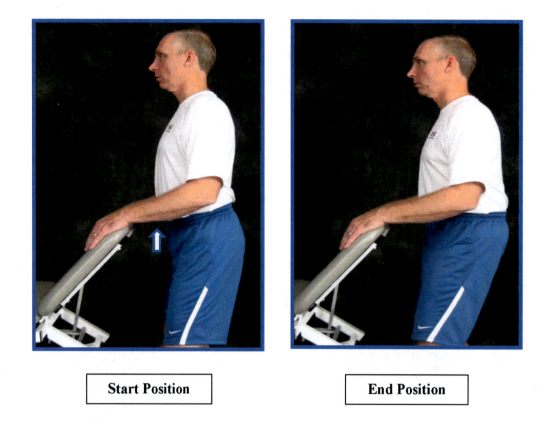

| Start Position | End Position |

Figure 18-49: Posterior Lumbopelvic Tilting – Standing:

In patients with more severe degenerative (acquired) changes in their lumbar spine, causing stenotic narrowing and resultant lumbar and LE pain, lordotic flattening (lumbopelvic tilting) will often reduce the intensity of discomfort experienced when standing and during ambulation. When pain is experienced during a stationary upright activity, the patient is instructed to use both the gluteal and lower abdominal muscle groups and to find a lumbopelvic angle which reduces their discomfort. During ambulation the instructional emphasis for lordotic flattening should center on use of the lower abdominal muscles only. Here the patient is instructed to pull their lower tummy upward and inward toward their belly button. It may not be practical to hold this isometric contraction for a long period of ambulation but it is practical to hold a slight posterior tilt for short times as a patient walks from item to item in a store or from room to room in their home. Again, posterior pelvic tilting while walking is accomplished by pulling the lower abdomen upward and inward. When standing still, bilateral glut contraction can assist the posterior rotation of the pelvis.

Therapeutic Exercise

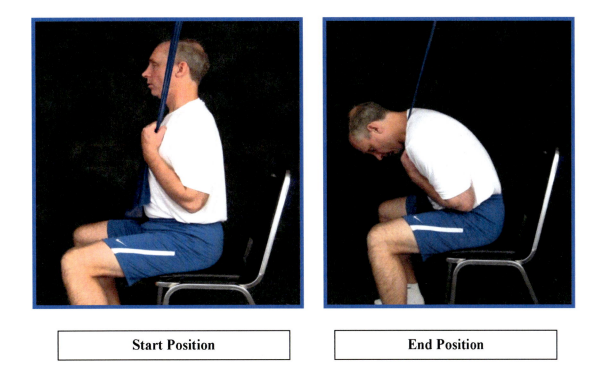

Start Position | End Position

Figure 18-50: Resisted Flexion / Assisted Extension - Seated:

This is an exercise technique which temporarily relieves pain impairments associated with acquired lumbar stenosis.[39] The patient is instructed to comfortably and smoothly "curl up" (flex) his or her spinal segments against elastic band resistance and then allow those same bands to assist the trunk back to an upright position. Often patients with this condition find that gently flexing their lumbar spine changes the amount of compressive load on pain sensitive posterior lumbar structures. Several sets of this motion are performed using the 30 second work and 30 second rest program. Note, place a knot in the middle of a large slice of blue or black elastic band. The knot is thrown over the top of a door and the door is securely closed. The patient has two movement options with this procedure. First, a slow flexion curl up can be performed close to the end range of lumbar flexion and this motion is immediately followed by assisted extension back to the upright position. Second, the patient may choose to perform a resisted curl up, stay in that position, and perform a small oscillatory resisted flexion/assisted extension motion maintaining a degree of flexion in all lumbar segments. This short amplitude oscillation should be performed for 30 seconds before returning to the upright position. The movement is repeated until the patient notes an improvement in their lumbar pain intensity.

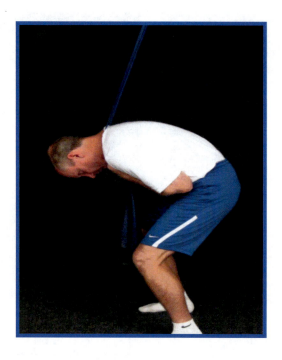

Figure 18-51: Resisted Flexion / Assisted Extension - Standing:

This is essentially the same exercise, but this version incorporates short arc squatting in order to add a LE strength-building component to the exercise procedure. In the same way the patient is encouraged to gently flex their lumbar spine against resistance (abdominal muscle training) and to simultaneously flex their hips and knees. Elastic band assisted extension will reduce the loading on the lumbar segments and associated soft tissues as the spinal extensor muscles will not need to contract as forcibly in order to return the patient back to the upright position.[39] It is not uncommon to find LE weakness impairments in patient with chronic lumbar stenosis. Patients presenting with lumbar stenosis and LE weakness will find this version of Resisted Flexion/Assisted Extension to be helpful. Note: elastic band assistance back to the upright position will also reduce loading on the LE joints as well. Multiple sets of 6-10 reps can be performed with a rest breaks as needed. A large slice of blue or black elastic band is typically used and knotted in the middle. The knot is thrown over the top of a door and the door is securely closed.

Therapeutic Exercise

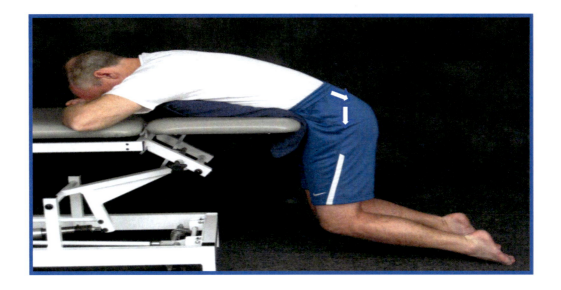

Figure 18-52: Lumbar Self – Mobilization, Forward Bending (Flexion)

I believe that this is by far the safest method for performing lumbar self-stretching in the direction of forward bending. Unfortunately, too many people still attempt to stretch their lumbar spine by touching their toes when in an upright position. Toe touching provides no support for the lumbar segments and places a large tensile load on many posterior anatomical structures including the sciatic nerve. By placing the patient's abdomen on the table, and incorporating additional pillows, the lumbar segments are well supported and extra or unnecessary vertebral translation is prevented. The patient is taught to let their pelvis "sag" into a posterior tilt, which will promote a reduction in lumbar lordosis. This will allow for safe stretching of a number of posterior soft tissue structures. Note how the back of the cervical spine is "lengthened" and how the cervical segments are protected in this position. This stretch may be held for 30 seconds and up to a minute. Patients with stiffness impairments limiting lumbar forward flexion and patients who experience low back pain in the upright (standing) position will find this self-stretching exercise procedure helpful.

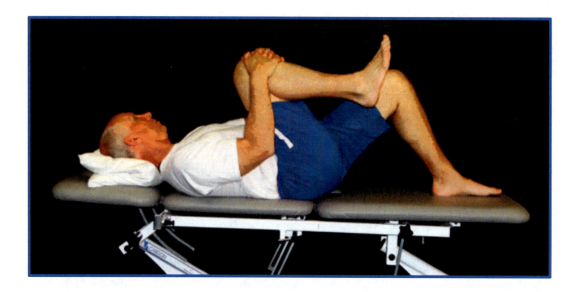

Figure 18-53: Lumbar Lordotic Flattening (Flexion)- Single Knee to Chest:

This exercise is an old as Physical Therapy itself. The single knee to chest exercise has a number of benefits. End range passive hip flexion will stretch the hip extensor muscles, the posterior hip capsule and this motion will, similar to 18-52, flatten our patient's lumbar lordosis. Lordotic flattening is particularly useful for pain impairments associated with loss of posterior disc space and acquired (degenerative) lumbar stenosis.

Therapeutic Exercise

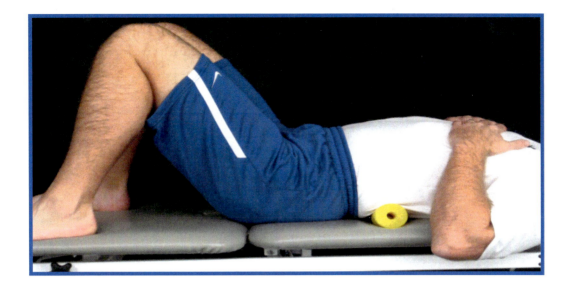

Figure 18-54: Lumbar Self – Mobilization Backward Bending (Extension) in Hook lying – Swimming Noodle:

Note the patient position for this extension self-mobilization (stretching) exercise. The patient is placed in hook lying with the hips flexed to approximately 60 degrees. For me, this is the clear position of choice for stretching impaired lumbar extension due to segmental stiffness and improving lumbar posture when the patient's lumbar region has taken on an overly kyphotic position due to advanced degenerative changes. Unlike the prone lying extension exercises, which forces excessive hyperextension through the lower lumbar segments, this version of lumbar extension self-mobilization will protect the lower lumbar segments. The patient is instructed to lie in a hook lying position and then perform a bridge in order to lift their lumbar region off the treatment table or their floor at home. Next, a swimming noodle with a wooden dowel inserted into the noodle is placed across the upper or lower lumbar region. Demonstrate and or instruct how to set his/her spine down onto the noodle and to focus on dropping their pelvis over the lower edge of the noodle. This will promote lumbar extension and anterior tilting of the pelvis. The noodle may be moved up or down the lumbar spine in approximately 1 inch increments across all five motion segments. Generally, this stretch is held for 15-30 seconds per segment.

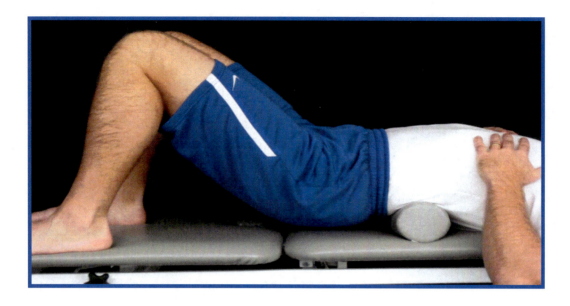

Figure 18-55: Lumbar Self – Mobilization Backward Bending (Extension) in Hook lying – Soft Foam Roll:

A three-inch soft foam roll may also be used to provide a less specific self-stretch as compared to the smaller swimming noodle. The patient is instructed to lie in a hook lying position and then perform a bridge in order to lift their lumbar region off the treatment table or a floor at home. Next, the soft foam roll is placed across the upper, mid or lower lumbar region. The patient is instructed to and guided by their therapist to set their lumbar spine and pelvis down onto and over the lower edge of the roll. This will promote lumbar extension with associated anterior tilting of the pelvis. Lumbar extension performed in this position will promote a more even sharing of lumbar segmental movement and pelvic movement, something that the prone based lumbar extension exercises do not. In prone lying, anterior tilting of the pelvis cannot occur and this will force excessive and unnecessary extension motion through the segments. Not a great idea, particularly in cases of early grade disc degeneration that causes discogenic based segmental hypermobility. Generally, this stretch is held for 15-30 seconds with a roll of this size placed in three spots, the upper, mid, and lower lumbar regions.

Therapeutic Exercise

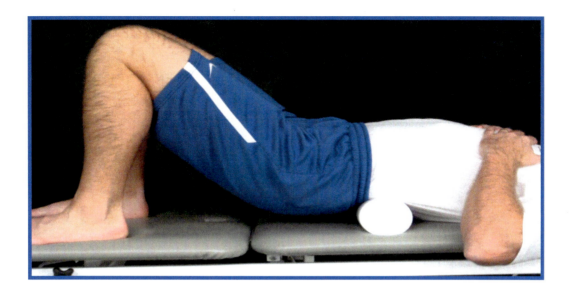

Figure 18-56: Lumbar Self – Mobilization, Backward Bending (Extension) in Hook lying – Firm Foam Roll:

Similar to the three-inch soft foam roll, a three-inch firm foam roll can be used for this exercise in some cases. In general, these firm foam rolls are not tremendously comfortable when used for this exercise except in patient cases where there is little to no low back pain and extension stiffness impairment, not pain, is the primary feature of the lumbar condition. Note the positioning of the patient's hips around 60 degrees of flexion is a key feature of these hook lying self-mobilization exercises. As the patient drops their pelvis downward over the lower edge of a noodle, roll, or wedge (18-56) the lumbar segments will be mobilized toward extension but not into hyperextension. In particular, the hook lying position and anterior pelvic tilting will prevent excessive compression of the posterior disc space at the L4 and L5 levels. Loss of disc height often occurs posteriorly. Understanding this, ask yourself why we would want to prescribe any exercise, which significantly closes down the posterior aspect of the motion segment. Generally, this stretch is held for 15-30 seconds with the roll approximately placed in the upper, mid, and lower lumbar regions.

Therapeutic Exercise

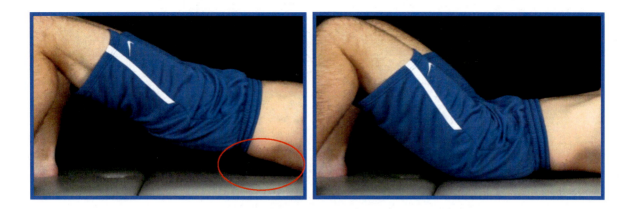

Figure 18-57: Lumbar Self – Mobilization, Backward Bending (Extension) in Hook lying – Thoracic Mobilization Wedge:

This is the last version of the self-mobilization exercises and is the most specific one. Again, the patient is placed in hook lying with their hips flexed to approximately 60 degrees. Indications for this exercise are extension movement (stiffness) impairment and improving lumbar posture when the patient's lumbar region has taken on an overly kyphotic position secondary to advanced degenerative changes. These hook lying extension self-mobilization exercises may assist in fluid redistribution within the IVD. This may be particularly useful in younger lumbar pain patients who have lost their lordotic position, particularly after spending time in forward flexed positions. Patients should first be instructed to lie in a hook lying position and then perform a bridge in order to lift their lumbar region off the treatment table or floor at home. Next, the wedge is placed such that the peaks of the wedge are in a caudal position and supporting the lumbar transverse processes of the cranial vertebrae of the segment to be stretched. The patient is instructed to set their spine down onto the wedge and to focus of dropping their pelvis over its peaks. This will promote a more specific segmental lumbar extension. The wedge may be moved up or down the lumbar spine in approximately 1 inch increments across all five motion segments. Generally, this stretch is held for 15-30 seconds per segment.

Therapeutic Exercise

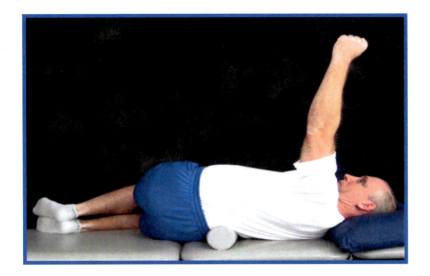

Figure 18-58: Lumbar Self – Mobilization, Constrained Rotation with Locking in Flexion and Side Bending:

I am not much for the idea of repetitive non-specific rotational self-mobilization of the lumbar spine. I believe large amplitude multi-segment lumbar rotation places too much tensile and compressive load through the lumbar discs and if performed too often and for too many years actually can damage the IVD. I believe this can be particularly problematic in the two lowermost lumbar discs. So, if a patient is demonstrating impaired trunk rotation and this impaired rotation is associated with a functional limitation, then this exercise above is how I would attempt to safely stretch the thoracolumbar segments into rotation. Note how that the lumbar spine is placed in flexion by virtue of the position of the hips. Next, note how a soft foam roll is placed in the lower lumbar region in order to right side bend the lower lumbar segments. Based on motion coupling, those same lower lumbar segments will be forced toward a right rotated position. As the patient is taught to slowly and carefully rotate their trunk to the left as shown above, the lower lumbar segments will not be able to follow into full left rotation and in effect based on the pre-positioning in flexion and right side bending, they will only follow the trunk rotation back to a mid-position. This will minimize the rotational load through the lower two discs. This controlled self-stretch may be held of up 30 seconds.

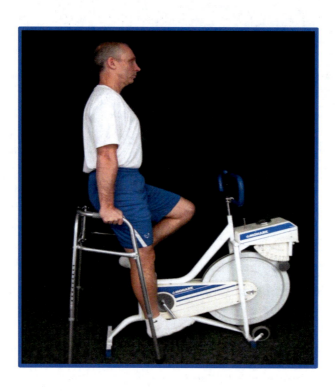

Figure 18-59: Aerobic Conditioning with Lumbar Self-Traction:

Patients with chronic low back pain, particularly those who have been off work for some period of time due to their lumbar problems often benefit from some form of aerobic conditioning. Stationary cycling provides a means to build aerobic capacity in some of our lumbar pain patients. Unfortunately, most stationary bikes offer little in the way of lumbar support. Patients with load sensitive lumbar conditions often do not tolerate a non-supported seated position. Symptom control while training aerobically in a seated position can be achieved if intermittent self-traction is applied. For example, during a 20-minute aerobic workout, the patient is instructed to intermittently press down onto a walker which is placed around and behind the patient. The patient uses their upper extremities to provide lumbar self-traction for several seconds and does so as often as necessary to prevent any increase in low back pain.

Therapeutic Exercise

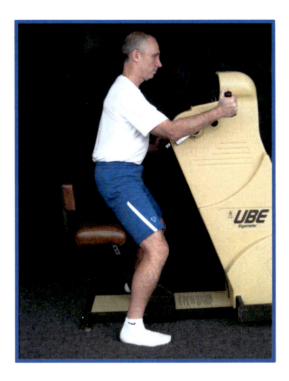 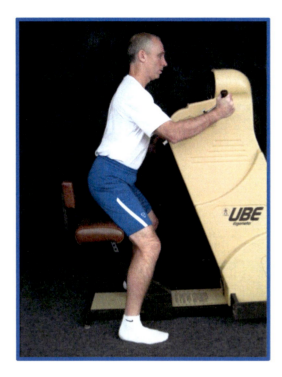

Figure 18-60: Aerobic Conditioning and Non-Symptomatic Lumbopelvic Positioning:

Along the same lines as exercise 18-57, the upper body ergometer can be used to improve aerobic capacity in our lumbar pain patients. The figures above demonstrate attention to lumbopelvic positioning during upper body aerobic training. In the figure on the left, the patient is aerobically training with their lordosis reduced, in other words they are training while intermittently performing and holding a posterior pelvic tilt. The figure on the right demonstrates a patient who may be more comfortable and dynamically more stable in a slight anterior pelvic tilt with a small degree of hip hinging to facilitate spinal extensor contraction. Clearly, the main point is this, have your patient find their most comfortable and most stable lumbopelvic position while training aerobically.

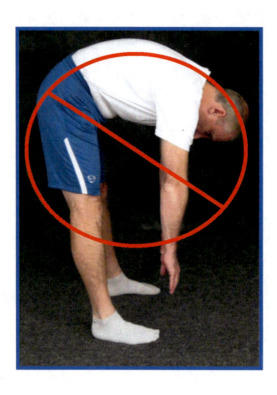

Figure 18-61: Lumbar Exercises with Injury Potential – Lumbar Flexion in Standing

It is reasonable to evaluate loaded (standing) cardinal plane lumbar motions during an examination in order to determine if there is a pain or movement impairment. Otherwise, there is little to no therapeutic value in the repetitive performance of these motions. Early in life when the lumbar discs (the spinal segment's primary stabilizing structure) are strong, the segments are able to tolerate the repetitive performance of motions like this. As the spine ages or in cases of pathological disc degeneration, typically caused by end plate damage and annular tearing, these same movements are not well tolerated, often cause discomfort and with long term repetitive performance can further damage the disc. In most cases there is nothing "therapeutic" about any of the following motions (18-59 – 18-65). Standing flexion places excessive tensile load on the posterior annulus fibrosis and sciatic nerve. We use this movement and end range position to provoke these tissues during an examination, why should we consider this a good therapeutic stretch?

Therapeutic Exercise

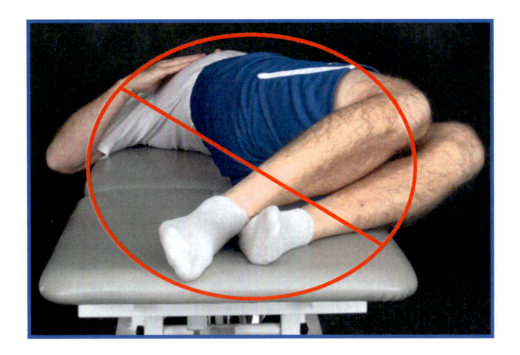

Figure 18-62: Lumbar Exercises with Injury Potential – Lumbar Rotation in Hook lying

In some circles this "therapeutic procedure" is known as the windshield wiper exercise. While lumbar facet orientation can vary a great deal, and in general the facet joints help to guide and constrain lumbar motion, these posterior joint may not constrain rotational movement quite as well at the two lower most lumbar segments. As a result, the L4 and L5 discs will be subjected to the greatest amount of compression (Nuclear portion) and tensile load (Annular portion) during rotational movement. So, my advice here is to not turn your wipers on! If your patient has low back pain secondary to discogenic instability/hypermobility, stay away from this exercise. Remember, significant and recurrent back ache and radiculitis involve disc degeneration and resultant segmental instability. It is only with late grade degeneration that segmental motion begins to decline. Large amplitude spinal ROM exercises can feed into the problem of excessive segmental motion secondary to disc degeneration.

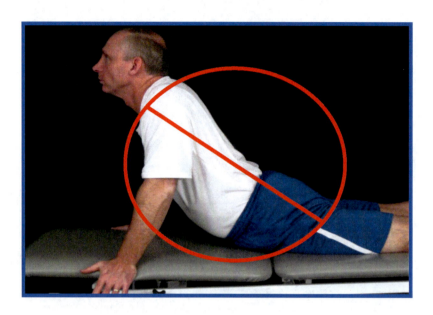

Figure 18-63: Lumbar Exercises with Injury Potential – Prone Press Up

I mentioned earlier in this chapter that most all significant orthopedic lumbar conditions involve disc degeneration and resultant discogenic instability/hypermobility. Some examples in this text have included disc degeneration with resultant segmental hypermobility, disc degeneration with radiculitis, degenerative spondylolisthesis, and acquired lumbar stenosis. It is my contention that only "younger" lumbar spines or lumbar spines without significant discogenic pathology are able to tolerate this motion. I would go as far to say that we could prescribe just about any movement pattern in patients with first time back ache and if there are no significant pathologic change in the discs that patient would improve. Apply this movement pattern to any patient with advanced grade degenerative disc changes and with any of the conditions mentioned above, and it is likely that they won't tolerate the repetitive performance of this movement or the end range lumbar position. Yes, early in life or in the early stages of a problem, the spine can handle prone based lumbar hyperextension. That does not mean that repetitive application of this movement/position is good for the lumbar segments if performed over time or when performed later in life or in more advanced stages of a disc condition.

Therapeutic Exercise

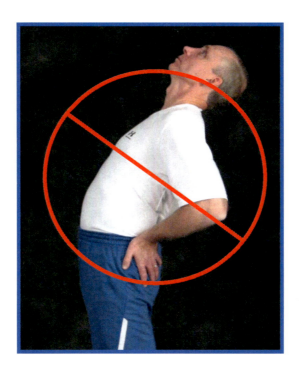

Figure 18-64: Lumbar Exercises with Injury Potential – Lumbar Extension in Standing

The performance of this motion in this position causes lumbar hyperextension and significant compressive loading to the posterior disc and lumbar facet joints. In standing, a good portion of the trunk weight is also loaded onto these important posterior structures. It is fairly well accepted that excessive compressive loading of joint cartilage elsewhere in the body is not good. I believe the same applies here. If this motion is performed too often, too much, or for too many years, I feel there is potential for this movement pattern to speed up the process of posterior disc degeneration and facet arthrosis. Think about this, some athletes are forced to stop competing in certain sports due in part to the repetitive hyperextension motions. Further, most all patients with symptomatic disc degeneration with and without hypermobility and or radiculitis never tolerate this movement during physical examination. Despite these common finding, the prescription of standing lumbar hyperextension in standing is still common place.

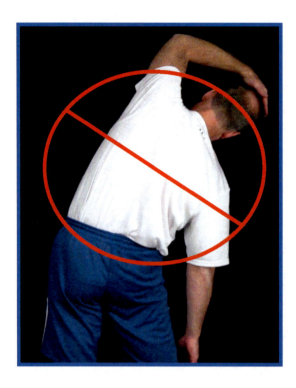

Figure 18-65: Lumbar Exercises with Injury Potential – Lumbar Side Bending in Standing

Lateral lumbar listing is a clinical sign which points toward asymmetric disc degeneration. Grade I-IV disc degeneration is most typically associated with increased segmental translation. This excessive vertebral translation does not just occur in the sagittal plane; it can also occur in the frontal plane during side bending motions. In cases such as this, the performance of repetitive loaded (standing) lumbar side bending may not be a good idea. To repeat the same concept, repetitive performance of this type of loaded lumbar motion early in life may damage the lumbar segments. It is fine to ask a patient to perform this movement during an examination when evaluating for a pain or movement impairments. Otherwise, the repetitive performance of this movement as a stretching exercise may actually, over time, injure the lower lumbar segments.

Therapeutic Exercise

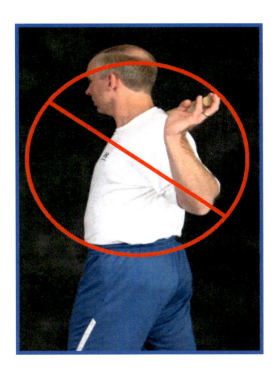

Figure 18-66: Lumbar Exercises with Injury Potential – Lumbar Rotation in Standing

Loaded lumbar rotation provides an excellent way to overly compress the nucleus pulpous and overly tension the annulus fibrosis. Typically, the L4 and L5 segments will move the most and often click or pop as a result of this movement. These sounds may be associated with transient relieve of backache or stiffness. The key word is transient. Chronic self-cracking or self-popping of a lumbar segment will likely have a long term deleterious effect on the segment. Think about it, the relief associated with self-popping (self-manipulation) never lasts, and most patients must continually self-manipulate. It is quite likely that the sound elicited during similar movement patterns (Figures 18-60 and 18-65) are coming from segments that already move well and likely already move too much. Remember, segments where the disc is beginning to degenerate typically show excessive angular or translational movement and are inclined to make more noise.

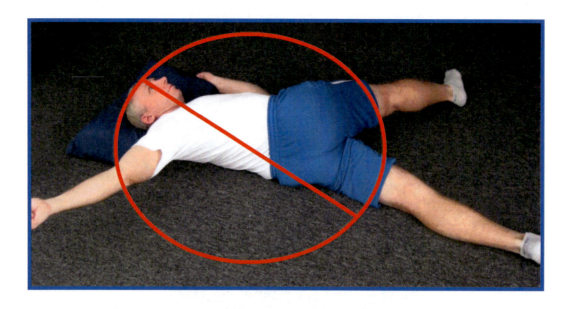

Figure 18-67: Lumbar Exercises with Injury Potential – Lumbar Rotation in Side Lying

Really nothing else to add here, other than to say, please consider my comments from figures 18-60 and 18-66). The individuals who can tolerate this movement are individuals who have fairly healthy lumbar segments. Like the other exercises with injury potential, I feel that individuals merely have to perform these motions long enough and in many cases they will eventually develop a lumbar problem. Because an exercise motion "feels OK" when an individual is young and has healthy discs, does not mean that same exercise motion is "OK" to continue to perform throughout life.

Therapeutic Exercise

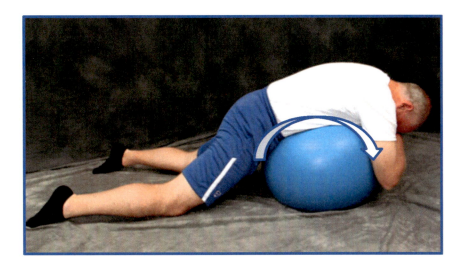

Figures 18-68: Swiss Ball Supported Spinal Stretching:

We have covered a number of different exercises in this chapter including this last segment which discusses how **not** to stretch your lumbar spine (Figures 18-61-18-67). Let's conclude this chapter by looking at how the large exercise ball can help our patients achieve a degree of soft tissue stretching without placing excessive compression, bending, or torsional loads on their lumbar motion segments and their disc in particular. First, remember that vertical positioning of the trunk will load your lumbar segments. Therefore, to protect your patient's lumbar discs reduce load in a more horizontal position over the exercise ball. The figure above shows supported multi-segment spine flexion. Note the gentle cervical, thoracic and lumbopelvic flexion Note how the knees are flexed to reduce tensile loading on the sciatic nerve and how the lumbar segments are supported as the Swiss ball gently presses the abdomen in a posterior direction. Also, see figures 18-52 and 18-53.

Therapeutic Exercise

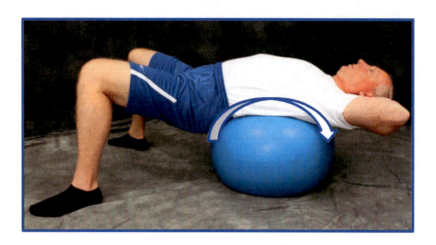

Figure 18-69: Swiss Ball Supported Spinal Stretching:

The picture above demonstrates general spinal extension by letting the pelvis sag down over the lower edge of the ball and the upper thoracic region sag down over the top edge of the ball. Note how the cervical spine is supported. This is a safe way to extend the spine and to promote good posture. Also, see figures 18-54-57.

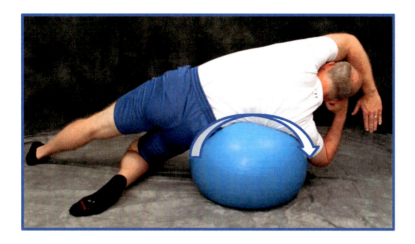

Figures 18-70: Swiss Ball Supported Spinal Stretching:

I discussed in figure 18-53, not to "crush" your patient's lumbar discs, facet joints and IVF with standing (loaded) side bending. The figure above demonstrates how to let the pelvis and upper back sag down over the bottom and top portion of the exercise ball and as a result, achieve a gentle and supported side bending stretch. Note how the lower most leg is flexed at the knee to increase base of support and note how the cervical spine is supported in a mid-position.

Epilogue

Well, that is it for the time being. I hope this text book gives clinicians a few new ideas for their exercise prescription and in some way helps the patients that you are responsible for. Readers may not agree with everything I have written, and that is OK. Disagreement may prompt further research. Continue to be creative with your exercise positioning, arc of therapeutic movement, speed of therapeutic movement, amount and type of motion assistance and amount and type of motion resistance. Respect your patient's orthopedic condition, the stage that condition may be in and how much time tissues have had to heal after an injury. Push patients to get stronger and more flexible, but not at all costs. Ultimately there may be a price to pay due to the over performance of loaded strength training and large amplitude multi-segment spinal stretching exercises. When your patient presents with joint pain or painful joint motion, make sure your therapeutic exercise motions are in fact therapeutic. In other words, the patient should be less painful when finished with their therapeutic exercise. An increase in pain or a "flare up" is NOT an acceptable reaction to therapeutic movement intervention. It is a sign that the exercise motion or exercise dose was incorrectly prescribed. Remember, it is OK for our younger patients and our athletic clients with healthy cartilage and healthy soft tissues to experience post exercise muscular discomfort. It is also OK for patients to experience mild stretching discomfort when self-stretching or self-mobilizing a shortened soft tissue structure. On the other hand, patients with varying level of degenerative change in their cartilage and discs or in patients who have experienced soft tissue injury, exercise that increases their level of discomfort in NOT therapeutic.

References:

1. Licht S. Therapeutic Exercise. New Haven, CT: Licht 1965.
2. Codmen EA. The Shoulder. Philadelphia: Harper & Row, 1934.
3. Delorme TL. Restoration of muscle power by heavy resistance exercises. J Bone Joint Surg Am 1945;27:645-650.
4. Kabat H. Studies in neuromuscular dysfunction XIII: new concepts and techniques of neuromuscular reeducation for paralysis. *Perm Found Med Bull* 1950;8:112-120.
5. Evjenth O. HambergAutostretching
6. DeLorme TL, Restoration of muscle power by heavy resistance exercises. J Bone Joint Surg Am. 1945;27:645-667.
7. Zinovieff AN. Heavy resistance exercise: the Oxford technique. Br J Physiol.1951;14:129-132.
8. Hurley B. Does strength training improve health status? Strength Conditioning J 1994;16:7-13.
9. McArdle WD, Katch FL, Katch VL. *Exercise Physiology*. 2nd ed. Philadelphia, Pa: Lea and Febiger;1986.
10. Lash JM, Sherman WM. Skeletal muscle function and adaptations to training. In: *American College of Sports Medicine: Resource manual for Guidelines for Exercise Testing and Prescriptioin*. 2nd ed. Philadelphia: Lea & Febiger;1993.
11. Anderson B, Burke ER. Scientific, medical, and practical aspects of stretching. *Clin Sports Med* 1991;10:63-86.
12. Jonagen S, Nemeth G. Griksson F. Hamstring injuries in sprinters: the role of concentric and eccentric hamstring muscle strength and flexibility. *Am J Sports Med* 1994;22:262-266.
13. Williams PE, Goldspink G. Connective tissue changes in immobilized muscle. *J Anat.* 1984;138:343-350.
14. Bandy WD, Irion J. The effect of time of static stretch on the flexibility of the hamstring muscles. Phys Ther 1994;74:845-850.

15. Bandy WD, Irion JM, Briggler M The effect of time and frequency of static stretching of flexibility of the hamstring muscles. Phys Ther 1997;77:1090-1096.
16. 14. Sullivan PE, Markos PD. Clinical Decision Making in Therapeutic Exercise. Norwalk Connecticut: Appleton & Lange;1995.
17. American Physical Therapy Association. Guide to Physical Therapist Practice, second edition. Phys Ther 2001;81:1-768.
18. Woolacot MA, Shumway-Cook A, Nashner LM. Aging and posture control: Changes in sensory organization and muscular coordination. IntJAging Hum Dev 1986;23:97-114.
19. Bowsher D. Nociceptors and peripheral nerve fibers, In: Wells PE, Frampton V, Bowsher D, eds. *Pain Management in Physical Therapy*. Norwalk Ct. Appleton & Lange, 1988.
20. Malone TR, Garrett WE, Zachazewski JE. Muscle: deformation, injury, repair. In: Zachazewski JE, Magee DJ, Quillen WS, eds. *Athletic Injuries and Rehabilitation*. Philadelphia: WB Saunders;1997:71-91.
21. Woo SL-Y, Buckwalter JA, eds. *Injury and repair of the musculoskeletal Soft Tissues*. Park Ridge, IL: American Academy of Orthopeaedic Surgeons;1988:133-167.
22. Salter RB. Textbook of Disorders and Injuries of the Musculoskeletal System. 2nd ed. Baltimore: Williams &Wilkens: 1983.
23. Buckwalter J, Rosenberg L, Coutts R, et al. Articular Cartilage: injury and repair. In Woo SL-Y, Buckwalter JA, eds. *Injury and Repair of the Musculoskeletal Soft Tissues*. Park Ridge Il: American Academy of Orthopedic Surgeons; 1988: 465-482.
24. Andriaacchi T, Sabiston P, Dehaven K, Dahner L, et al. Ligament: injury and repair. In : Woo SL-Y, Buckwalter JA, eds. *Injury and repair of the musculoskeletal Soft Tissues*. Park Ridge, IL: American Academy of Orthopeaedic Surgeons;1988:103-132.
25. Paris SV, Loubert PV. Foundations of Clinical Orthopedics. St Augustine, Fl: Institute Press, Division of Patris Inc;1999: 195-211.
26. Messier SP, Loeser RF, Hoover JL, Semble EL, Wise CM. Osteoarthritis of the knee: effects on gait, strength, and flexibility. *Arch Phys Med Rehabil*. 1992;73:29-36.
27. Brandt KD, Slemenda CW. Osteoarthritis epidemiology, pathology and pathogenesis. In: Schemacher HR Jr, ed. *Primer on the Rheumatic Diseases*. 10th ed. Atlanta: Arthritis Foundation;1993:184-187.

28. Roddy E, Zhang W, Doherty M. Aerobic walking or strengthening exercise for osteoarthritis of the knee? A systematic review. *Ann Rheum Dis* 2005;64:544-548.

29. Ettinger WH, Applegate W, Rejeski J, Morgan T, Shumaker S, Berry MJ, O'Toole M, Monu J, Craven T. A randomized trail comparing aerobic exercise and resistance exercise with a health program in older adults with knee osteoarthritis. JAMA 1997;277:25-31.

30. McConnell FM, Bell M. Exercise for osteoarthritis of the hip or knee. Cochrane Database Syst Rev. 2003;3:CD004286.

31. Bautch JC, Clayton MK, Qili C, Johnson KA. Synovial fluid chondroitinsulphateepitodes 3B3 and 7D4, and glycosaminoglycan in human knee osteoarthritis after exercise. Ann Rheum Dis 2000;59:887-891.

32. Roos EM, Dahlberg L. Positive effect of moderate exercise on glycosaminoglycan content cartilage: A four month, randomized, controlled trial in patients at risk for osteoarthritis. Arthritis and Rheumatics 2005;52:3507-3514.

33. Creighton D, Kondratek M, Krauss J: Use of anterior tibial translation in the management of symptomatic patellofemoralchondrosis in older patients - A case series. The Journal of Manual and Manipulative Therapy 2007; 15(4):216-223.

34. Dai L: Disc Degeneration and Cervical Instability: Correlation of MRI with radiography. Spine 1998; 23(16): 1734-1738.

35. Miyazaki M, Hong SW, Yoon SH, Zou J, TwoB, Alanay A, Abitbol JJ, Wang J: Kinematic analysis of the relationship between the grade of disc degeneration and motion unit of the cervical spine. Spine 2008; 33(2): 187-193.

36. Fujiwara A, Lim T, Hong H S, Tanaka N, Jeon CH, Andersson G BJ, Haughton VM: The Effect of Disc Degeneration and Facet Joint Osteoarthritis on the Segmental Flexibility of the Lumbar Spine. Spine 2000; 25 (23): 3036-3044.

37. Iguchi T, Kanemura A, Kasahara, K A, Doita M, Yoshiya S: Age Distribution of Three Radiologic Factors for Lumbar Instability: Probable Aging Process of the Instability With Disc Degeneration. Spine 2003; 28 (23) 2628-2633

38. Creighton D: Positional Distraction, A radiological confirmation. The Journal of Manual And Manipulative Therapy 1993; 1(3): 83-86

39. Creighton D, Krauss J, Marcoux B: Management of lumbar spinal stenosis through the use of translatoric manipulation and lumbar flexion exercises: A case series. The Journal of Manual and Manipulative Therapy 2006; 14(1): E1-E10.